American Pandemic

American Pandemic

The Lost Worlds of the 1918 Influenza Epidemic

NANCY K. BRISTOW

OXFORD
UNIVERSITY PRESS

OXFORD

UNIVERSITY PRESS

Oxford University Press, Inc., publishes works that further
Oxford University's objective of excellence
in research, scholarship, and education.

Oxford   New York
Auckland   Cape Town   Dar es Salaam   Hong Kong   Karachi
Kuala Lumpur   Madrid   Melbourne   Mexico City   Nairobi
New Delhi   Shanghai   Taipei   Toronto

With offices in
Argentina   Austria   Brazil   Chile   Czech Republic   France   Greece
Guatemala   Hungary   Italy   Japan Poland   Portugal   Singapore
South Korea   Switzerland   Thailand   Turkey   Ukraine   Vietnam

Published by Oxford University Press, Inc.
198 Madison Avenue, New York, New York 10016

www.oup.com

Oxford is a registered trademark of Oxford University Press

Library of Congress Cataloging-in-Publication Data
Bristow, Nancy K., 1958-
American pandemic : the lost worlds of the 1918 influenza epidemic / Nancy K. Bristow.
p.   cm.
Includes bibliographical references and index.
ISBN 978-0-19-981134-2 (hardback)
1.Influenza—United States—History—20th century.
2. Epidemics—United States—History—20th century. I. Title.
RA644.I6B75   2012
614.5′180973—dc23   2011039800

*To the memory of my great-grandparents, my family's past
and to my nieces and nephews, our families' futures*

TABLE OF CONTENTS

ACKNOWLEDGMENTS

As I have tried to write the history of the people who lived and died in the pandemic I have felt a deep gratitude to the voices of the past that have made such work possible. This gratitude carries with it a tremendous sense of responsibility to do justice to the stories they have shared. I feel a similar sense of both gratitude and responsibility to the countless people and institutions whose support made this book possible. Perhaps the best part of bringing this work to print is the opportunity to thank them publicly for their help.

Parts of this manuscript were originally published in "It's as Bad as Anything Can Be': Patients, Identity, and the Influenza Pandemic,' in *Public Health Reports*, vol. 125 (2010, Supplement 3: Influenza Pandemic in the United States), and "You can't do anything for influenza': doctors, nurses and the power of gender during the influenza pandemic in the United States," in *The Spanish Influenza Pandemic of 1918–19: New Perspectives,* eds. Howard Phillips and David Killingray (London: Routledge, 2003), 58–69, 262–266. I thank both publishers for allowing me to reprint portions of those essays here.

I am deeply grateful for the sustained financial support of the University of Puget Sound, which has come in the form of sabbatical leaves, Martin Nelson Summer Research Grants, and a John Lantz Senior Sabbatical Fellowship, and to the National Endowment for the Humanities, which provided generous support with a fellowship in 2003–2004. I also owe a great debt to Oxford University Press, and to all of the talented people there who have handled my work with exceptional professionalism. I am particularly grateful to Niko Pfund for his continuing support of my work, and to Susan Ferber, editor extraordinaire. I thank her for her remarkable insights, her persistent patience, and her ability to help me see the forest as well as the trees. This is a much better book because of her. I also thank the anonymous reviewers who read this book in draft form and provided superb guidance to me. I hope they can see the positive results of their efforts here.

Because primary sources on the pandemic are notoriously difficult to find, I have been unusually reliant on the genius of archivists and librarians. I am deeply indebted to several: Mitch Yockelson and Bill Creech at National Archives I; Tab Lewis at National Archives II; Ken House at the National Archives in Seattle; Deborah Osterberg at the National Archives in San Francisco; Kathy Goss at the Hazel A. Braugh Records Center of the Red Cross; Steve Bartell at the New York City Municipal Reference and Research Center; Richard Sommers, David Keogh and Pam Cheney at the U. S. Army Military History Institute; Jeffrey Anderson at the College of Physicians of Philadelphia; Maureen Burton and Andrew Basden at the National Library of Medicine; Scott DeHaven at the American Philosophical Society; Helen Sherwin at the Nursing Archive at Boston University; David Klaassen at the Social Welfare History Archives at the University of Minnesota; Lois Hendrickson and Penny Krosch at the University Archives at the University of Minnesota; Susan Sutton at the Minnesota Historical Society; Jill Costill at the Indiana State Library; Regina Rush in Special Collections at the University of Virginia; Michael G. Rhode at the Otis Historical Archives at the Armed Forces Institute of Pathology; Betsy Weiss at the Barbara Bates Center for the Study of Nursing at the University of Pennsylvania School of Nursing; Dolores Judkins and Jeff Colby at the Oregon Health Sciences University Library; Gail Rodgers Redmann at the Historical Society of Washington DC; Joellen El Bashir and Ida Jones at the Moorland-Spingarn Research Center at Howard University; as well as the staffs at the Library of Congress, the Idaho State Historical Society Archives, the Bancroft Library at the University of California at Berkeley, the Still Picture Branch of the National Archives, Sterling Library at Yale University, Schlesinger Library at Radcliffe University, the Washington D.C. Public Library, the Schomburg Center for Research in Black Culture, and the Columbia University Oral History Project. For their help with images I am very grateful to Scott Anderson at the Sharlot Hall Museum; Colleen Holt at the Jerome, Arizona Historical Society; Beth Alvarez at the University of Maryland; Coi Drummond-Gehrig at the Denver Public Library; the folks at Digital Services at the University of Virginia, and Susan Sutton at the Indiana Historical Society. Many of these people went far beyond what I could have asked for. I also offer special thanks to Peggy Burge at Collins Memorial Library at the University of Puget Sound for her expertise and her ceaseless support of my research and my teaching.

I am especially appreciative of the scholars who work on the history of the 1918 pandemic, both those who did the path breaking that made my work possible and those who have provided me with a community of colleagues. This book has been improved immeasurably through opportunities to present pieces of it at conferences, including the Organization of American Historians Annual Meeting in 2005, and the American Association for the History of Medicine

Meetings in 2001, 2002, and 2004. Three special conferences dedicated to influenza were profoundly influential in shaping this work. I would like to offer special thanks to Howard Phillips and David Killingray for "Spanish Influenza After Eighty Years—Reflections on the Influenza Pandemic of 1918–1919" at the University of Cape Town in September 1998, to Alexandra Minna Stern and Howard Markel for the "Workshop on the History of the 1918–1919 Influenza Pandemic in the United States" at the Center for the History of Medicine at the University of Michigan in May 2009, to Michael Bresalier and Patrick Zylberman for "After 1918: History and Politics of Influenza in the 20th and 21st Centuries," at the Ecole des Hautes Etudes en Santé Publique in Rennes, France in August 2011, and to all of the scholars who helped to make these conferences models of intellectual engagement and exchange. I also thank Jeffrey Anderson for his help with the blues, James Armstrong for inspiration and conversation, Jeffery Taubenberger for the remarkable tour of his laboratory, Howard Phillips for his ongoing support of my work, James Higgins for leading me to *They Came Like Swallows* and for sharing his work on cemeteries, and Carol Byerly for her exemplary scholarship, her intellectual generosity, and her friendship. Ed Linenthal deserves special thanks for a long conversation in the Mississippi Delta that reshaped my thinking about the issues of forgetting and remembering.

Closer to home, my colleagues at the University of Puget Sound have enriched my intellectual life in ways too many to count over the last twenty-one years. I am especially grateful to all of my colleagues in the History Department—David Smith, John Lear, Katherine Smith, Jennifer Neighbors, Benjamin Tromly, Suzanne Barnett, Theodore Taranovski, and the late Walter Lowrie—for providing me with my first intellectual home and sustaining my belief in our work as historians. I owe special thanks to two departmental colleagues—William Breitenbach and Douglas Sackman—for their intellectual and ethical guidance, their expansive support of my work, and the model of humane professionalism they have provided. I should add that this book would not have made it to print without Doug's continued encouragement. I would never have made it through my first week, let alone twenty-one years, at the university without the support and expertise of Florence Phillippi. More recently, the African American Studies Program and the Race and Pedagogy Initiative have deepened and broadened my sense of what it means to be a teacher-scholar, and I thank all of my colleagues in the community and at the university for helping me grow. In particular, I thank Dexter Gordon for his leadership and his belief in possibility, Alice Coil for her brilliance, her skill, and her humor, and Margaret Birmingham for her wonderful good spirit and her effectiveness. I owe a very special debt to Grace Livingston, who has remade my life at the university over the last several years, providing intellectual mentoring and pedagogical inspiration that have expanded my imagination and my heart. And then there are my students. Those who have inspired me are simply too numerous to name here. I do hope that each of them already knows how profoundly they have shaped my work and understands how meaningful their determination to truly understand the past has been for me. This new generation has much to offer our world, and I gladly put the future in their hands.

I continue to be exceptionally fortunate in my friends, who have encouraged me, supported me, and proven remarkably forgiving of me. My life is immeasurably richer for having them alongside me in my journeys. I want to thank especially for their support during this project Ruthanne and Ed Rankin, Pat Krueger, Mike Honey, Mary Ellen Hughes, Rob Wells, Heather Bruce, Bruce Adams, John and Amy Hanson, Suzanne Holland, Deborah Rosen, Priti Joshi, Rob Shaeffer, and Margaret Moulton.

My family has been a part of this project from the beginning, and has provided support of every type imaginable, not only for this work but throughout my life. To my extended family of Bristows, Jacksons, Landyes, Tewksburys, Moores, and Smiths I offer my humblest thanks for their love and support. If I have sometimes wavered in my belief in myself, my family has always been there to shore me up. The model of humanity they have provided me has been a guide throughout my life, and their love has been my sustenance. Guy, Nancy, Jay, Lori, Chris and Sally Jackson have long been my dear friends, and I thank them for embracing me as a part of their family. I also owe a never-ending debt to my brothers Mike and Jim Bristow, who have had my back and cheered me on my entire life and are my oldest friends, to my sister-in-law Willow Dean, whose strength and heart know no bounds, to Karen England for her amazing model of kindness and caring, and to Gwen Fyfe, who remains as dear to me as ever. Liza, Coho, Pearl, and Pauli have been my constant companions and have buoyed me with their steady reminder of the value of simple things and the expansiveness of love.

My parents' support has been essential to this project and to my life. Their belief in me gave me the courage to pursue my chosen paths and their moral compass has guided me along it. My father, J. David Bristow, did not live to see this book in print, but I can only hope that his model of integrity and compassion come through in its pages. My mother, Kathleen Bristow, continues to inspire me daily with her deep strength, her remarkable engagement with the world, and her boundless embrace of life and of our family. I still hope that I might grow up to be at least a little like them both.

My great-grandparents were the inspiration for this book, and it is dedicated to them. I knew them only through their wonderful son John, but have kept their picture with me throughout this project as a constant reminder of the human costs of the pandemic. Like millions of Americans caught in the storm of influenza, their particular story is lost to us. My hope is that this book gives voice, in some small way, to their experiences in the dark days of the pandemic.

I have also dedicated this book to my nieces and nephews: Allison, Lydia, Patrick, Sara and Jamie Jackson, Paul McGown, Christie Farson, Katie and Brian Kehrl and their children Harper and Gardner, Ryan and Brett Fairbanks, and John and Lizzy Bristow. Each of them is a remarkable person who makes me believe in a future brighter than the past. I love them more than I can say. I owe special thanks to Sara Jackson for brightening our lives, our home, and my university with her remarkable presence over the past five years, and to Lydia Jackson and Paul McGown, who have made our lives much richer with their move to the Northwest.

My greatest thanks, as always, must be to Gordon Jackson. My best friend for so many years now, he has become the finest part of who I am. Wherever he is, it will always be my home. My gratitude for the life we have built together is beyond measure, as is the joy it brings me.

American Pandemic

Lost Worlds

According to family lore, in the fall of 1918 John Bristow, an adolescent of 14 or 15, was orphaned in Pittsburgh, Pennsylvania. His mother Elizabeth had died quickly and unexpectedly of influenza. While attending funeral services a few days later, his father began feeling ill. Within days, John lost his only remaining parent. In the course of a week he had become both an orphan and an adult. (See Figure 0.1) Even the comforts of home were taken away, the family's few possessions removed by relatives during the second funeral. With both parents gone, John went to work. Little more is known about this catastrophic event in young Bristow's life, an event that was repeated millions of times during the fall and winter of 1918–1919 as the worst influenza pandemic in recorded history raged around the world.

Experts today estimate that as many as one-third of humans around the globe, perhaps 500 million people, and over one-quarter of Americans, roughly 25 million people, were infected by this new incarnation of influenza, incorrectly dubbed Spanish influenza by its contemporaries. Striking with unprecedented ferocity, the pandemic caused no fewer than 50 million deaths worldwide.[1] Attacking in four waves, influenza hit first in the spring of 1918, but it attracted little public notice among Americans who expected annual influenza outbreaks. The wave of disease began to garner attention as it moved to the European battlefields during the late spring and summer. Then, in late August, the pandemic exploded in its second wave, striking simultaneously on three continents and spreading rapidly throughout the world. A third wave followed close behind, attacking in the winter as many communities were still recovering from the autumn crisis. In early 1920 influenza would strike in one more wave, or perhaps the first seasonal outbreak of this new influenza strain.[2] The second wave of the pandemic was the most costly, when morbidity rates in most communities ranged between 25 and 40 percent. Though other influenza pandemics had killed only .1 percent of the infected, this attack wielded a shockingly high mortality rate of 2.5 percent, largely the result of bacterial pneumonia. Some 675,000

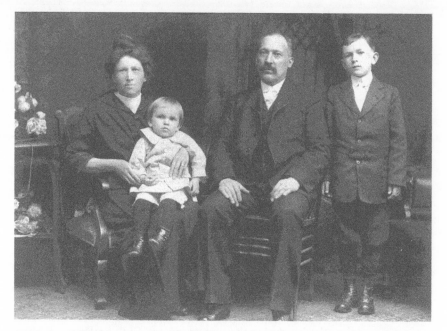

Figure 0.1 The Bristow family, approximately 1913. From left: Elizabeth, William, John Sr., John Jr. Both parents are believed to have died in the fourth wave of the pandemic in 1920.

American perished, half a million more than normally died from influenza each year.[3] The impact was severe enough to lower life expectancy for Americans in 1918 by twelve years.[4]

High rates of infection and death were made all the more startling, and ultimately more disruptive, as Americans recognized just who it was who was sickening and dying. Influenza is traditionally associated with an age-specific mortality chart shaped like a "U," the result of high death rates among infants and the elderly. Infection rates during the 1918 pandemic remained consistent with this model as children evidenced the highest rates of illness. Mortality rates, though, defied previous patterns associated with influenza as 99 percent of excess influenza deaths occurred among Americans younger than 65. The result was a W-shaped mortality chart (see Figure 0.2) that reflected the surprisingly high death rates for adults between 20 and 40, a population that suffered almost half of the pandemic deaths in the United States.[5] John Bristow's parents, my great-grandparents, were two of those victims.

Oral histories offer up only fragments of my great-grandparents' story. John and Elizabeth Bristow were immigrants from Northern Ireland. Settling in Pittsburgh, John moved houses for a living. In 1905 their son John was born, and some years later a younger brother, William, followed. Elizabeth had family living nearby when the epidemic struck. Beyond these simple details, threads of

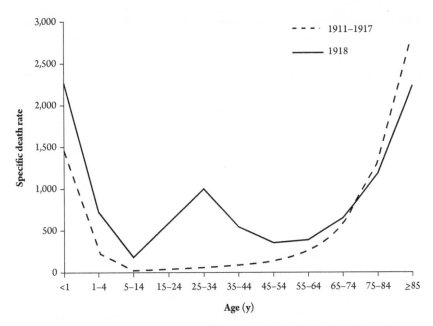

Figure 0.2: This chart graphs the difference between influenza's usual "U"-shaped mortality patterns and the "W" pattern that emerged in 1918. "Figure 0.2. 'U' and 'W'- shaped combined influenza and pneumonia mortality, by age at death, per 100,000 persons in each age group, United States, 1911–1918." Jeffery K. Taubenberger and David M. Morens, "1918 Influenza: The Mother of All Pandemics," *Emerging Infectious Disease* 12 (January 2006): 19.

information too sparse to weave into a recognizable tapestry of their lives, little else is known. Did John and Elizabeth immigrate together, or did they meet in the United States? What had they left behind in Ireland, and what were their hopes for their lives in America? How did they imagine their children's futures? The contours of their lives and the facts of their deaths, as well as the consequences for John and William, are largely lost with the passage of time and memory. As my brother Jim, who through sheer coincidence named his children John and Elizabeth, suggested when I asked him to recount what he knew of our great-grandparents, "I know nothing of them. My history starts with their dying in the flu epidemic of 1918."[6]

It was the desire to develop some understanding of what the Bristows might have experienced in those difficult days of 1918 that first motivated my research into the pandemic. This work soon led to a surprising discovery. John and Elizabeth Bristow, it seems, did not die in 1918; both of their names appear in the 1920 census. Rather than succumbing to the second deadly wave of influenza in the fall of 1918, they were likely victims of the 1920 outbreak, which continued to show many of the epidemiological markings of the 1918 pandemic. The specific details of my family's experience of the influenza crisis are little clearer today than when I began this book, replaced by my broader purpose of constructing a social and cultural history of the influenza pandemic in the United States as a richer backdrop for understanding the experience of millions of Americans—some of them remembered as members of our families, others of them now nameless and faceless—whose lives were forever changed by this cataclysm.

At a time when race, class, gender, region, age, religion, and other social identifiers shaped lives of great difference and disparity in this country, to imagine a comprehensive account of all Americans seems audacious at best, arrogant at worst. And yet it is precisely this diversity of experience that makes a fuller exploration of the pandemic both necessary and meaningful. Despite the widespread nature of the incident, sources reflecting the full reach of its impacts are notoriously hard to locate. While the public health responses to the epidemic are easy to track, citizens' reaction to those responses are more difficult to identify. While physicians' recommendations for treatment are readily available in the medical press, their private responses to the meaninglessness of their efforts were rarely spoken or recorded. And the virus's significance in the private lives of Americans—those who suffered its scourge as well as those who tended the ill, those who died in the epidemic and those who were left behind to mourn—is much more elusive. This book is an effort to piece together fragmentary sources to hear voices previously unheard and elucidate the range of ways Americans experienced the pandemic.

It has long been an article of faith among historians of the United States that the epidemic of Spanish influenza was one of the great forgotten episodes of American history, an argument made most notably by Alfred Crosby in his 1976 book, *Epidemic and Peace*. Crosby noted that though "the destruction wrought by Spanish influenza is memorialized in reams of published statistics in every technologically advanced nation that was not in a state of chaos in 1918," the epidemic "never inspired awe, not in 1918 and not since."[7] Except for a few rare exceptions, Crosby explained, Americans simply forgot the medical disaster of 1918, excluding it almost entirely from both popular periodicals and academic textbooks in the decades to come.[8] When Crosby's book was reissued in 1989, its new title, *America's Forgotten Pandemic: The Influenza of 1918*, highlighted the nation's failure to remember, and in subsequent years countless authors have repeated this claim.[9]

There is important truth in this rendering of the epidemic: the public culture of the United States did turn its back on the memory of this event. But such a characterization of the epidemic's impact also neglects the complexity of a national memory that includes not just the public and shared narratives but also the private recollections of individuals and families. A few voices, including

Crosby's, have introduced this corrective.[10] The national amnesia posed "a mystery and a paradox," Crosby offered, because the nation had in fact remembered the epidemic at the level of "intimate" recollection.[11] This book foregrounds this point, arguing that for millions of Americans, both those who suffered from influenza and those who lost loved ones to the disease, the 1918 pandemic lived on in vivid memories and in lives indelibly marked by those experiences.

My family offers one example of this more private remembering. In the summer of 1995 my father and I took our last backpacking trip together. While we hiked from the Columbia River to Mt. Hood in Oregon I learned for the first time that John and Elizabeth Bristow had died in the influenza pandemic. I had long been fascinated by the influenza outbreak and had even considered pursuing its history for my doctoral dissertation. I had also known my grandfather well as a child and was aware he had been an orphan. Even so, I had managed to pass the first thirty-seven years of my life without making the connection between these histories. My family, it might seem, was following a pattern of forgetting common among Americans. Such a conclusion, though, glosses over what was actually a quiet process of remembering. Though I did not learn the story of my great-grandparents' deaths during the pandemic until well into adulthood, my grandfather had not neglected to tell it to others. In the summer of 2004, as I interviewed members of my immediate family—my mother, my brothers, my niece and nephew—I discovered that while the youngest Bristows did not know this history, others certainly did.

On the basic facts family members seem to agree. My grandfather John was orphaned suddenly when his parents died in the influenza pandemic in Pittsburgh. Other details emerge only sporadically, perhaps apocryphally, and always with uncertainty. The confusion surrounding the timing of the Bristows' illnesses and deaths—when did they succumb to influenza?—highlights the fallibility of our shared memory. Among various family accounts other discrepancies emerge. My brothers and I had always understood that my grandfather lost everything when family members ransacked the family's home during the funeral of his second parent, and we believed that my grandfather had raised his younger brother after the loss of his parents.[12] "The only thing left behind was John and his younger brother," Jim clearly remembered.[13] Recalling with relish our grandfather's ingenuity, he detailed how he had purchased a blind horse and cart from which he sold fruits and vegetables. "They could go out when many of the other street vendors were unwilling," my brother conveyed with some pleasure, "because the horse didn't know, couldn't see anything . . . and wasn't scared of slipping on the streetcar tracks."

While my brothers and I have long cherished this heroic vision of our grandfather looking after a helpless younger sibling, my mother's version of the story differs in significant details. John, according to her account, was 15 years old when influenza struck and he did not raise his younger brother but saw William placed in an orphanage. My mother's story also casts the looters of the family home in an entirely new light. "When your grandfather came home from the funeral," she explained, "the house had been totally cleaned out by the other members of the family. And they took John . . . into their home, with all his stuff of course. And so he lived with these brothers [of Elizabeth Bristow]."[14] While these various accounts offer significant contradictions, the one thing we do know is the cause of John and Elizabeth's deaths and the importance their passing held in the life of my grandfather and his brother.

If the pandemic was not forgotten, but rather lived on in individual and family memories and in countless lives remade by personal trauma and family loss, such a finding only heightens the need to explain our nation's public amnesia. As I have worked on this book, I have benefited from the work of others who have wrestled with this dynamic of forgetting and remembering as it appeared in personal, community, and national reactions to other tragedies. When people respond to catastrophe, shared ways of describing and ultimately of understanding such an event emerge, so-called preferred narratives of a culture's response to crisis.[15] In recent decades, study of collective memory has focused on how nations, as well as smaller cultural groupings, have remembered their past, recognizing the purposefulness of memory-making and the important relationship between a culture's depictions of its past and the circumstances of its present.[16] Preferred narratives emerge as those stories that best fit a culture's beliefs about itself and about its past, present, and future. This book explores the preferred narratives that emerged both during and following the epidemic, seeking to illuminate the public amnesia about the pandemic that contrasted starkly with its profound private impact. What made it possible for a culture to forget an event so significant and so fully remembered in the lives of so many people?

Some have argued that the rapid onset and sudden departure of Spanish flu caused its fleeting presence in American memory. A further epidemiological explanation maintains that it was the pandemic's particular virulence among young adults, and the corresponding limits of its impact on the nation's leadership class, which allowed it to be so easily forgotten.[17] While it is true that the pandemic did not produce lasting social or cultural change and that the disease's epidemiological patterns contributed to that outcome, this was not because influenza traveled too fast to affect Americans or because they were unimpressed with its impact. A horrifying disease that bore little resemblance to the common yearly influenza, pandemic Spanish flu shocked Americans even as it disrupted the most basic patterns of their lives. Rather than leading to deep change, though, the disorder seemed instead to reinforce the status quo, leaving little cultural mark of the epidemic's impact. Confronting an unfamiliar disease and circumstances that were anything but familiar, many Americans clung to established norms amidst the chaos. Social identity shaped Americans' pandemic experiences in the most powerful ways, health care professionals as well as patients, men as well as women, whites as well as people of color, middle and upper classes as well as the working class. Men and women viewed the events through gendered lenses and responded in ways that fit with expectations about their masculine or feminine identity. Race and class hierarchies, in turn, shaped the behaviors of those who most benefited from them, ensuring that some people in the country suffered from not only influenza but also the indignities and inequalities of the American caste system.

This is not to suggest that all Americans responded to the epidemic by acting out their prescribed social roles. The crisis of the pandemic allowed for substantial challenges to the existing cultural norms. For instance, practitioners of alternative medical systems called into question the efficacy of allopathic (mainstream Western) medicine and found a desperate and sometimes sympathetic public willing to engage in practices ranging from folk cures to chiropractic. Similarly, targets of white, middle-class "uplift" during the crisis, the poor and people of color in particular, often resisted such interventions and relied instead on the standards and practices of their own communities. Yet these challenges to existing social categories only highlighted both how rare, and ultimately how powerless, such efforts were. Though Americans often tried alternative treatments during the epidemic, their expectations of modern medicine—that it would cure patients easily and efficiently—survived the crisis, as did the growing authority of mainstream health care professionals. Even less disturbed were traditional racial and class hierarchies. The race riots and failed labor strikes of 1919 would soon demonstrate just how little impact the epidemic had had on white supremacist thought or on the basic belief that economic opportunity was open to all. It may be that this confirmation of the established and the traditional helped to ensure that the epidemic would pass easily from public attention. Acting to reinforce rather than unsettle the social and cultural status quo, the influenza crisis remade individual lives but not Americans' communal life.[18]

This conservative approach to the circumstances of the pandemic was mirrored in Americans' reaction to the growing power of government evidenced during the emergency, and during the war more generally.[19] Though willing to accept public health officials' guidance in the early weeks of the crisis, as weeks and months passed and these officials proved unable to contain influenza, Americans grew restive under their control. Only the passing of the epidemic prevented a more significant challenge to their authority. The epidemic, then, was one more chapter in the tale of Americans' rejection of the Progressive era and the enhanced role of the state it had encouraged. As the epidemic waned, so, too, did Americans' willingness to accept governmental intervention in their daily lives. One part of Americans' broader turn to conservative politics in the post-epidemic era, the influenza crisis again fostered not change but the rein-forcing of traditional patterns in American public life.

Those public consequences the epidemic did have, in turn, were often made invisible by broader forces shaping American life. Most obviously, World War I and the coming of peace kept the American people's attention focused away from the pandemic.[20] An exploration of the language Americans employed to narrate their experiences in the pandemic reveals how completely the two events were joined in their minds and memories. The military conflict trumped the ep-idemic in public discourse, keeping the pandemic both literally and figuratively relegated to back pages and small type.[21] The war and the epidemic were soon conflated into a single struggle in many Americans' minds, with influenza deaths subsumed under the broader category of wartime losses and the pandemic recast as a chapter in the epic tale of World War I.

Some commentators have dismissed the issue of public amnesia altogether, suggesting that because such a response is easily explained by human nature or the dynamics of national memory, it is of little importance. H. L. Mencken, the noted essayist and social critic, noted that the epidemic "is seldom mentioned" and that "most Americans have apparently forgotten it," but argued that such a response was "not surprising." He explained, "The human mind always tries to expunge the intolerable from memory, just as it tries to conceal it while cur-rent."[22] More recently, the popular historian of the flu epidemic, John Barry, con-curred, arguing that the nation's forgetfulness "may not be unusual at all," that such is the nature of memory.[23] Such claims may underestimate how frequently natural disasters, including epidemics, have preoccupied the recorders of human history. Most famous, of course, must be Thucydides' description of the ravaging of ancient Athens by the plague, an account that has served as both inspiration and model for centuries of accounts.[24]

In turn, if Americans, or human beings, are prone to forgetting their commu-nities' worst moments, the very commonality of this response makes under-standing it all the more important. Those who have written about other incidents of trauma offer a useful starting place for understanding both the causes and consequences of this public amnesia. Rape survivor Susan Brison described "the massive denial of those around me," a reaction she came to understand as the result of their unwillingness "to imagine the victim's shattered life." Such imagin-ings, she understands, would undercut "their illusions about their own safety and control over their own lives."[25] Not entirely dissimilar has been the reaction of Western cultures to the narratives of Holocaust survivors, too often remade into what historian Lawrence Langer calls "narratives of evasion."[26] Though the epidemic was a very different kind of event, this desire to shut down a narrative of helplessness, evident with other kinds of trauma, may help to explain Ameri-cans' unwillingness to retain a public memory of the pandemic. Certain kinds of stories, it seems, are not deliberately told by a culture or retained as part of its conscious history. The specifics of the flu pandemic's story, and of American culture in 1918–1919, exaggerated this tendency toward evasion. The influenza pandemic was, simply put, the wrong narrative for its time and place. To remember the pandemic would have required Americans to accept a narrative of vulnerability and weakness that contradicted their fundamental understandings of themselves and their country's history.

Some have suggested that it was the familiarity of epidemics generally, and of epidemic influenza more specifically, that led to the nation's amnesia.[27] Americans were certainly more familiar with epidemics in the early twentieth century, but this argument fails to acknowledge the buoyant optimism in the power of science that had come to characterize Americans' perceptions of modern medicine by 1918. The return to pandemic conditions was a terrible surprise, a shocking descent into a past from which Americans hoped they had escaped.[28] Progressive-era Americans were fixated on progress, growth, and development, and they wanted to believe that experts could solve whatever problems they might face. Beliefs about American health care mirrored this pattern. By 1918 doctors, nurses, and public health experts trusted in their ability to protect the American people from the kind of epidemic that had menaced the nation in the nineteenth century, and laypeople shared this optimism.

Though they proved unable to prevent the epidemic, in its aftermath health professionals replaced the anguished narrative so many Americans held to privately with an optimistic narrative more in keeping with their professional self-image. From this perspective, the epidemic was first and foremost an opportunity—for the fields of public health, medicine, and nursing and for the nation.[29] Forgotten was the failure of public health leaders to mobilize the nation in advance of the approaching scourge. Ignored was the inability of modern medicine to protect Americans from influenza, pneumonia, and death. Denied was the reality that the influenza pandemic was the worst health disaster in recorded history. As this narrative came to dominate the public accounts of the epidemic, the painful memories so many Americans held in their hearts were erased from the public discourse. This erasure of their stories left them to suffer privately, and often silently, exacerbating the tragedy of the epidemic.

The social and cultural history that follows is focused especially on the experiences of Americans as they endured the influenza pandemic and on the public and private narratives they created to explain and give meaning to those experiences. Chapter One traces the history of influenza in the decades immediately preceding the 1918 epidemic. When Americans confronted the epidemic in 1918, most had some familiarity with influenza, and many remembered the last pandemic of 1889–1890. Despite influenza's continuing threat, the growth of scientific medicine and its repeated successes in controlling infectious diseases led professionals in medicine and public health to confidently articulate the promise of their work. Influenced by germ theory and often aware of the bacteriological revolution, the lay public, in turn, developed a complex understanding of influenza. Sharing, to some extent, the optimistic outlook of health care professionals, they domesticated influenza, understanding it as a troubling, but ultimately familiar, annual visitor. Such narratives did little to prepare Americans for the impending cataclysm.

Chapter Two moves into 1918 and the intimate world of the influenza patient, investigating the meaning of the epidemic in the lives of its most immediate victims, as well as the network of family, friends, and neighbors that surrounded them. While the virus did not discriminate among its victims, American culture certainly did. This chapter details the profound impact of gender, class, and race in shaping responses to the pandemic. The continuance of familiar social norms served for some as a bulwark against the unfamiliar storm of the pandemic, ensuring that existing social hierarchies would be reinforced during the crisis, though some Americans resisted them. The chapter also explores how Americans tried to make sense of the pandemic. While some found Christian purpose in the chaos and others a renewed commitment to democracy, for most it was the war that best served as a metaphor for interpreting their experiences. Framing the struggle with influenza as a martial contest, Americans employed the rhetoric of war to describe the epidemic and in doing so imbued not only the battle but also its costs with heightened meaning.

The next two chapters turn to health care professionals. Chapter Three focuses on the efforts of public health officials and practitioners as they sought to control the epidemic and on the responses of citizens to the new interventions in their lives they faced as a result. From prohibitions on common drinking cups to mandated school closures and public masking, public health officials asked Americans to accept new intrusions in their public lives, while educational materials urged changes in private behaviors as well. Narrating their efforts to tame the influenza outbreak as a classically Progressive reform program, public health officials reminded Americans of their responsibilities as citizens of a nation at war. Americans were initially receptive, hoping to protect themselves from the worst of the crisis by relying on professional guidance. As the scourge proved immune to the measures employed by health officials, citizens resisted restrictions and offered new challenges to the authority of the public health leadership.

Chapter Four examines the experiences of doctors and nurses who provided health care during the epidemic. Though these two groups of medical professionals worked together closely during the crisis, their narration of their experiences differed dramatically, again suggesting the power of social identity in shaping reactions to the pandemic. Adhering to standards that measured performance on the basis of masculine qualities of skill and power, physicians defined their success in terms of patient survival. In the context of the pandemic, such a standard was difficult to meet, and doctors often felt starkly disappointed in themselves and their profession. The challenges posed by folk medicine, patent medicine hucksters, and alternative medical practitioners only enhanced the sense of crisis the epidemic posed to mainstream physicians. Nurses, on the other hand, seemed to thrive during the epidemic. Challenged to serve others, and to do so with a caring, self-sacrificing, and domestic touch, nurses found confirmation of their professional skills and feminine identities during the epidemic.

Chapter Five shifts to the aftermath of the epidemic and the experiences of the various participants in the months following its conclusion, exploring the competing narratives that emerged as these groups attempted to make sense of the calamity. While physicians were certainly chastened by the pandemic, their voices nevertheless joined the triumphal chorus of public health practitioners and nurses looking to a bright future in the years that followed. More generally in the public sphere, too, laypeople shared with health care professionals this narrative of opportunity and promise. While Americans neglected the pandemic in the public sphere and soon erased it from the national narrative, millions of Americans continued to remember the ways in which their lives were forever changed by the influenza crisis of 1918–1919. The book concludes with an epilogue that illuminates the cost of public amnesia and its divergence from so many Americans' private memories.

In December 1918, W. A. Brooks, the Acting Chief Surgeon for the State of Massachusetts, posited, "Probably the real history of the epidemic of the so-called 'Spanish Influenza' will never be known. Perhaps it is just as well that all of its horrors should not appear in print."[30] This book suggests, instead, that we owe the victims of the pandemic and ourselves a fuller understanding of the tragedies of 1918, an understanding that might help us better serve each other when the next crisis comes.

1

"Influenza has apparently become domesticated with us"

Influenza, Medicine, and the Public, 1890–1918

In late 1889 reports of influenza in Europe reached the United States. From Antwerp to Rome, from London to St. Petersburg, Europeans were awash in the disease.[1] The *Chicago Tribune* announced in an article entitled "Everybody Is Sneezing" on December 15, "Nothing since the Eiffel tower has absorbed so much public attention as this aggravating and mysterious malady that . . . today holds not less than a hundred thousand Parisians in its annoying but happily harmless clutches."[2] Though reports might acknowledge the scale of the epidemic, most initially maintained a reassuring tone for their readers.[3] Thus an editorial in the *New York Times* asserted on December 11, "Nothing could well be more ludicrous than the spectacle of whole nations trembling before the advance of an influenza."[4]

As the epidemic reached American shores in late 1889 and spread across the country in the first days of the new year, many commentators continued to downplay its risks. On December 19 the *New York Times* detailed an outbreak in Charles Street Jail in Boston, noting that though they wavered on whether the outbreak was connected to the European epidemic, "the health authorities do not think there is any particular cause for fear." Paraphrasing a report from the professional weekly, the *Medical Record*, the article predicted, "North America . . . does not seem to be very favorable to the development of epidemic influenza in its worst forms, and it is not likely that we shall have a severe visitation." Though conceding that the disease might offer a threat to "children or the aged," the article concluded, "The disease is not dangerous" and "very slightly, if at all, contagious."[5]

Even as experts reassured the American public, reports from Europe described a deteriorating situation. By the end of December the *New York Times* printed an alarming headline declaring "Influenza's Fatal Phase" in Europe. A story from Paris the next day explained, "The influenza is spreading and is very fatal. The large number of deaths is exciting grave apprehensions."[6] As the pandemic's range expanded and its death toll grew, headlines across the nation soon announced its widening and worsening reach in the United States. "Gaining a Foothold Everywhere."[7] "First Fatal Case in Chicago."[8] "West Virginia Has It."[9] "All Baltimore Seized."[10] "It Has a Firm Grip on Milwaukee."[11] "Sickness in Oregon."[12] "Raging in Dakota."[13] "La Grippe—The Disease Has a Firm Hold in San Francisco."[14] "It Is Spreading—The Influenza Is the Biggest Thing in Atlanta Just Now."[15] "Rough on the Indians."[16] And then, definitively, "The Fatal Influenza."[17] What had once been Europe's problem had quickly made itself America's problem.

On January 1, 1890, New York health officials, acknowledging the prevalence of influenza in New York and linking it to the "Russian Influenza" believed to be plaguing Europe, issued "An Official Warning." The announcement asked both the healthy and the sick to look after themselves and urged those with "colds" or "influenza" to "seek medical aid at once."[18] "It was only the other day that we were congratulating ourselves upon the lowest death rate recorded in the vital statistics of the city," the *New York Times* editors reminded readers, "and on the last day of the year the mortality is greater than has ever occurred before, except in the extreme heat of Summer." Though uncertain the epidemic disease was really influenza, the paper conceded that "whatever it is, it is doing serious mischief." Given the new danger, the editors concluded, "It is plain that nobody who is attacked can afford to delay for an hour to invoke medical advice."[19]

Once it struck, influenza spread swiftly to disrupt businesses and public services across the country. In Philadelphia and New York the police departments were hard hit.[20] In Detroit, policemen were joined in their illness by the "clerical and working force" of most stores and factories in town.[21] In Atlanta the post office employees were "prostrated," while in San Antonio the telephone exchange suffered.[22] At the Clinton prison in New York, the inmate workforce was "weakened" by hundreds of cases, and the state penitentiary in Missouri suffered a similar fate.[23] In Milwaukee "many business houses" were "short-handed," and in "public offices a number of clerks" were sick.[24] In Providence, Rhode Island, "all court business" was "suspended."[25] In Colfax, Illinois, "deplorable conditions" emerged as the town was attacked by the epidemic even as the few doctors in town suffered from influenza or traveled elsewhere to attend to sick family members.[26] At the Tillamook lighthouse off the coast of Oregon, "one of the keepers" came "down with the dread disease," while both Los Angeles and Pittsburgh reported stricken workers on the railroads.[27] In Astoria, Oregon, influenza acted as a "sort of opiate on matters in general," particularly for the young.[28]

Despite Americans' alarm over the march of influenza in the winter of 1889–1890, it was by no means the first flu pandemic. Hippocrates is sometimes credited with being the first to detail an outbreak in 412 BCE.[29] Because the influenza virus was not definitively identified until the 1930s, historians' accounting of previous epidemics and pandemics is an inexact science, but estimates suggest as many as ninety-four epidemics between 1173 and 1875 in Europe, with perhaps as many as fifteen reaching pandemic proportions since 1500.[30] In the Americas, contact with Europe brought influenza along with other epidemic diseases. Influenza may have attacked Hispaniola as early as 1493, the result of infected animals on Columbus's vessels.[31] In the 1550s influenza again crossed the Atlantic to devastate Native Americans.[32] By the eighteenth century influenza epidemics in the American colonies were commonplace. Outbreaks of influenza continued to plague the young nation with multiple epidemics preceding that of 1889–1890.[33] The epidemic of 1889–1890, though, was especially severe, both because of the emergence of a new strain and because, with the advent of industrialization and urbanization, it could "move with the speed of trains and steamships" to invade the populations of overcrowded cities.[34]

When Americans confronted the pandemic in 1918, then, many of them had experience with influenza. In addition to a history of influenza outbreaks reaching back centuries, anyone older than thirty or so could remember 1889–1890 and had lived through countless less dramatic appearances since. How did this familiarity with pandemic incursions of influenza shape Americans' understanding of the dangers in 1918 and influence their responses to this new crisis?

By 1890, allopathic medicine, or what is commonly referred to today as "western" or "mainstream" medicine, had gained the dominant place in American health care.[35] Alongside these physicians, public health leaders had achieved significant successes in disease prevention in recent decades. While neither profession was fully institutionalized into American life, both were in ascendance. Both were also imagining the nature of disease and of their authority over it anew, changes encouraged by the rise of bacteriology. For public health and medical professionals alike, however, influenza represented a complex problem. Both cause and cure remained unknown, and health care providers could do little more than treat the symptoms and hope for their patients' recoveries. The epidemic of 1890 exposed the limitations—in terms of knowledge and effectiveness—of both medicine and public health, and debates flourished in the scientific press about causes, consequences, prevention, and treatment during the outbreak. Despite this uncertainty, both fields remained hopeful that each year brought the nation further from an age in which infectious disease could rampage unchecked through their communities.

Among laypeople, in turn, influenza produced contradictory responses. On the one hand, it was a familiar illness, easily downplayed as more inconvenient than dangerous. On the other, Americans recognized that influenza was capable of raging around the globe in pandemic proportions. While Americans acknowledged the dreadful possibilities of influenza and admitted their powerlessness before it, particularly during epidemic attacks, these depictions rarely dominated public discussions. Lay Americans shared with health care professionals an optimistic vision of modern medicine and "domesticated" influenza as a well-known and ultimately insignificant presence. As a result, when reports of epidemic influenza appeared in the fall of 1918, Americans could not imagine the horrors to come.

Public Health and Medicine at 1890

On the eve of the 1889–1890 pandemic, health professionals faced their responsibilities with new confidence, a result of the new field of bacteriology and the support it provided for both the scientific method generally and the principles of germ theory specifically. Such developments seemed to promise practitioners a future in which they would know and fully understand the causes and transmission of disease. Germ theory—the idea that illness is the result of infection by specific microorganisms that reproduce themselves—was familiar to many Americans by the late nineteenth century.[36] In fact, the essential idea of contagion, that people were infected by human carriers of disease, had persisted as a theory for hundreds of years.[37] In the middle of the nineteenth century it had competed with several other theories, including most notably environmental, moral, and hereditary explanations. Perhaps most popular of the competitors was miasma theory, which held that disease was caused by toxic air, by "some kind of putrefaction in the atmosphere, or by some climactic influence, or by noxious fumes from decaying organic materials."[38] By the 1880s preoccupation with the atmosphere had evolved into an updated "zymotic" theory, which connected the spontaneous emergence of infective agents to filth or decay but based its claim in the modernizing field of chemistry.[39]

Atmospheric explanations for disease coexisted with the belief that external symptoms of health or sickness reflected an individual's moral state.[40] Such understandings provided comfortable excuses for the prevalence of illness and high mortality rates among particular populations, as the privileged classes could associate poverty and illness with what they perceived as the natural immorality of immigrants, people of color, and the poor. Hereditary explanations, based in rudimentary understandings of genetics, joined this mix of ideas.[41] For instance, tuberculosis, widely known as "consumption," was often believed to result from lungs predisposed to the illness through inherited weakness.[42] Populations suffering most obviously from poor health conditions were understood by some practitioners to be inherently weak, an idea that fit neatly with moralistic and environmental explanations for disease.

By the middle of the nineteenth century, interest in the cause of disease heightened as a result of the worsening conditions of American cities and the corresponding decline in American health. Though Americans' physical well-being had always been closely tied to their social and economic status—with Native Americans, enslaved Africans and their descendants, the poor, and urban dwellers faring especially badly—until the nineteenth century some Americans, particularly those living in New England and in isolated rural communities, experienced more robust health than Europeans. As the American economy became increasingly commercial and industrial and the urban landscape became overcrowded, dirty, and filled with the desperately poor and the recently arrived, this changed, producing lowered life expectancy and rising death rates.[43] With streets often buried beneath a city's garbage and human waste sitting in open drains, conditions in urban areas were often appalling. Yellow fever, cholera, diphtheria, typhoid, typhus, measles, whooping cough, influenza, and countless other illnesses swept through American cities with some regularity.[44]

Such conditions prompted new interest in reforms that might protect and improve American health. In the early days of the nation, public health was largely a local affair, centered primarily on urban areas and closely tied to assumptions about the need to control the immorality of the poor.[45] Even into the early years of the nineteenth century, when a public health movement swept through Western Europe, American health reformers remained focused on individual habits and particular populations.[46] Eventually, though, the worsening conditions of the cities prompted a growing anxiety among the middle and upper classes.[47] Adherents of environmental and moral theories joined forces to advocate for broad-based public health reforms in what became known as the "Sanitary Movement." Given their assumption of the link between moral and physical filth and disease, these reformers, known as "sanitarians," focused their energies on cleanliness and clean living, hoping to uplift morals even as they cleaned up homes and neighborhoods.[48] The United States Sanitary Commission, founded during the Civil War to protect the health of the soldiers, boosted the reputation of public health as it demonstrated the powerful possibilities of sanitary principles.[49]

In the aftermath of the war, reformers worked to institutionalize public health in American life. Though many cities had municipal health boards, often established in the midst of epidemic emergencies, it was the establishment of New York City's Board of Health in 1866 that revolutionized urban health efforts. The result of activists at the local, state, and national level and encouraged by public health reformers, physicians, journalists, and other citizens, the city's health department provided one of the only urban health agencies available during the cholera epidemic that hit the nation shortly after the Civil War. Other major cities, including Chicago, St. Louis, and Cincinnati, soon established health boards based on its example. Though the corruption of machine politics, insufficient budgets, political in-fighting, resistance from competing agencies, and a general tendency toward laissez-faire government slowed the pace of change, between 1870 and 1890 enormous progress was made in the establishment and success of public health efforts in the nation's cities. State and national coordination of public health efforts emerged alongside these municipal efforts. Louisiana established the first state Board of Health in 1855, a weak forerunner to the more powerful Massachusetts Board of Health founded in 1869. California (1870), Minnesota (1872), Michigan (1873), and others soon followed. Though these boards often remained relatively weak and insubstantial, they had become numerous by 1890.[50] At the federal level, too, public health forces mobilized. The United States Federal Marine Hospital Service, founded in 1798 to provide care for sailors, had gained expanded responsibilities over the course of the nineteenth century, including the building of separate hospitals for its patients, but these efforts were rife with corruption and the hospitals themselves were poorly managed. Beginning in 1869, reformers worked to improve both the organization of the Service and the quality of its physicians.[51]

Governmental public health efforts were complemented by a range of efforts in the private sector, including voluntary organizations such as the Red Cross and others dedicated to the eradication of a specific disease, life insurance companies interested in prolonging the lives of their customers, and new philanthropic groups.[52] Perhaps most importantly, in 1872 reformers created the American Public Health Association (APHA), which would prove a vital step in the professionalization of public health work.[53] With all of these pieces in place, in the decades immediately preceding the epidemic of 1890 public health reformers instituted a range of new measures—the construction of sewers, the routine removal of trash and cleaning of streets, the creation of safe water supplies, and education on hygiene and cleanliness—and claimed substantial victories in the fight against disease.

Many of these reforms were motivated by sanitarians' moralistic vision, but germ theory was rising in status by 1890. After experimentation led by Louis Pasteur and Robert Koch in the 1860s and 1870s in Europe produced evidence for the validity of germ theory, bacteriologists working in laboratories not only made clear the connection between specific microorganisms and specific diseases but succeeded in identifying the infectious agents responsible for illnesses that had long troubled Americans, including tuberculosis and cholera.[54] As the public health leader Charles V. Chapin declared in 1885, "What was theory has become fact."[55]

Though public health workers and physicians had different professional objectives—with public health workers emphasizing disease prevention and physicians committed to patient treatment and cure—they found a shared sense of promise in germ theory.[56] An article published in *Forum* in 1890, likely by Cyrus Edson, Chief Inspector of Infectious Diseases for New York City (and later its Health Commissioner), illustrated this new optimism. Germ theory had allowed scientists to gain new understanding of the "most common and most fatal" diseases, he noted. "Until recently," he explained further, "we knew the infective diseases only by . . . symptoms; now we know some of them by the appearance of the germs that cause them. We know the conditions under which they thrive and multiply."[57] Though these discoveries would prove most useful in terms of disease prevention, in the heady years following these early discoveries scientists' hopes extended to control and cure.[58] Edson concluded, "Sanitary art, now become sanitary science, stands an able protector against these [diseases]. Armed with the effective weapons she places in our hands, we no longer dread such fearful visitations. Yet this science is but in its infancy. When it has reached its full growth, the filth diseases, now already called the 'preventable diseases,' will be things of the past."[59] On the eve of the 1889–1890 pandemic, public health and medical leaders described their professions as poised to prevail over countless diseases that had once plagued Americans.[60]

Scientists Confront the Challenge of Influenza

With the outbreak in the winter of 1889–1890, influenza challenged the optimism and confidence of medical practitioners and exposed the continuing theoretical rifts among them.[61] Even the name of the illness was disputed when influenza struck that winter. Though the term "grippe" was generally used interchangeably with "influenza" in this period, some scientists understood the two to represent distinct biological entities.[62] Others were not even certain that the disease in question was influenza. Most common was the suggestion that dengue, not influenza, was ravaging the nation, an idea encouraged by ongoing conflation of the two illnesses by some medical professionals. Illustrating this confusion, the authoritative *Index Medicus: A Monthly Classified Record of the Current Medical Literature of the World* listed "Influenza and Dengue" together in its subject listings.[63] A correspondent for the *Journal of the American Medical Association* (*JAMA*) referred to the epidemic malady as "la grippe, influenza, dengue, horse distemper, 'it,' the great unknown."[64] As Dr. C. F. Ulrich suggested, "This strange disease enjoys as many titles as a European nobleman."[65]

The confusion over terminology reflected deeper and more complex disagreements about the nature of both influenza and infectious disease, even among those who could agree that a particular disease—influenza—was responsible for the epidemic. Given the prevalence of the disease and the ready availability of cases to observe, the symptoms would seem easy to enumerate. Among the symptoms Dr. William Porter listed in a lecture to the St. Louis

Academy of Medicine were "a sudden attack, a chill, more or less complete, a succeeding fever, frequently severe pains, general prostration, more or less dryness of the throat and nares [nostrils], often followed by free catarrhal secretions, with convalescence in from five to seven days." Yet Porter soon acknowledged that there were "many variations," which took their cues from "the personal characteristics of the patient."[66] Further, though many agreed with the standard course outlined by Porter, other physicians associated many additional problems with the disease as well. Some identified ear and eye trouble, while others noted "cardiac depression" and "neuralgic or rheumatic pains."[67] The medical literature frequently ascribed insanity and suicide, as well as other types of mental illness, to influenza as well.[68] For some observers, influenza seemed to pose a challenge to every aspect of an individual's health. Morell Mackenzie, an internationally known specialist of diseases of the nose and throat, explained, "Influenza is the very Proteus of diseases, a malady which assumes so many different forms that it seems to be not one, but all diseases' epitome."[69] The editors of *JAMA* concurred: "Not a single organ or tissue of the body has escaped its ravages."[70] For others the differences in symptoms were explained by distinguishing among varying types of influenza, often described as "catarrhal, abdominal, and nervous" forms of the disease.[71]

The experts' differences of opinion were still more obvious in arguments over the etiology, or cause, of influenza.[72] Today we know that influenza is caused by a virus, a causal agent too small to be seen with the technology available in either 1890 or 1918. It was not until 1931 that Richard Shope of the Rockefeller Institute identified the virus responsible for influenza among swine, initiating renewed interest and an upsurge of research on influenza, leading to the 1933 isolation of a human influenza virus.[73] Since that time, we have learned a great deal about the virus and the circumstances that give rise to pandemic strains, knowledge that helps explain the difficulties scientists faced as they sought to make sense of the outbreak in 1890. Like other living creatures, viral strains survive by reproducing. However, viruses lack much of the molecular machinery required for making new copies of themselves and must invade the cells of a host and commandeer some of its cellular machinery for viral replication, often sickening the host, sometimes humans, in the process.

There are three main types of influenza, Types A, B, and C, and influenza viruses are further distinguished by the genetic character of their hemagglutinin and neuraminidase proteins. Within Type A influenza, the type that create pandemics, there are sixteen known hemagglutinin, or "H" subtypes, and nine known neuraminidase, or "N" subtypes. This system allows virologists to unambiguously describe an individual virus. To take a well-known example, a virus with the Type 5 hemagglutinin form and the Type 1 neuraminidase would be designated "H5N1."

The influenza virus is remarkably adaptable, and an outbreak is often characterized by the coexistence at any given time of several different strains. Though a viral infection produces future immunity for a specific infecting virus, the influenza virus is continuously changing due to random mutation. This leads to what is termed "antigenic drift," limited but frequent changes in its genetic make-up that allow the virus to elude the immune system of previously infected hosts. A pandemic-causing virus usually results from a different process, what is known as "antigenic shift," a more dramatic transformation of the influenza virus caused when a single cell hosts two separate and distinct strains of influenza and the viral reproduction process recombines the two parental strains into a new hybrid virus. Pandemic strains arise through antigenic shift occurring when an influenza strain normally infecting humans is combined with one that normally infects animals. No significant immunity may exist to this new virus, because it has never before circulated among the human population. Though Type A pandemic strains appear to originate first among birds, Type A can also infect many other mammals, including not only humans but also pigs, cats, horses, and whales, thus providing multiple reservoirs for new viruses potentially able to infect humans. Generally when a new virus emerges, it spreads from animal to human hosts without producing human-to-human infections and the strain remains isolated. When further changes in the virus facilitate human-to-human infection, though, pandemics can result.[74]

Because the influenza virus was still decades away from discovery in 1890, advocates of germ theory had a major problem to contend with when they applied it to influenza. Although bacteria had been isolated as the cause of some diseases, viruses remained only a theoretical concept. As a result, physicians often admitted that their knowledge of the cause of epidemic influenza was still quite limited. As the editors of *JAMA* explained in January 1890, "We have as yet no positive knowledge; rather, we have everything yet to learn."[75] A year later the same journal would report, "There yet remains much to learn regarding this somewhat remarkable affection," and in 1892 would continue to acknowledge the "uncertainty" regarding influenza's "nature and treatment."[76] Though assigning blame for influenza to an unseen microbe required a leap of faith, this was a leap many physicians were nevertheless willing to make by 1890.[77] Despite their admission of the ongoing ambiguity of the epidemic's origin, the editors of *JAMA,* for instance, continued to argue for "bacteriological studies" as a means to understand influenza and the epidemic.[78]

Others, though, rejected germ theory, pronouncing it a flawed idea that distracted scientists from focusing on sounder possibilities for influenza's source. Noting that "we are not sure that any disease is caused by a living germ," Dr. A. C. Davidson complained in 1891 in the pages of the *Southern Medical Record,* "Many modern etiologists seem to have lost sight of every factor in the product of any morbific process except the death-dealing germ." He continued,

With them heredity, diatheses, the vicissitudes of weather and other meteorological conditions, elements of decomposition, impure atmosphere, gluttony, insufficient and unwholesome food, inebriety and other environments, potent factors in the formation of disease, are entirely overlooked. Having their gaze fixed upon the one ignis fatuus, they become oblivious to all things else in heaven, earth or sea.[79]

For those who rejected germ theory, more traditional explanations for epidemic influenza were still readily available. Miasma and zymotic theories remained persistent voices in medical discussions during the outbreak.[80] One Tennessee physician pointed to the traditional notion of the "medical constitution of the air" as the crucial factor in the epidemic.[81] Even the *JAMA* editors would acknowledge the prevalence of "heavy fogs" during the outbreak.[82] Some physicians would cite humidity as a factor, others cold conditions or "warm climates," and still others "atmospheric ozone."[83]

Understandably, physicians reached widely varying conclusions about the best treatment as well. The editors of *JAMA* suggested what they viewed as appropriate treatment in December 1891:

In the treatment of la grippe, the first most necessary thing is to require the patient to go to bed, and to there remain until convalescence is assuredly established. A nutritious diet of easy digestion, eggnog and red wines, strychnine, quinine and sedatives are indicated. Small doses of calomel and bicarbonate of soda rubbed up with a little sugar of milk, to excite the glandular functions and keep the alimentary canal freely open, with rest of body and mind, is the course of treatment.[84]

This treatment regimen, with its emphasis on rest, diet, and pain control, corresponded to that posed by many other physicians. At times physicians disagreed, for instance regarding the proper use of antipyrin[e], a drug designed for fever reduction and pain relief.[85] Alcohol and caffeine, too, were promoted by many physicians, but denounced by others.[86] Some physicians offered different treatments depending on the stage of illness, while others focused on the dominant symptoms to determine treatment.[87]

Allopathic treatments, in turn, were challenged by several alternative medical systems, including, for instance, osteopathy, chiropractic, homeopathy, naturopathy, Thomsonianism (a system based in the centrality of the body's vital energy and a belief in nature's power to cure), and hydropathy (which emphasized water as the principle curative element). These schools of medical thought, called "the medical sects" or "irregulars" in the nineteenth century, offered keen competition in an era in which allopathic medicine often offered both frightening treatments and limited results.[88] Though allopathy had gained substantial power by 1890, the epidemic opened renewed opportunities for alternative medical practitioners.

Homeopathy, for example, was one of the oldest of the medical sects and quickly articulated a potent challenge to the allopaths during the 1890 epidemic. Having emerged in Europe in the early nineteenth century in response to the "therapeutic excesses" of the regular medical practitioners, homeopathy had made its way to the United States by the end of the 1820s.[89] Its founder, Samuel Hahnemann of Germany, built the practice of homeopathy on what he termed "the law of similars," the essential notion that "like cures like." In practical terms this meant that patients were best treated with drugs that would create those symptoms associated with the disease from which they suffered.[90] His complementary "law of infinitesimals" suggested that "the smaller the dose, the more effect in stimulating the body's vital force," encouraging treatment with miniscule doses of the prescribed medication.[91] Homeopathy offered not only less frightening treatments than allopathy but also opportunities for self-treatment, apparently impressive success rates, and a "holistic" approach to illness.[92]

Recounting a monthly meeting of the Homeopathic Clinical Society of Chicago, a report on the epidemic "poured hot shot into the ranks of the disciples of allopathy." The homeopaths blamed "the large number of deaths" on the "over-medication" of patients by regular practitioners.[93] An essay in the *North American Journal of Homeopathy* in 1891 by Dr. George Allen reinforced this position, arguing boldly, "Regarding the medical treatment [of influenza], it should be strictly homeopathic." Allen asserted further, "A study of the comparative results obtained by the two schools of medicine in the treatment of this disease, shows overwhelmingly in favor of the homeopathic system." The homeopathic approach, he reassured readers, would allow for the successful recuperation of patients and the dodging of secondary complications, known as "sequelae."[94]

The allopaths fought back, reaffirming what they viewed as the importance of expert medical care during the epidemic. The editors of *JAMA* worried about the "mental perversities" often associated with epidemics, in particular "the idea that the epidemic is to be treated by 'common sense,' or by nostra which have been largely advertised, or by specifics which are known to the laity mainly through their frequent mention in the daily press." Such a response, they contended, led people to believe "it is wholly unnecessary to seek skilled assistance." Hoping to stem the tide of such foolishness, the editorial concluded, "It is serious enough to cope with an epidemic and its sequelae, without having matters complicated by ignorant and reckless experimental therapeutics."[95] The challenge of the epidemic, then, did not undercut the importance of medical expertise, this writer concluded, but rather highlighted its value to the ignorant public, vulnerable to the competition of alternative practitioners.

The Public and the Domestication
of Epidemic Influenza

When the epidemic hit in the winter of 1889–1890, laypeople in the United States were, like the health care professionals, divided in their understandings of the cause, treatment, and prevention of disease. They had long suspected that infected individuals might spread disease by their "breath, spit, skin particles, and bodily evacuations," and even their infected belongings, and had acted on those beliefs most obviously when they avoided contact with the ill, fled cities during epidemics, or scrubbed a sickroom after a crisis passed.[96] But such behaviors might as easily express an embrace of miasma theory. Indeed, the Sanitary Movement had already encouraged Americans to eliminate the sources of zymotic disease by removing filth, cleaning up water systems, and modernizing sewers and household plumbing. By 1890 germ theory had not necessarily supplanted these earlier ideas. Laypeople often found germ theory a useful addition to their beliefs, seeming to offer a scientific basis and a fuller explanation for their accepted views and habits related to disease.[97]

When the pandemic broke out, the debates among scientists and practitioners about the nature of disease were covered in the pages of newspapers and popular magazines. What was causing influenza and producing it in epidemic form? Was this outbreak the same as seasonal flu? The answers in the popular press ranged widely. The example of a single newspaper illustrates how confounding the scientific coverage in the popular press might be. On December 28, 1889, the *Chicago Tribune* ran an editorial that stated directly, "Influenza is always with us when the proper meteorological conditions exist, its severity depending upon their extremes."[98] Six days later, the same paper carried a story on "the source of la grippe" which declared that Russian influenza was caused by "an infusorial parasite."[99] Four days after that, a front-page story began, "Something is epidemic in Chicago. It may not be influenza. It may not be la grippe. It may not be an importation from Russia or anywhere else. But, whatever it is, it is here."[100] On January 12, five days later, the *Tribune* ran an editorial reporting that scientists were anxious to understand the cause of influenza and arguing for the importance of germ theory in that search: "It is believed that the air we breathe and the water we drink swarm with microbic life too minute for our eyesight, aided by the microscope, to perceive."[101] The very next day, though, the same paper suggested the possibility that "the microbes which are causing the prevailing influenza owe their existence to our unusually mild winter" and went on to link the weather conditions to sun spots.[102] The day after that the paper announced that "it has recently become evident to medical men that the ailment known as la grippe or Russian influenza is propagated by microbes" but also suggested that "the microbe is the first living thing which makes its appearance in organic matter undergoing the process of decomposition," seemingly arguing for germ theory even as it described a process associated with miasma and zymotic theory.[103] Articles interviewing local physicians only complicated the information transmitted to Chicagoans on the nature of influenza and its epidemic incarnation, as local practitioners offered a wide range of opinion on the causes of the epidemic.[104]

Acknowledging the unknown cause of influenza, many commentators tried to convince the public that there was neither a preventive nor a "specific" treatment for influenza and urged instead that people act with prudence, patience, and common sense.[105] Such pleas, though, carried little weight in a country swarming with influenza. Quinine and whiskey, often used in the treatment of colds, served as the treatment of choice for many.[106] Others turned to folk and herbal remedies. The *Eastern Oregon Republican* published a "remedy for La Grippe" that included going to bed without supper, covering up well, and drinking a heated mixture of "one pint fresh lager, four ounces stick cinnamon, four ounces rock candy, four eggs, fresh." All that remained was for readers to "get up in the morning, take a warm bath with soap, rub down with a good towel and you can go to work a well man."[107] Patent medicine hawkers saw in the epidemic a sterling opportunity for profits and offered their wares to a desperate public. Leading with a provocative headline asking, "Is Grippe Contagious?" Paine's Celery Compound reassured readers that "no one is ever afflicted with it if his or her nervous system is in good condition" and quoted "the celebrated Dr. Vandervoort of New York" who maintained that "nothing . . . can so quickly or surely put the body in shape to resist the ravages of this disease as Paine's Celery Compound."[108] Hunnicutt's "Throat and Lung Cure of Mullein, Tar, Wild Cherry and Honey" pitched itself as the "sure cure for Russian Influenza" and reminded readers "it contains neither opiate nor minerals of any kind."[109] Of course, such products were precisely the kind of "treatments" medical leaders had warned against.

Confronted with epidemic influenza, lay Americans struggled to understand and make sense of the crisis. Sometimes press coverage emphasized the frightening scale of the battering, noting influenza's wide and indiscriminate reach. Headlines described the disease as the "Ubiquitous Grippe" and "The Great Leveler," and stories noted "from emperors to potboys, no one has been exempt."[110] Nobody, it seemed, was safe from the limitless reach of influenza. "It spares no one," the *Chicago Tribune* explained. "In Russia the Czar on his throne and the Nihilist at work on a bomb were alike sufferers. It will be equally impartial in New York. Jay Gould and the street laborers, Mr. Cleveland and Gov. Hill will have the same cough, catarrh, and vertigo. It will be one of those few occasions when all men are equal."[111] Felling victims regardless of their social, political, or economic positions, influenza also seemed to strike without regard to geography or climate. "It spares no region nor latitude. . . . It is ubiquitous, pouring its miasm on lake, mountain, marsh, or city in winter or summer, in dry seasons or wet, without impartiality," explained one report in late 1889.[112] The popular press announced again and again "new cases without number," noted "the list of its victims is increasing," and conceded that these victims were "dying by the hundred."[113] Recognizing themselves as largely helpless against such a disease, Americans sometimes described themselves as powerless against such a scourge. "There are no means for avoiding it," the *New York Times* announced simply a few months into the pandemic.[114]

Remarkably, despite this situation some Americans dismissed the power of both influenza and its epidemic presence. A few local commentators reassured their neighbors that their particular community would escape the scourge because of its special characteristics. Southern Californians, for instance, celebrated, and attempted to sell, their health-giving climate and repeatedly articulated their confidence that it would protect them from any serious consequences from the disease.[115] Far more common than this local exceptionalism were broader efforts to minimize the strength of the epidemic altogether. Some reports simply denied its existence, suggesting the reported influenza outbreak was nothing more than an attempt to dress up the common cold with a more exotic façade. In late December 1889 the *Atlanta Constitution* quoted a local physician who said of the "colds pervading the city," "We can call these influenza, if we please. The truth is, the name is largely a fad or fashion. Its [sic] another way of having a cold—a sort of excuse for sniffling."[116] During the first week of January 1890, even the Registrar of Vital Statistics in Chicago, W. M. Tomlinson, claimed, "This whole thing is simply a mania. There is no epidemic. Whenever a person catches a little cold he thinks he has 'la grippe.'"[117]

Such blanket denials of the pandemic became more difficult to maintain as Americans faced spiraling infection and death rates. Even so, many observers continued to downplay the danger by drawing connections between the epidemic situation and the commonplace cases of the flu that struck every winter. As a local farmers' newspaper in Des Moines reported, "La grippe is. . . . a fashionable title for an old disease."[118] Or as the *San Antonio Daily Express* explained, "A study of the history of la grippe inclines THE EXPRESS to believe with Solomon, that 'there is nothing new under the sun.'"[119] Reminding Americans that influenza was a familiar disease with a lengthy local history and a predictable course, commentators "domesticated" the epidemic, returning it to the realm of the known. Noting just how old influenza really was, accounts of the epidemic often went on to describe the history of the disease and its epidemic appearances, both globally and in the United States, both in the distant past and in recent centuries, and suggested what might be expected from the epidemic under "ordinary conditions."[120]

If influenza was familiar, it might also be framed as inconsequential.[121] When it reached Atlanta in early 1890, the city's leading newspaper dubbed the local version the diminutive "little grip." "In Atlanta," the paper explained on January 25, "Prince Grip counts his subjects by hundreds, for almost everybody has had it, is just taking it, or tells you of somebody of his acquaintance who has joined the ranks of the great grip majority." Though the paper advised people not to "laugh it off," the article retained a light tone in giving advice if one took sick: "When you feel the first grip of the grip humor its grip and the grip will soon quit gripping"[122] This appeal to humor was widespread. A piece in the Marshall, Michigan, *Daily Chronicle* suggested, "A correspondent suggests that one of the surest cures for the grippe is to get thoroughly scared and think you are going to die before morning. That will generally start a copious perspiration and next morning you will be much better, having frightened away pneumonia and saved the funeral expenses."[123] *Harper's Weekly* used the pandemic as an opportunity to poke fun at drunkard husbands and their witless wives in a cartoon on January 11 that suggested the symptoms of "the grip" bore a striking resemblance to the illness incurred during late nights at the Masonic or Odd Fellows' halls.[124] (See Figure 1.1.) The *Chicago Tribune* even carried a column, "Between Sneezes," on December 29 that featured snippets of humor from newspapers around the country, and followed with a similar column mixing humor and advice on December 30.[125] Between them, these columns also suggested the broad use of humor around the country, including items from papers as varied as the *Philadelphia Times*, the *New York Herald*, the *New Orleans Picayune*, the *Detroit Journal*, the *Peoria Transcript*, the *Grand Rapids Eagle*, the *Cincinnati Times-Star*, and the *Minneapolis Times*. Influenza's familiarity allowed for a calm, even jocular, treatment, stripping the epidemic of its frightening demeanor.

The clearest evidence of domestication was the way the disease and its current attack became a shared reference point, a part of the cultural lexicon. Journalists could employ the reference in commentary on subjects ranging from theatre reviews to animal husbandry, from race relations to electoral politics, and know that any reader would understand it as an example of wretchedness and omnipresence.[126] Perhaps the most popular embrace of influenza as a commonplace in the culture was its use to sell products. Not surprisingly, ads for products such as patent medicines, winter clothing, and firewood emphasized their products' capabilities against influenza.[127] For instance, the Golden Eagle Clothing Company advertised its wares as "the doctor's prescription" for a "poorly-clad boy" who was "suffering with la grippe." "The doctor," the ad explained, "has influenz-ed his mother to purchase one of those $2.50 all wool boys' suits."[128] More telling were efforts to use the epidemic as a familiar reference in the selling of products entirely unrelated to the illness. "Kerchew! Achew!–Hew -!-!-!-!

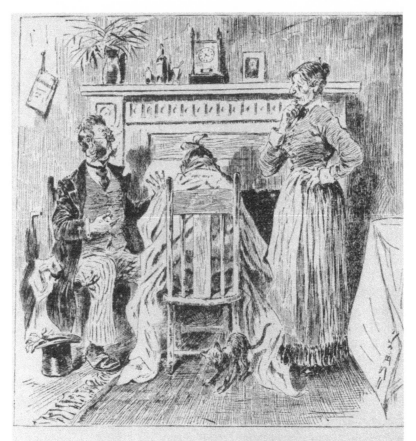

"What's the matter with him, Doctor?"

"Him! He has all the symptoms of the prevailing ailment—he's got the grip."

"La, sakes, that's nothing! He said he'd got that ten year ago, when he come home one night from a Masonic or an Odd-fellers' meetin'; only he didn't take on quite so bad as this. Reckon I'll hev ter keep him in nights agin."

Figure 1.1 Americans wove influenza into the culture during the pandemic of 1890. In this cartoon, *Harper's Weekly* used influenza to poke fun at drunkard husbands and their witless wives. "What's the matter with him, Doctor?" *Harper's Weekly* 34 (January 11, 1890), 23.

Most every one has the Grippe in some form, and we would like to get Our Grip on your purchase of Furniture, Carpets, Mantels, Etc.," suggested an ad in the *Atlanta Constitution* in February 1890.[129]

As Americans suffered through the pandemic of 1889–1890, they showed a remarkable ability to accept influenza as a common feature of their lives. Practiced by its annual appearances, Americans had developed defense mechanisms, domesticating influenza by integrating it into the culture and reassuring themselves that even in pandemic form it was something well known.

Medicine, Public Health, and Influenza
Between the Pandemics

Almost three decades separated the crisis of 1890 from the attack of Spanish influenza in 1918. The pandemic of 1890 had offered bacteriologists new opportunities to practice their science with first-hand evidence drawn from the crisis. This work and the studies that followed advanced the cause of germ theory but failed to identify influenza's causative agent. On the eve of the epidemic of 1918, the debate surrounding influenza's cause had largely shifted to a search for the particular disease agent. This debate did little to quell the professionals' optimism about their ability to control disease.

This expanding confidence was encouraged by the continued discoveries of the bacteriologists. In 1891 scientists cured their first case of diphtheria and by 1894 American scientists William Park and Anna Williams of the New York City Health Department had made broad use of the antitoxin possible.[130]Scientists continued to identify the microorganisms responsible for troublesome diseases, and by 1918 they had discovered the microbes responsible for dysentery, malaria, scarlet fever, leprosy, bubonic plague, typhoid, yellow fever, gangrene, bacterial pneumonia, whooping cough, and syphilis. Such successes confirmed the accuracy of germ theory for scientists and seemed to open up a limitless future for their work.[131] Though bacteriologists would make much larger leaps in preventing disease than in curing it, the turn of the century marked a period of remarkable development in American scientific medicine.

In these years, the understanding of influenza remained closely tied to the experiences of 1889–1890. In the immediate aftermath of the epidemic many recollections were not particularly positive. Treatment remained symptomatic, and physicians were forced to admit their inability to cure or shorten the course of the disease.[132] E. J. Blair, a physician from Monmouth, Illinois, expressed his exhaustion with the persistent symptoms of influenza among his patients. Noting that cases seemed to continue "week after week, month after month," he wondered in 1892, "When will this condition of things cease?"[133]

If the epidemic had illustrated some of the gaps in medical knowledge, leaders in the profession were hopeful that those gaps would soon be closed.[134] Research by bacteriologists and pathologists made possible by the pandemic resulted in a flurry of publications in medical journals. Two authoritative texts based on research in Europe—by Franklin Parson in 1891 and Otto Lichtenstern in 1896—played an especially prominent role in the thinking of American medicine in the years between the pandemics.[135] While scientists had evidence to prove that influenza was an infectious disease, and knew that the pandemic of 1890 had brought very high infection rates and seemed to cause unusually high mortality rates among young adults, this knowledge raised as many questions as it answered.[136]

Discussions among the scientific elite in the years between the pandemics focused especially on the issue of the particular disease agent responsible for influenza. In 1892 Dr. Friedrich Johann Pfeiffer, a highly reputable scientist at the Institute for Infectious Disease in Berlin, announced that he had identified the bacterium responsible for influenza based on research with patients in the 1890 epidemic.[137] In the years between the pandemics many physicians made the case for what came to be known as "Pfeiffer's Bacillus" or the *Bacillus influenzae*.[138] Perhaps most tellingly, the leading medical textbook, William Osler's *The Principles and Practice of Medicine*, began listing influenza as a "Specific Infectious Disease," rather than an "Infectious Disease of Doubtful or Unknown Etiology."[139]

Though many scientists accepted this solution to the influenza puzzle, others soon argued that bacteriological research undermined Pfeiffer's claim. Even Osler complicated the place of the *Bacillus influenzae*, noting its regular presence in humans and its association with other diseases.[140] When a significant wave of influenza struck in 1915–1916, numerous researchers found little evidence that Pfeiffer's microorganism was actually causing the disease.[141] As Dr. Isaac A. Abt of Chicago fretted in 1916, "If one asks, What is the etiology of grip: what have the studies shown? he finds there is a great deal of confusion. Bacteriologists find every organism. It makes us think that the grip infection is very elusive and difficult to find, or else the bacteriologists have not solved the question."[142] Dr. Joseph A. Capps and Dr. A. M. Moody shared this concern, noting, "If physicians are generally agreed on the existence of a grip epidemic, it is equally true that bacteriologists have failed to agree on the causative organism."[143] While some scientists seemed willing to consider the possibility that Pfeiffer's bacillus still played some sort of role in epidemic influenza, perhaps as a "secondary invader," opponents often rejected the causal agency of the bacillus altogether, sometimes offering alternative microorganisms, such as the streptococcus or pneumococcus bacilli, to explain the illness.[144] Though scientists still found themselves in disagreement regarding the causal agent for influenza, such debates demonstrated the broad acceptance of germ theory by 1918.

In the area of treatment far less had changed. Doctors still had little therapy to offer their patients and acknowledged their inability to do more than treat symptoms and look after the patient's comfort.[145] Without a specific treatment, physicians acknowledged their inability to cure influenza and cautioned against supposed cures. As the *New York Times* summarized one physician's position, "There was no remedy for the grip and . . . all that was left for the patient to do was to suffer and bear it."[146] Even as medicine counted its successes, then, influenza continued to elude its reach.

Germ theory offered considerably more in the area of preventive medicine and public health.[147] Though few public health measures were employed in the 1890 epidemic, by 1918 the public health movement was truly on the rise, in the midst of what historians call "the 'golden era' of the American public health movement."[148] Laissez-faire politics dominated much of the last quarter of the nineteenth century in the United States, but in the early twentieth century the reform activism of Progressivism opened up new opportunities for public health professionals. Dedicated to the essential systems of the United States, Progressives sought to repair the damage done to democracy and capitalism through machine politics and monopolies, and turned to the power of what they envisioned as a newly reformed government to wield control over the broad range of problems industrialization was leaving in its wake. To solve those problems, Progressives turned to experts, valuing the knowledge and perceived rationality of professionals trained in their fields. Progressivism was never entirely consistent and reformers' visions were frequently framed by their context, by their economic, racial, gender, geographic, religious, and social positions in the culture, producing seemingly contradictory impulses. Despite these contradictions and divisions, though, Progressivism dominated American public life in the first two decades of the twentieth century and led to substantial reform on the local, state, and federal levels, the result of both private and public initiatives.

The problems of urban health were a natural focus for Progressives, who expanded public health efforts at all levels of American government in the decades between the pandemics.[149] Increasingly the "New Public Health" came to dominate American thinking about health.[150] Emphasizing the bacteriological approach, public health leaders advocated for a range of programs to control disease, including, for instance, research laboratories that could lead to identification and diagnosis, hospitals to handle infected patients, legislation to make mandatory the reporting of certain diseases by physicians, the collection of statistics related to health and disease, and health education programs to spread knowledge to the masses.[151] In 1902 Congress acknowledged that the Marine Hospital Service had become the dominant player in federal public health efforts and changed its name to the United States Public Health and Marine Hospital Service. In 1912 its name was shortened to the United States Public Health Service (USPHS), a change reflecting its new responsibility for research and information distribution among civilians.[152] The United States Army also took a leading role in the arenas of research and disease prevention, expanding the work of its Medical Department. Progressive activism in an array of arenas prompted a variety of other federal initiatives supporting public health efforts, including for instance the creation of both the Food and Drug Administration and the Children's Bureau.[153]

In the years preceding the 1918 pandemic, despite the continued ignorance regarding influenza's causes, public health advocates directed considerable attention to its prevention. Milton J. Rosenau, a Harvard scientist of substantial reputation and soon the director of the USPHS Hygienic Laboratory, explained in 1916, "It makes comparatively little difference to us from the standpoint of preventive medicine, from the standpoint of the health officer, whether this disease is due to the bacillus influenza. . . . If we know how they [causal agents] are spread we may be able to control them."[154] If Americans would fully embrace public health measures, some argued, even a goal of entirely eliminating influenza was within reach. Colonel William C. Gorgas, well known in the years before the 1918 epidemic for his work improving health in the Canal Zone and soon to become the Surgeon General of the Army, suggested in 1913 that influenza "could be abolished everywhere if people became convinced that it was worth while [sic] to take the requisite trouble."[155] Though influenza could not be treated, public health leaders noted that the advances in bacteriology made it possible for Americans to fight its spread.[156]

During the winter of 1915–1916, scientists, public health officials, and physicians found themselves again facing influenza in epidemic proportions. Responding to the upsurge in cases, public health leaders emphasized preventive measures, encouraging Americans to think about how to avoid the flu rather than cure it and emphasizing the responsibility of the healthy to avoid infection and those already sick to avoid infecting others.[157] In their suggestions about prevention, local public health leaders continued to couple their acceptance of germ theory with earlier notions about the nature of disease. The New York Times illustrated such a combination in December 1915 when it published the local Health Department's recommendations for "those who wish to avoid the grip germ." The article detailed measures individuals might employ to avoid infection: "Beware the office towel. Don't breathe through your mouth. Don't be a spitter. Give careful attention to ventilation. Keep in the open air as much as possible. Dress warm, but not so warm as to be susceptible to the cold air. Sleep with your windows open. Don't forget your handkerchief."[158] While some of these behaviors—avoiding public spitting or using a handkerchief—were clearly based on germ theory, others reflected earlier ideas about disease, in particular notions popularized by the sanitarians. Though public health experts played a growing role in American life in the early years of the twentieth century, they sometimes found themselves frustrated, nevertheless, by what they viewed as ignorance and the inappropriate behaviors it produced.[159]

In April 1917 the United States entered World War I, providing new responsibilities and new opportunities for the public health forces. Under President Woodrow Wilson's wartime leadership, the federal government's role in Americans' lives grew in several ways. Much of this growth was directly related to the prosecution of the war, to the nation's effort to mobilize, train, transport, and support an army overseas. Even as he asked Congress for a declaration of war on

April 2, the president laid out a program for the conflict that included expanded taxation to pay for it, a draft to fill the ranks of the army, and a program of "enforced loyalty" to mobilize the citizenry.[160] Over the next eighteen months, these basic provisions for the war effort expanded exponentially, as the nation's Progressive leadership attempted to fulfill what John Dewey referred to as "the social possibilities of war."[161] From the Committee on Public Information to the National War Labor Board, from the Food Administration to the Council of National Defense, Progressives asked Americans to shape their behaviors to fit the needs of a nation at war.

Many health care professionals hoped that wartime efforts and opportunities might bring improvements to American health as well. For the military these hopes were closely tied to recent history. The Spanish American war, in which more soldiers died from disease and tainted food than from battle wounds, had had a chastening effect on military medical officers. In its aftermath they had worked hard to improve the health conditions of the American fighting force, and by the beginning of the war they believed they were seeing results.[162] Army Surgeon General William Gorgas, for instance, celebrated the good health of American troops during the skirmishes on the Mexican Border in 1916. Though outbreaks were not unknown during that campaign, Gorgas noted that such dangers had been "promptly checked."[163] A public health official shared this upbeat view of the possibilities science provided to eliminate the medical chaos formerly associated with war. "Those pestilences once considered as the inevitable accompaniment of military movement," he explained in an article in *Military Surgeon* in 1917, "have been shorn of terror by the hand of science."[164]

As young draftees reported for service, though, public health leaders discovered a civilian health crisis. Thanks to the recent advancements in both medicine and public health, military recruits in World War I faced more rigorous and more complete medical examinations than ever before. The results alarmed public health activists as they watched the disqualification of what they understood as too many potential fighting men.[165] Irving Fisher, the Yale professor of political economy and a Progressive who had advocated for a federal role in public health, described the problem in the *American Journal of Public Health* in August 1918: "We find that one man out of three, medically examined, is rejected." According to Fisher, the draft's revelation of the nation's poor health constituted a new challenge for public health leaders, and one from which they could not turn away. The unique circumstances of war, it seemed, had revealed a much greater responsibility. "We should, during the war, certainly after the war," he concluded, "take the lesson of war to heart, and in systematic fashion try to conserve human life."[166]

Military medical officers took that charge seriously, and worked hard at the task of what the historian Carol Byerly describes as "building a healthy army."[167] Employing tactics ranging from mandatory vaccinations to mosquito abatement, the military's medical leadership set out to keep the troops in good health.[168] In turn, concerns about the potential military costs of venereal disease prompted Wilson to establish the Commission on Training Camp Activities, a civilian agency responsible for protecting the men in uniform from sexually transmitted diseases.[169] It was never only the soldiers whose health mattered in this war, though. In the modern, industrialized war, production capabilities on the home front were an essential component of the war effort, raising the stakes for civilian health as well.[170] These wartime exigencies made it easy for public health advocates to conflate their work with the war effort.[171] In a typical and aptly titled article, "Health at Home to Help the Army," Frank Stockbridge made the case for this link. Though national health was always important, Stockbridge maintained, in time of war it was vital. "It is just as much the Government's duty to keep the industrial army fit as it is to sustain the fighting forces in the field. It is just as much our war—this war on diseases that threaten our efficiency in the greater war on the Mad Dog of Europe—as is the conflict raging overseas," he urged.[172]

Alongside new responsibilities, the war offered opportunities as well, as Americans might recognize the urgency of public health needs and accept a heightened governmental role in their lives.[173] By 1918, public health leaders believed they were seeing significant progress in their efforts to mobilize public interest in Americans' health and support for public health reforms. As one observer noted in the pages of *Survey* magazine in April 1918, "So far from arresting public health progress, the war has suddenly defined America's public health problem. . . . Into a year there has been packed the progress of a decade."[174]

Confident in their ability to engage the citizenry, public health leaders also expressed a new confidence in the ability to control epidemics. A lead article in the *American Journal of Public Health* in May 1918, detailed this story in a forty-year retrospective on the APHA. Proceeding from discovery to discovery and heralding the heroism of the organization's leaders, the article celebrated the accomplishments of the APHA specifically, and of public health and science more generally. "To make the solitary places of human life glad, to see not alone an individual, a community, a nation, but a whole world freed from the Damoclean sword of death ever hanging imminent in smallpox, cholera, yellow fever or plague and other infections, as tuberculosis," the article suggested, "is to give the worker in public health a sense of potent influence over the lives of his fellow men and of close association with every one who works for human betterment and for the uplifting of mankind."[175] The rhetoric of masculine potency suggests how expansively public health leaders envisaged their new possibilities.

By the eve of the epidemic, then, American scientists, physicians, and public health experts had begun to imagine a world free of infectious disease, a world in which their own labors could protect Americans, indeed citizens of the world, from the plagues that had hounded earlier generations, a world in which "epidemics" were "now a thing of the past."[176] In such a world the New York City Health Department declared, "Public health is purchasable" and "within natural limitations, a community can determine its own death rate."[177]

Influenza and the American Public Between the Pandemics

The developments in the fields of bacteriology and public health did not go unnoticed by the lay public.[178] The rising acceptance of germ theory, already evident prior to the 1890 pandemic, continued to spread and Americans increasingly understood influenza as an infectious disease. In 1899 Finley Peter Dunne's popular "Mr. Dooley" wrestled with the "grip bug" and illustrated popular conceptions of germ theory.[179] A humor column based on the trials and tribulations of a bartender in Chicago, "Mr. Dooley" offered opportunities for commentary on a range of issues. By 1899, when Mr. Dooley came down with the flu, he had followers nationwide.[180] "Th' doctor says I swallowed a bug," Mr. Dooley explained, "Ah lah grip bug." Describing the doctor's account of how his ingestion of the "mickrobe" had led to his illness, Mr. Dooley continued, "'Ye took wan in an' warmed it,' he says, 'an' it has growed and multiplied till ye'er system does be full iv thim,' he says, 'millions iv thim,' he says, 'ma-archin' 'an' counther marchin' through ye.'" Though Dooley proposed "insect powdhre" as the cure, the doctor instead sent him home to rest and wait out the illness. The rest of the column detailed how "th' mickrobes had fun with" Dooley, drinking, dancing and generally carousing through his body, placing germ theory at the center of the joke on the hapless Mr. Dooley.

Earlier ideas about the cause of disease remained popular as well, though, and it was not uncommon for Americans to combine a basic acceptance of germ theory with earlier ideas about the cause and cure for influenza.[181] Miasma theory, with its emphasis on climatic and atmospheric conditions, continued to serve as a popular explanation.[182] Some commentators suggested the power of "regular meals, regular sleep, regular work, the avoidance of all excesses and plenty of fresh air" in avoiding influenza, implying that clean living was requisite to good health.[183] Others continued to argue for various folk cures. An ad for Sunkist lemons in 1917, for instance, laid claims to being "an old-time prescription, and one your doctor will endorse today," and recommended "hot lemonade and a warm night's sleep" to help with "grippe and colds."[184] Similarly, a "Special to the New York Times" touted evaporative oil of turpentine as "an influenza preventive," while an article in the 1907 Los Angeles Times suggested the value of cinnamon as a treatment and a later article argued for the power of "the oil contained in the onion, chives, radish, and horse-radish."[185] Patent medicines, too, continued to seek consumers' attention and dollars with outrageous claims for their curative capabilities.[186]

Americans also continued to embrace contradictory narratives about the meaning of influenza in their lives, continuing to express its possible danger while also persisting in their domestication of it. The recognition of influenza's seriousness was signaled directly as the disease appeared in official listings of causes of death in individual cities and states and in the nation as a whole. Agencies as varied as the United States Census Bureau and the New York City Department of Health, as well as insurance companies, compiled statistics on influenza's role as a commonplace killer.[187] Though coverage of influenza in the popular press waxed and waned in the ensuing years according to the disease's apparent virulence and prevalence, throughout the decades separating the 1890 and 1918 pandemics journalists reminded Americans of the dangers associated with influenza. Using a headline that emphasized awareness that "Influenza Is Not a Harmless Disease," the *Atlanta Constitution* reminded readers in 1913 that "when influenza, commonly called La Grippe or just plain old 'grip,' went around the world in 1889–90, many were inclined to look upon it as a harmless kind of fashionable disease"; but the article argued that this was "a viewpoint that was speedily changed in those localities where hospitals became charnel houses."[188] In the *Los Angeles Times* influenza remained "the dread disease,"[189] "the Scourge of the Closing Years of the Nineteenth Century,"[190] or simply "the monster disease."[191] In 1913 the *New York Times* suggested that the significant role of influenza in American death rates was well known by "everybody who reads the papers nowadays."[192] Much of the coverage of influenza in the popular press between 1890 and 1918 emphasized "epidemic" visitations of the disease and their particular perils.[193] It was during those purported epidemic outbreaks, such as the significant outbreak in 1915–1916, that influenza garnered the greatest public attention for its threat to Americans' health and for its status as a killer.[194]

As during the 1890 pandemic, though, not every description of influenza acknowledged the dangers associated with it. Familiarity, it seems, might also create a relaxed attitude about influenza, leading Americans to dismiss it as an ordinary, and ultimately harmless, problem. In January 1916, *McClure's*, a popular magazine, published a short story with the simple title "Grippe!"[195] With the nation again mired in epidemic conditions of influenza, such a title might have introduced a harrowing account of the disease's impact, a cautionary tale about the dangers the epidemic posed. While the story contained appropriate references to the need to treat a case of the grippe with care and fostered a strong public health message about prevention, the piece was largely about the growing affection between a too-busy lawyer and a "girl" doctor practicing in a rural backwoods. The story begins when the hardworking young lawyer, Westervelt, takes off for a few days of country motoring. Sneezing on his way out of town, Westervelt soon falls ill to "the insidious germ which had taken up its tenancy in Westervelt at five in the morning."[196] When he stops for the night in the small hamlet of Milton, the innkeeper warns him that only one of the three local physicians is available. While making clear that this doctor would not be appropriate if "anything *serious*" were the matter, the proprietor reassures Westervelt that "the doctor'll take care of a cold all right."[197] The reasons for the local man's hesitation are soon clear to the reader as a beautiful young woman arrives and announces that she is, in fact, the doctor. Diagnosing her patient with "grippe," the doctor must convince him that she is capable of his care, and in doing so she suggests how little there is to fear from influenza. "'Of course you're at liberty to send for another doctor,' she said calmly, 'but—even the silly, prejudiced people here in the country admit that I can cure a case of grippe.'"[198] Published in the midst of the 1915–1916 influenza epidemic, this story nevertheless suggested that while female doctors were sometimes dismissed as incapable, even *they* could handle a case of influenza.

This contradictory imagery of a dangerous but domesticated disease was again nowhere clearer than in advertisements. The disease and its attendant dangers remained a perfect sales pitch for products ranging from medicinal whiskey to heating systems.[199] Ads for patent medicines continued to warn of the dangers of influenza and then reassured readers that their product could prevent or cure the dreaded malady. Johnson's Tonic portrayed a man literally wrestling with grippe, depicted here as a skeleton, and warned, "Grippe—You may recoil with horror, but you cannot escape!" and "Grippe—He kills young and old, rich and humble alike," and then concluded, "Johnson's Tonic cures GRIPPE."[200] Or, as another ad warned, "Danger Follows Attack of Grip—Many People Are Left in a Wretched Condition After the Influenza Passes," before offering an easy prescription: "Dr. Williams' Pink Pills for Pale People contain just the elements needed to build up the blood and restore the lost color and vitality."[201] As they had in 1890, advertisements in the succeeding decades continued to domesticate influenza's threat, placing it constantly before the public and suggesting its dangers were easily handled with the purchase of a product.

Medical experts recognized that Americans did not always take influenza seriously and scolded them for this mistake. As an 1894 story in the *Los Angeles Times* explained, "Physicians say that since its advent the grippe has destroyed more lives than cholera, smallpox, or typhoid, or consumption, and yet it scarcely attracts the attention of the public or sanitarians."[202] Similarly, an article entitled "Grip Don'ts," written by a student from the University of Missouri and later published in *JAMA* in 1916, led with the suggestion, "Don't laugh at the grip. It is a deadly and dangerous thing."[203] These criticisms only confirmed that many Americans, though aware of influenza, did not take it particularly seriously. As a paraphrase of a report by the Chicago Health Department concluded in 1901, "Influenza has apparently become domesticated with us."[204]

When influenza arrived in the spring and fall of 1918, Americans faced it with confidence. The careful hopefulness of science in 1890 had been replaced by a bolder optimism as scientists expressed certainty about a future free of infectious disease. The American public shared in this growing hopefulness and embraced scientific advances with enthusiasm, though sometimes combining this embrace with a persistent loyalty to earlier theories and practices. A familiar disease, influenza had struck in epidemic proportions in 1890, had continued its annual visitations in the intervening years, and despite the outbreak in 1915–1916, was considered by many a common, everyday, and largely harmless disease. Though scientists continued to contend over its etiology, prevention, and treatment, germ theory and its related discipline of bacteriology had gained the dominant place in American medicine's thinking about disease generally and influenza specifically. The resulting successes had spread a new mood of scientific optimism throughout the culture. Such a view did little to prepare Americans for the uncommon virus that wreaked its havoc on the nation, and the world, in 1918.

"The whole world seems up-side-down"

Patients, Families, and Communities Confront the Epidemic

On September 12, 1918, Edith Potter enrolled in the fourth grade at Chemawa Indian School in Salem, Oregon. Her father, Frank Potter, a member of the Nome Lackee tribe in California, was dead. Her mother, Jessie Barker, had signed papers consenting to her daughter's enrollment at the boarding school and obligating herself to "abide by all the rules and regulations for Indian schools."[1] Traveling from her home in Covelo, California, the 15-year-old Edith was anticipating at least three years away.

Founded in 1880, Chemawa was only a year younger than the inaugural off-reservation boarding school, the famed Carlisle Indian School, and was based on the same premises—that the seemingly intractable "Indian problem" would be solved by assimilation, that children were the best hope for such a process, and that only removal from their families and their reservations, and thereby all exposure to their cultures and traditions, would enable these Indian children to become true Americans. By 1918 the Chemawa Indian School was self-supporting and sat on 441 acres, much of this land having been purchased through the proceeds of the students' labor. Like other off-reservation boarding schools, Chemawa operated according to strict military regimentation. Students split their days between work and schooling, with both geared to preparing them for lives as laborers.[2]

Shortly after her arrival at Chemawa, Edith passed a medical examination, but just a few weeks later, on October 18, the Superintendent of the school, Harwood Hall, wrote to the Superintendent at Round Valley Agency in Covelo with worrisome news. "Edith Potter is quite sick," he explained. "Will you please advise her mother?" Though she was suffering from "a very bad case of the grippe," Edith was "in no danger as yet" he reassured, and concluded, "We are doing all possible for her and believe and hope we can ward off the pneumonia."[3]

Edith Potter's was one of over 500 cases of Spanish influenza suffered by the children at Chemawa Indian School that fall. The epidemic "unsettled the entire school," forcing a month-long quarantine and halting all academic work for three weeks.[4] Just hours after the first letter was written to her mother, a telegram went out warning that though "everything possible [was] being done for her," Edith was "seriously ill with influenza."[5] The next day, October 20, another telegram was sent to California, this time with the tragic news that Edith Potter had "died of influenza this morning." She would, of necessity, be buried that same day.[6]

The following week Superintendent Hall sent Jessie Barker a copy of a form letter personalized with Edith's name and details about her funeral.[7] The correspondence expressed condolences and explained what had happened, while also highlighting the institution's responsible handling of the epidemic. "This disease which has taken thousands upon thousands throughout the country," Hall maintained, "was no worse here than elsewhere," and "it was not due to Chemawa or its location," he assured her. He noted that influenza had been brought to the school "by new students coming in." Once the illness struck, he comforted Edith's mother,

> Absolutely everything possible was done in the way of medical care and nursing. The sick was never left alone for one minute, someone was administering to their needs and looking after them and I want you to feel that in this sickness that your daughter has had as good attention as she possibly could have had in any hospital or home. I have spared neither expense, nor time nor trouble. Altogether I feel we have done just as well as could be done.[8]

Sharing his sympathy with the grieving mother, Hall also described the funeral and burial. "A nice casket was furnished and a protestant minister conducted the services in the presence of all students," and a marker as well as "flowers in abundance" were placed on the coffin and grave.

Such news did little to relieve Jessie's sense of loss. Hoping to bring her daughter's body home for burial, she was frustrated to learn this was impossible and was forced to settle for a promise that in a year's time she might again take up the issue. Thirteen months later, with the aid of the Round Valley Superintendent, Jessie Barker sought the return of Edith's body.[9] The request met a largely unsympathetic response. "Inasmuch as the County Health Officer was in attendance on the influenza cases and is thoroughly acquainted with the condition of the body of Edith Potter after death," Superintendent Hall wrote, "I am a little inclined to think he will recommend against its removal, for you know there are very stringent regulations in regard to care of corpse being removed and a metallic sealed metal casket will have to be provided at considerable expense." Though he agreed to pursue the case, he concluded nevertheless, "I think it would be foolish to take it up at the present time."[10]

Because only fragments of their story have survived in the public record, the outcome of Jessie Barker's efforts to reclaim her daughter's body remains unknown. Yet even this incomplete account reveals many of the themes that emerge in the history of those who experienced the influenza pandemic most closely—the patients who became ill and the families and communities that suffered alongside them. Most obviously, as in Edith Potter's case, influenza struck quickly and without warning, ravaging its victims and often bringing death to the patient and sorrow to his or her loved ones in just a few days. Racing through communities, the epidemic spread anxiety along with the influenza virus, devastated both those who took sick and those who cared about them, and disrupted the most precious patterns of Americans' lives. When death struck, governmental policies and community disorder often hijacked families' efforts to care for the deceased, as public chaos compounded private trauma.

The influenza virus itself was not selective in its victims, belying notions of gender, class, and racial superiority. The well-to-do were as sick as the poor, European Americans as sick as other ethnic and racial groups, men as sick as women. Anyone might become ill; anyone might provide comfort. But if the influenza virus did not discriminate among its victims, American culture was not so equitable. Economic circumstance and social norms framed the impact of the disease, as well as the choices people made as they responded to it and the meaning with which both the sick and their caregivers infused their experiences.

Edith Potter, for example, confronted the epidemic from the confines of the Chemawa Indian School, the result of a federal policy designed to eliminate her "savage" Indian identity and replace it with a "civilized" American prepared for democratic citizenship. Though such goals motivated the school's administrators, other consequences of federal Indian policy operated more subtly in enrollment decisions made by Indian parents and children.[11] Poverty, sometimes exacerbated by the loss of a parent or abusive family situations—all consequences of the wars against Native Americans and the reservation policies that followed—took children away from their families and sent them to the Indian schools.[12] Edith Potter and her mother likely had little idea how her enrollment might affect her health. The Indian schools were breeding grounds for disease, which Indian families soon discovered as reports of tuberculosis and of regular epidemic visitations of measles, pneumonia, mumps, meningitis, trachoma, and influenza reached them.[13] Though health reforms were implemented after 1910, World War I distracted federal attention, and health conditions at the schools again worsened. In the months preceding the epidemic, Indian students at Chemawa suffered from a range of health problems, including tonsillitis, appendicitis, "eye trouble" (potentially trachoma), scabies, "stomach trouble," and tuberculosis, and every month at least a few children were sick enough to be hospitalized.[14] When the pandemic hit, the boarding schools were just the latest example of the longtime spread of disease and death among the indigenous people of the United States.[15] Though their situations ranged widely, the social identities of other Americans also created particular contexts for the germ's invasion.

Despite the disruptions caused by the epidemic, or perhaps precisely *because* of them, Americans often reacted with a keen adherence to social norms, which may have provided an antidote to the sense of instability wrought by the epidemic for some. Both women and men frequently reacted to influenza publicly and privately with sentiments and behaviors consistent with gender expectations. Class, too, affected Americans' choices during the pandemic. As poverty compounded the difficulties faced by working-class families, they often found themselves confronting charity organizations and social workers who saw in the epidemic opportunities for "uplift." Such struggles were exacerbated by racial and ethnic differences as aid workers viewed their clients through the lens of white supremacy and as people of color resisted the assumptions of racial hierarchy. While some Americans embraced social norms as a coping mechanism, others found meaning in their rejection of such norms.

Facing a familiar foe in an unfamiliar guise, Americans worked hard to make sense of their experiences, relying on a range of descriptions and explanations in this effort. Not surprisingly, many emphasized the sheer power of the disease and their helplessness before the scourge. Others, though, rejected such a narrative and described their experiences in ways that allowed them to exert some sense of control over the situation or to imbue the pandemic with meaning. African American leaders, for instance, sometimes viewed the crisis as a unique opportunity to challenge dominant racial norms and to call for a restructuring of American race relations. Others, too, found democratic meaning in the nation's common struggles and saw in it a model of the nation's best self. Religion proved a popular lens, too, with Americans seeing variously God's judgment or His mercy in the trials of the crisis. Most common in Americans' choice of images for the disease outbreak were martial representations, a familiar rhetorical device made more complex in the context of World War I. In the midst of the inexplicable, Americans turned to familiar idioms to express a belief that the deaths in the epidemic were not only heroic, but also meaningful.

Facing a New Foe

The mild first wave of the epidemic swept through the United States in early 1918 largely unnoticed and unheralded, indistinguishable from the annual irritant.[16] Because influenza was not yet reportable, the disease gained public notice only when individuals died from it, and even then their records frequently referenced pneumonia, rather than influenza. The spring wave did not even gain a mention in the 1918 index for the *Journal of the American Medical Association,* which would track the autumn and winter waves of the epidemic closely. It was in the military camps that the spring wave was most readily apparent.[17] While some observers noted how quickly and effectively the disease spread, and others how it was sometimes followed by a particularly troublesome form of pneumonia, even among the troops the spring wave of influenza garnered only minimal attention. A few pathologists found peculiarities in the postmortems of springtime victims, particularly lungs filled with liquid and showing signs of hemorrhaging, but this seemed more noteworthy after the fall epidemic struck. Also evident was the unusual mortality pattern of this influenza, which struck healthy young people especially hard.[18] Yet these telltale signs of a looming danger went largely unheeded.

In Europe the disease was not initially severe, but its impact was nevertheless significant given the ongoing war. By April it had spread to the British Expeditionary Force as well as the German troops, and by May to French soldiers. Soon the citizens of Italy and Spain were also sick. Because the Spanish government had not imposed wartime censorship and allowed reporting on the country's struggles with the disease, observers named the illness Spanish influenza, a tag that stuck. By June the disease had reached Britain, and though it began departing the battlegrounds by July, it continued to ravage civilians in much of Europe. As influenza raged around the borders of the United States—in Puerto Rico and Cuba, in Hawaii and Panama—Americans were relatively flu-free that summer, preoccupied by the war but not by influenza. Yet over the course of just four months this new influenza had become pandemic.[19]

Influenza returned to American shores in its second wave on August 27. It arrived relatively quietly among two or three sailors at Commonwealth Pier in Boston, but it proved highly contagious. Within a few days the numbers of sick skyrocketed, and by the end of the second week influenza had infected 2,000 sailors in the First Naval District. The first civilian to be hospitalized in this new wave entered Boston City Hospital on September 3. Days later influenza hit Camp Devens, north of Boston in Ayer.[20] Simultaneous explosions occurred in Brest, France, and Freetown, Sierra Leone, and soon influenza had circled the globe. Apparent isolation did nothing to protect communities against the virus, which spread with horrifying efficiency. From the outback of Australia to the villages of the Inuit above the Arctic Circle, influenza struck hard. Meanwhile, influenza moved quickly from its Boston landing to infect the remainder of the United States. By the end of October 1918, from Buffalo to Birmingham, from Pittsburgh to Portland, Americans were drowning in a sea of disease.[21]

This influenza brought different, and often horrifying, symptoms. While perhaps one-fifth of the infected escaped with mild cases, accompanied by only the usual aches, fever, and cold-like symptoms, the remaining victims endured illnesses that bore only scant resemblance to a regular case of the flu, suffering very high fevers and pulmonary edema. An article in the *Journal of the American Medical Association* early in the epidemic described the onset as "very sudden," as patients sometimes moved from "an apparently well condition almost to prostration within one or two hours." Though a few victims noted a preceding sore throat or general malaise, for most the attack came without warning. With a quickly developing fever ranging from 101 to 105 degrees, the patient also suffered from "severe headache, weakness, general malaise and pains of varying severity in the muscles and joints, especially in the back." Acknowledging the severity of discomfort, the report concluded, "The patient feels as though he had been beaten all over with a club."[22] Other observers focused on the "great prostration" and "chilliness" that accompanied the onset, the "drowsiness" and the occasional "nervous symptoms."[23] For some these symptoms passed without complications in a week or so, but for others they only grew worse, bringing sneezing, nasal congestion, irritation in the eyes, and a cough prompted by infection in the larynx and the airways to the lungs.[24] Delirium and unconsciousness often followed. Perhaps the most "conspicuous feature" of this new influenza was the "bloody exudate" that filled the lungs, the "peculiar and intense congestion of the lungs with hemorrhage into the lung substance."[25] Many of the fatal cases were marked by belabored breathing, nosebleeds, a bloody or sputum-filled cough, a high fever, and a blue or purple discoloration of the extremities and the face as patients literally drowned from fluid in their lungs.[26] As one physician explained, "It is only a matter of a few hours then until death comes, and it is simply a struggle for air until they suffocate. It is horrible."[27] In autopsy, patient's lungs were frequently found to be "like the lungs of the drowned."[28] Others suffered what appeared at first to be a standard influenza infection, but an infection that soon paved the way for pneumonia, which ravaged the lungs and again brought death to many.[29]

The Distress of the Patients

Franklin Martin kept a diary for his wife during a postwar tour of Europe and detailed his encounter with Spanish influenza. On January 12, 1919, on board ship returning home, he noted that he had "felt chilly all day and after noon went regularly to bed."[30] Though he went to lunch the next day, he was still cold, and returned to bed that afternoon, and despite "all the blankets I could get was still cold."[31] With a fever of 105, his condition grew still worse. "About 12 o'clock I began to feel hot. I was so feverish I was afraid I would ignite the clothing. I had a cough that tore my very innards out when I could not suppress it. It was dark; I surely had pneumonia and I never was so forlorn and uncomfortable in my life." Fearing the worst, Martin planned his own funeral and worried over his cremation and the proper placement of his ashes. "Then I found that I was breaking into a deluge of perspiration and while I should have been more comfortable I was more miserable than ever." Daybreak found him in a wretched state: "When the light did finally come I was some specimen of misery—couldn't breathe without an excruciating cough and there was no hope in me."[32] Martin, though miserable, would survive his illness.

Others shared Martin's experience with Spanish influenza. One soldier who claimed he had only "had a slight touch of it" nevertheless maintained, "It certainly is the worst sickness I ever had."[33] Clifford Adams of Philadelphia made his agony still clearer, declaring, "I got to the point where I didn't care if I died or not."[34] The American poet, Robert Frost, wrote in early 1919, "The only way I can tell that I haven't died and gone to heaven is by the fact that everything is just the same as it was on earth . . . I was sick enough to die and no doubt I deserved to die."[35] Or as another victim stated succinctly, "I was never so sick in my life as I was then."[36] (See Figure 2.1.)

In addition to the pain and discomfort, patients felt the impact of their illness on their cognitive and emotional states. Though the physician Harvey Cushing suffered a high fever, it was the loss of feeling in his extremities that seemed most troublesome. "More or less in bed owing to my hind legs, which are in a chronic

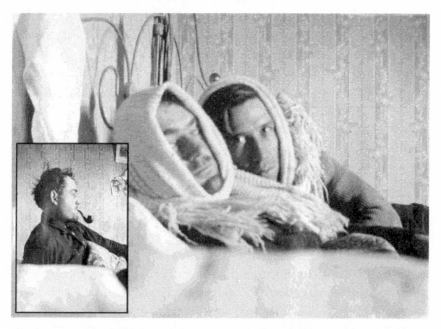

Figure 2.1 Patients suffered severe symptoms, as evidenced in the faces of Charles Kinsman (inset) and Frank Wilson in Mayer, Arizona. Photo of Charles Kinsman (inset) and Frank Wilson. Photo courtesy of Sharlot Hall Museum Library and Archives, Prescott, Arizona. Collection unknown.

state of being asleep up to the knees and threaten to leave me in the lurch," he recorded in his diary.[37] Eventually his hands would become numb as well, and he would suggest "that shaving's a danger and buttoning laborious. When the periphery is thus affected the brain too is benumbed and awkward."[38] Other patients described a descent into delirium. "Time was a blur as I was lying in that little upstairs room and I . . . had no sense of day or night, I felt sick and hollow inside," one patient explained.[39] Or another maintained, "You were sick as a dog and you weren't in a coma but you were in a condition at the height of the crisis you weren't thinking normally and you weren't reacting normally, you sort of had delusions."[40] Some patients died in a day, though most endured a longer illness—perhaps three or four days, a week, or ten days of crisis. For those who survived, good health might not return for months, and some found that their health never fully returned.[41]

In a country already suffering a shortage of nurses and doctors due to the war, professional medical aid could be nearly impossible to find during the epidemic. When influenza broke out in Philadelphia, for instance, 26 percent of the city's doctors were in the ranks of the military; an even higher percentage of nurses were absent.[42] In cities and towns across the country the shortage of medical help was severe.[43]

Hospital beds were in short supply as well. Over the course of the nineteenth century, the hospital had shifted dramatically from an institution of last resort to a symbol of scientific medicine and the centerpiece of modern health care. Increasingly hospitals served the ill from across economic classes and did so in rapidly expanding numbers.[44] During the epidemic, Americans desperately sought out hospital beds only to find them filled to capacity. City and state governments struggled, with the aid of the Red Cross, to provide hospital services on an emergency basis. In Massachusetts, public buildings such as schools and town halls, as well as some private buildings such as churches, were converted into hospitals, while district health officers oversaw the development of open-air hospitals throughout the state.[45] (See Figure 2.2.) In South Carolina the Bureau of the Public Health Service moved quickly to sanction the creation of emergency hospitals to treat the most common, and most costly, sequelae of influenza, pneumonia.[46] In Washington, D.C., overcrowding of the city's residents quickly prompted the opening of an emergency hospital in a space donated by the War Department for the purpose.[47]

Even those who gained access to a hospital often found that overcrowding and the exhaustion of resources undercut the quality of care. As one soldier described his experience at Camp Devens, "I spent 5 days in the base hospital on a cot in a hallway (no beds or rooms available) no medication—no doctors—no nurse."[48] A navy nurse confirmed such circumstances. "We didn't have time to treat them. We didn't take temperatures; we didn't even have time to take blood

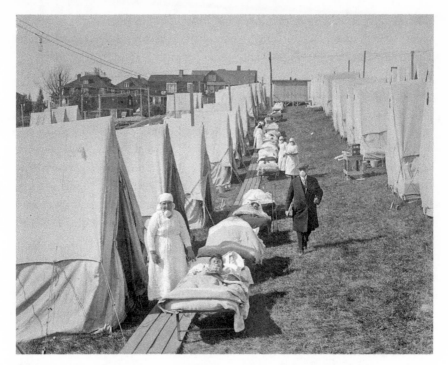

Figure 2.2 Massachusetts established outdoor emergency hospitals in several communities, including this one in Brookline. (165-WW-269B-19), Still Picture Branch, NA.

pressure," she noted. Recalling conditions among the patients, she continued, "There was a man lying on the bed dying and one was lying on the floor. Another man was on a stretcher waiting for the fellow on the bed to die," and further, "The ambulance carried four litters. It would bring us four live ones and take out four dead ones."[49] Others recalled being hospitalized in tents. In Gust Westby's case, his two-month hospitalization with pneumonia took place in an "unheated" tent where he suffered from "very few covers, no mattresses."[50]

Even such rudimentary facilities rarely proved numerous enough to serve all of those who sought care. Frequently finding themselves reliant on family care-givers, patients found their distress significantly worsened when those family members took sick. "The demands were so great," a nurse in Boston explained, "that often there was no one available, so that the sick had to care for the sick as best they could. Often a small boy or girl of seven or eight years would have to care for mother and father, perhaps several brothers and sisters."[51] Such stories— of families immobilized by influenza, of the ill or the very young struggling to take care of their sick relatives—appear repeatedly in accounts of the epidemic.[52] William B. Bean, who would go on to a distinguished career as a professor of medicine, was a child during the epidemic and the first in his family to come down with the illness. Though recovering quickly, he soon found himself "the only one who was in any way mobile" as his parents and siblings suffered with the disease.[53] "I managed to provide the family with milk and eggs and that was about all I could do except toast the bread and give them cereal," he recalled years later.

"Many distressing scenes were witnessed by the nurses," explained a report on the Emergency Nursing Service in New York City during the epidemic. "In one family two children were found dead, and the father and mother and three other children so ill that they were unconscious of the fact."[54] A report from the Red Cross in Baltimore noted that in many cases "not only two and three sick patients in one bed at a time but a dead body as well. And in not a few cases, three or four dead bodies were found in homes which had been there for several days because the families were unable to procure an undertaker for various reasons."[55] An account of the Red Cross in Coatesville, Pennsylvania, reported "distress in some homes, where fathers and mothers have died, leaving as many as nine little ones," and continued, "Oftentimes, we have found a family of five children with all of the little tots ill and alone."[56] As influenza devastated the country, patients often suffered its symptoms with only the aid provided by children or others sick with the disease. The consequence, in many cases, was agony.

Families, Communities, and the Crisis of the Pandemic

For those who remained healthy, the epidemic carried its own "torments of Hell" as they worried over the condition of their loved ones, and deaths left them "prostrated with grief."[57] With 4 million men and thousands of women serving the American war effort, separation made the anguish worse as relatives worried from afar and relied on uncertain mail services for news of the condition of loved ones.[58] When distances and resources allowed, family members sometimes rushed from homes to far-off bedsides, hoping to provide aid and avert disaster. Many arrived to find relatives near death or already gone. "We have had a great many sad, distressing, incidents," a Red Cross report from Camp Dodge in Iowa explained. "Women have travelled for days to get here, only to find a dearly loved son, husband, or brother has passed away."[59] The report continued,

> In the wards were more relatives beside the cots of a dead or dying boy, still and stunned by the suddenness of it, or grief stricken and inconsolable. In one ward I saw a mother on her knees beside her boy, holding his hands while he passed away. Another with her arm across her boy's

dead body, her head bowed upon his cot. Fathers would stand with bowed heads waiting for the end. Mothers fainted or became hysterical. A father went insane.[60]

Those who could not travel to their children's sickbeds fared little better when death struck. Mary Murphy, like Edith Potter, was enrolled at Chemawa Indian School in Oregon when she contracted influenza and died. In a letter to the Superintendent, her mother, Annie, wrote that though she was "satisfied with the care you took of her," she was, nevertheless "more than grieved to loose [sic] her." "I would have felt better if I could have seen her," she concluded. Determined not to suffer another such loss, Murphy expressed her intentions to bring her other girl, Maggie, "home as soon as I can" because "I worry a great deal by her being so far away."[61]

If parents suffered desperately with the loss of a child, children left without parents often found themselves without home or family. Accounts of the epidemic detail again and again the tragic circumstances of young children left orphaned and the difficult problem they created for extended families and communities already reeling from the impact of influenza. By November 8, New York City counted 31,000 children from 7,200 families who had lost one or both of their parents.[62] In some cases, if the children were old enough, they faced early adulthood, taking charge of their own lives and those of their siblings. In other cases, though, orphans became the responsibility of extended families or of their broader communities.

Across the country, communities adjusted to the crisis in countless ways, adapting their communal life to weather the influenza storm. Some of the changes were relatively straightforward and demanded little of community members. On October 7 the president of Yale University postponed the reception for faculty he had planned for later in the month, and the next day the mayor of Seattle canceled the Puget Sound Shipyard League's championship baseball game.[63] That same week, the town outside Camp Bowie in Texas placed a prohibition on "picture shows" and in Kelso, Washington, the Boys' and Girls' Club Fair was canceled, as was a Teacher's Institute in nearby Kalama.[64] In the coming weeks, community singing was postponed throughout Minnesota, classes were canceled at Washington University in St. Louis, Hampton University in Virginia put off its fiftieth anniversary celebration, and at Dartmouth College, Chapel was abandoned alongside classes and Dartmouth Night was postponed.[65] Other changes heightened the disruption brought by the flu. In Virginia, the State Board of Health demanded the strict enforcement of the ban on common drinking cups and focused energy on the problem of shared communion cups.[66] Coal mines in Kentucky shut down, and the Supreme Court of the United States chose to remain in recess rather than open its new session.[67] In Monroe County,

Pennsylvania, cars and trucks were "commandeered" to provide vehicles for "physicians, nurses, the sick and the dead."[68]

Soon Americans found themselves dealing with complex, and sometimes painful, changes in their routines and rituals as they confronted the myriad problems created by the epidemic. For many communities it was the massive numbers of dead bodies that posed the greatest challenge. According to one resident of a Kentucky mining community, "Every, nearly every porch, every porch that I'd look at . . . would have a casket box a sittin' on it."[69] Similarly, a physician at Camp Devens in Massachusetts conveyed to a fellow physician just how severe the situation he confronted was:

> It takes special trains to carry away the dead. For several days there were no coffins and the bodies piled up something fierce, we used to go down to the morgue . . . and look at the boys laid out in long rows. It beats any sight they ever had in France after a battle. An extra long barracks has been vacated for the use of the morgue, and it would make any man sit up and take notice to walk down the long lines of dead soldiers all dressed up and laid out in double rows.[70]

Sick soldiers described similarly grim circumstances in their camps. Gardner Jackson, though not sick with influenza, found himself in a combined flu and scarlet fever ward at Camp Hancock. "I'll never forget that first night there, with guys dying," he recalled over forty years later. His experience there was "a rough one," he explained, "because the morgue of the camp was right outside of this particular ward where we were, not more than twenty-five yards away. The guys were dying of flu at such a terrific clip that they just couldn't handle all the corpses. They were piled all outside, around the darn little morgue building. It was really quite a gruesome experience."[71] People were simply dying too quickly, and in too great a number, for communities to handle them in accordance with popular custom.[72] Again and again accounts of the epidemic described bodies "piled up like cords of wood," awaiting the respectful treatment normally accorded the dead.[73] The problems causing such delays were manifold. Often there were not enough caskets available; other times a shortage of undertakers delayed preparation for burial.[74] Morgue space was a common problem as well, as was a shortage of gravediggers. And finally, in some cases bodies sat unclaimed by families too sick to shoulder responsibility for their dead.[75]

All these problems came together in Philadelphia, one of the cities hit hardest by the epidemic. A Red Cross report on Philadelphia admitted, "It was the old case of 'War and Pestilence' in most emphatic form. Even the established means of disposing of the dead broke under the strain; and decomposing human bodies rotted in crowded mortuaries."[76] When the epidemic exploded there, the city morgue was unprepared to deal with the scale of dead the city produced. As another report detailed the situation:

> The one morgue in the city with a maximum capacity for the care of thirty-six bodies, contained several hundred. These were piled three and four deep in the corridors and in almost every room, covered only by sheets which were often dirty and blood-stained. Most of these bodies were unembalmed with no ice near them and in a temperature not even chilled. Their extremities were uncovered, and plainly visible. Some bodies were mortifying and the stench was nauseating. In the rear of the building, the doors were open and bodies lying all over the floor, a spectacle for gaping curiosity seekers, including young children.[77]

Conditions at emergency hospitals were often "equally serious, with no apparent remedy in sight" and private residences contained frightful conditions as well.[78] Undertakers, fearful of the risk of providing services in such a crisis, sometimes refused service without payment in advance, and in other instances they were accused of profiteering.[79] One Philadelphian remembered in vivid detail the screams of neighbors as their young son was taken away by a patrol wagon. Explaining their reaction, she recalled, "They used to just pick you up and wrap you up in a sheet and put you in a patrol wagon." Hoping to provide even the most primitive casket for their son, the parents pleaded to be allowed to provide a wooden macaroni box for their young child. "Please, please, let me put him in the macaroni box. Let me put him in the box. Don't take him away like that," they begged.[80] Though the city would act quickly to correct all of these conditions, the solutions continued to reflect the grim circumstances of a city awash in bodies. Some corpses were buried quickly with the understanding that they might be disinterred later, while others sat in newly established city "repositories" when burial was delayed.[81] Eventually the city would be forced to bury some of its dead in mass graves. In one example, first with the labor of students from St. Charles Borromeo Seminary and then with the aid of steam shovels, trench graves were dug at Holy Cross Cemetery in nearby Yeadon to receive the overflow of dead and decaying bodies of the city's southern and western neighborhoods which were overwhelming every effort to get them properly buried.[82]

Even in the best scenarios, families often did not feel that they had been able to put their loved ones to rest in a fashion that met their expectations. Funerals often came under public health restrictions, forcing Americans to adjust a ritual sacred in the minds of many. Though efforts were made in Philadelphia to reassure families that the bodies of the epidemic's victims were well taken care of, restrictions on funeral proceedings must have undercut such comforting. Because the crisis was so severe in that city, orders required that services for anyone dying of influenza were private and should be attended by healthy "immediate adult relatives" only. Further, the bodies of the deceased were not, under any circumstances, to "be taken into any church, chapel, public hall, or public building for the holding of public services."[83] Similar rules applied in other cities and towns throughout the country.[84] (See Figure 2.3.) Even in those cases when a family was well enough to attend to their lost loved one, as was the case for Jessie Barker, community circumstances and public policies often prevented survivors from engaging in the rituals traditionally associated with death.

Confronted with such unfamiliar circumstances, citizens reacted in a variety of ways to the stresses their communities faced; indeed, within single neighborhoods behaviors could range drastically.[85] Many Americans served selflessly during the epidemic, providing assistance in countless ways to friends and strangers alike and helping sustain their community's stability. As the Southeastern Chapter of the American Red Cross remembered about its work during the epidemic, "The greater part of the work was done 'unofficially', without reports, without mention, sometimes without recognition, either expected or desired, by

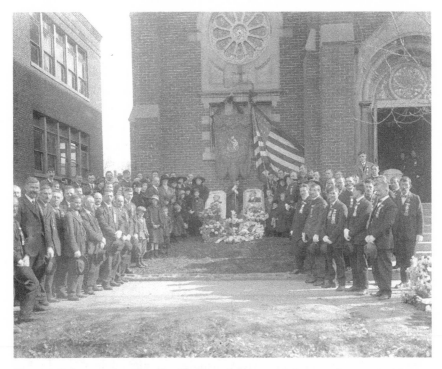

Figure 2.3 Some cities allowed public funerals but moved them outdoors, as in this double funeral in the Slovenian community of Indianapolis. The additional casket in the doorway illustrates the scale of death that communities faced. (P0069), Haughville Collection, Indiana Historical Society.

unselfish men and women who helped for the joy of the helping."[86] The Superintendent of Washington, D.C., schools reported the same response among his teachers. "To a most unusual degree," he noted, "these people wherever possible gave the service they were qualified to render without any other thought than that of helping in a real time of need."[87] While it is tempting to dismiss these reports as self-serving promotions, individuals sometimes expressed just this kind of commitment in more private correspondence as well. As one woman explained her desire to volunteer at the local emergency hospital, "I do think in a time like this . . . we should throw aside personal fear and help."[88] Indeed, thousands of Americans did step up to do the work of keeping their communities functioning during the epidemic.

These efforts were often coordinated by the American Red Cross (ARC), the most significant aid organization during the epidemic. Founded in 1881 by Clara Barton, by the eve of the epidemic the ARC was accountable to the United States Congress through its 1900 congressional charter and served as the nation's official disaster relief agency. While it included important governmental representatives in its governance structures, the ARC was both philosophically and practically based in the tradition of American voluntarism. In turn, though a national office in Washington, D.C., served as the headquarters for the organization, its structure of divisions and chapters reflected substantial localism in its operation. With the advent of the war, President Wilson established a War Council to conduct Red Cross operations, putting the organization more fully under governmental control. By the time the epidemic hit, the ARC had grown to fourteen divisions with 3,684 local chapters, 12,700 staff members, 20 million members, and 8 million women volunteering under its banner.[89] With its local chapters already working hard on war service, the Red Cross was ideally situated to shift some of its focus back to disaster relief, and during the epidemic it was the most common mechanism by which thousands of Americans participated in their community's struggles against the epidemic—sometimes as paid employees of the Red Cross, more commonly as volunteers. The work ranged broadly, from establishing and provisioning emergency hospitals to driving ambulances, from delivering fresh meals to nursing the sick in their homes, from creating and circulating educational pamphlets to surveying and serving community social needs in the aftermath.[90] (See Figure 2.4.).

Other organizations and groups also volunteered their members' time and energy to aid in their communities' struggles, and volunteers came from across the social and economic spectrum. In Roanoke, Virginia, for instance, the Ladies' Auxiliary of the local YMCA "handled the diet kitchen" for the Red Cross, while Boy Scouts helped out "running errands, and helping to deliver the meals," and the pastor of Greene Memorial Methodist Church "formed an organization in his church, which has done for families of the congregation the same

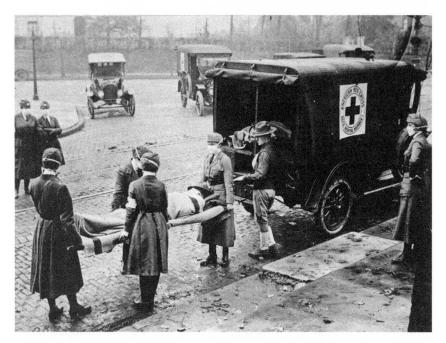

Figure 2.4 The Red Cross served in several roles during the pandemic. Here the Red Cross Motor Corps transports the ill in St. Louis, Missouri. (165-WW-269B-3), Still Picture Branch, NA.

sort of work done for the city at large by the Red Cross and the health office."[91] In Washington, D.C., with schools closed, teachers "engaged in many types of health work, including diet work, nursing, nurses' aid, transportation, Red Cross work, and general office work."[92]

Businesses often contributed to fighting the crisis as well, providing much needed services while keeping prices down. Outside Camp Dodge, in Des Moines, Iowa, businesses reportedly offered "splendid cooperation," providing desperately needed supplies, without profit, to the stricken camp.[93] Others proclaimed their determination not to profit from the crisis as well. The Owl Drug Company in Pasadena advertised, "Prices have not been advanced and will not be advanced under any circumstances."[94] Similarly, a civilian undertaker, called upon to assist at Camp Hancock, took great pride in his work and in the service he had provided to the government. Organizing embalmers from among the enlisted men, handling "628 bodies without a complaint," and saving the government "about $8000 in the transaction," he declared with some vehemence, "I will not be called a profiteer."[95]

Such an effort to avoid the profiteering label suggests there were others who gladly turned to the profits the crisis made possible. Businesses sometimes sought unapologetically to exploit the epidemic situation. As one florist acknowledged during the epidemic near Camp Jackson in South Carolina, "The demand for flowers frequently was so great that all the florists in this community exhausted their supply daily. Prices of everything were very high then, and I made money rapidly."[96] Both undertakers and health care professionals were sometimes accused of profiteering.[97] The Health Director of Washington, D.C., for instance, publicly decried the behavior of what he termed "the coffin trust," which he accused of "preying on unfortunate families" in a manner that "in this direful time is nothing short of ghoulish in spirit and unpatriotic to the point of treason."[98] A citizen in Philadelphia remembered a case of such profiteering by a local undertaker, who "used to get the people and take them out and pile them in the garage . . . and give the coffin to somebody else," but was eventually caught because of the smell emanating from his garages.[99] The rumors of a "coffin trust" in Washington, D.C., were significant enough to prompt an investigation in the nation's capital that confirmed the overcharging taking place in that city.[100] Doctors and pharmacists in New York City also faced investigation, in this case by the district attorney, for the "heartless, selfish, and unpatriotic" practice of profiteering.[101]

If some community members disregarded civic responsibility for the sake of profit, others did so out of fear, avoiding contact with influenza sufferers in hopes of preserving their own health. When the Red Cross in Kelso, Washington, advertised its need for local women to serve as nurses during the epidemic, their first request met with complete silence; not a single resident responded to the call. Even the threat of conscription prompted only one volunteer to step forward.[102] Similarly, nurses' accounts of the epidemic frequently noted the unwillingness of neighbors to pitch in to help a suffering family. As one nurse recounted of her experience in Luce County, Michigan, "One poor woman had nursed her husband and her three boys through serious cases of the 'flu', and then came down with it herself. . . . Not one of the neighbors would come in to help." At times even relatives could not be counted on to lend assistance. This same nurse continued, "I stayed there all night, and in the morning telephoned to the woman's sister. She came and tapped on the window, but refused to talk to me until she had gotten a safe distance away."[103] Though in this case the sister was shamed into helping, such results were not always assured. In Boston, visiting nurses reported again and again that the neighbors "were afraid to come to nurse," "were too frightened to go near them," and "could not be prevailed on to lend a hand."[104] In Perry County, Kentucky, a nurse reported people "starving to death not because there is a shortage of food but because the well are panic stricken and will not approach houses where the influenza exists."[105]

As these examples suggest, as Americans lived and died through the epidemic, their realities were shaped by the reactions of those around them, by the choices that individuals and institutions made in the midst of the crisis. This was not the familiar influenza of the past, and its consequences—from the

unparalleled suffering of the ill to the desperate conditions their numbers produced, from the horrifyingly high death toll to the cascade of dead bodies,
from the legions of orphans left behind to the burden on social and cultural
institutions—were as disruptive as they were surprising in homes, neighborhoods, towns, and cities across the nation. Such instability might have loosened social boundaries, freeing Americans to act outside their accustomed
roles as they confronted the exigencies of the epidemic. In the end, though,
social identity mattered deeply to many Americans as they struggled to shape
and understand the reality they endured.

Gender and the Pandemic

As women and men reacted to the influenza crisis, they often enacted their prescribed gender roles so effortlessly, and in ways so deeply ingrained, that the difference in their reactions can be hard to see. And yet, as they described their
experiences, gender norms encouraged subtle differences in the emotional exposure women and men allowed themselves. Throughout the pandemic women
seemed comfortable expressing their feelings, repeatedly sharing their concern
about the health of family and friends and, when bad news came, expressing their
grief openly.[106] As one woman suggested in a letter in October 1918, "These are
uncertain days. Before you know, people are sick. You hear of their death & it just
makes you so depressed & worried."[107] Or as another woman wrote in January
1919 after receiving "very sad news" in "the most depressing letter I think I ever
received," "I've been very 'blue' ever since."[108] Women also admitted the power of
the epidemic. When families stayed healthy, women took little credit and
acknowledged that influenza might still reach them, and even made plans for such
an eventuality.[109] Once stricken, women did not hesitate to detail the severity of
their condition or their helplessness in the face of the disease.[110]

This feminized response to the epidemic was common even among uncommon women. On March 13, 1919, Amelia Earhart wrote to comfort a friend,
Kenneth Griggs Merrill, who was recovering from a recent bout of influenza. "I
was sorry to hear about the Flu attack," she began. Acknowledging her own feelings about the disease, Earhart continued, "I hate and fear it, somehow more
than a little. Having seen so much of it, I suppose, has prejudiced me—with the
very uncertainty of treat-ment adding to the prejudice."[111] Earhart had had ample
opportunity to observe the disease, having worked on an influenza ward in
Toronto during the influenza epidemic there, and then contracting what she
understood to be influenza.[112] A woman soon heralded for her unusual courage,
Earhart nevertheless openly acknowledged how frightening she had found both
her own illness and that of others.

Men's responses to the epidemic—as both observers and as patients—often revealed a strikingly different set of gender expectations that required them to hide such strong emotions. The differences should not be overstated, of course. Worrying during the epidemic was never only women's purview, and men some-times openly expressed their concern for the well-being of loved ones and the anguish they felt as the epidemic took its toll.[113] But men frequently projected instead an image of masculine detachment.[114] Recording graphic details of the horrors they observed, men frequently did so with little emotional commentary. Male accounts routinely described circumstances in which victims "were dying faster than the bodies could be taken care of," or noted "they can hardly get enough coffins for the men dying," but did so with a seeming distance.[115] An obit-uary in a soldier newspaper seemed to command such a reaction. Recounting the loss of Private Henry E. Montague after a two-week illness that began with influenza and led to pneumonia, the paper described in detail both his last days and his funeral procession. While suggesting his unit might "well be proud that one of the men went West so cleanly," the article also reminded readers that this was, nevertheless, "no occasion for pathos or bombast."[116]

As men distanced themselves emotionally from the sickness and death sur-rounding them, they also sought to radiate courage and control. A private in a training camp in Tacoma, Washington, writing home to his mother, admitted his "latent fear" of influenza, given his own "weakness" with "la grippe," but assured her he was "trying to work on it."[117] "What the trouble is with me," he reiterated, "I am afraid all the time and I must study hard to overcome it." Though clearly frightened by the pandemic, this soldier felt compelled to stand strong before the catastrophe, and to overcome, or at least hide, any fear he felt. Others refused to admit such fear. Another soldier, Greg Auger, wrote home in November, "Of course I'm not immune but I'm not at all afraid of catching it." Auger followed up this reassurance with a further suggestion that even if he did get sick, he would soon recover. "Keeping fit is one of my best watchwords," he maintained, "because here's one boy that's figuring on coming back to the states in excellent condition."[118] Others would share Auger's expressed confidence. As one fellow wrote in mid-November, "To begin with, I haven't had Flu, Don't expect to get it, Don't want it, Have no use or time for it."[119] Another recalled his "perfect health record" and hoped to avoid it.[120] Still others suggested that even if they did take sick, they would suffer only mild cases.[121]

Once sick, men continued to express their command over the disease through accounts of their steady improvement and certain recovery.[122] One soldier, Joseph Turbyfill, wrote home to his wife repeatedly during his illness and con-tinually checked his complaints with reassurances of his returning health. "I am awfully weak and feel pretty no count but in ten days I will be out at work again," he wrote on October 22.[123] On October 25 he would assert, "Don't you worry about me one little bit my Clara, for I am alright in every way. . . . I'll soon be fat & strong again."[124] Three days later he would declare, "Dear, from this letter you see that I am feeling pretty good and not . . . sick. Why, except for a little feeling of delicacy . . . I feel like a regular guy today." Turbyfill even predicted his own recovery: "Remember you are not to worry about me for I am absolutely well when you read this."[125]

In his lengthy reassurances to his wife Turbyfill also intimated his own frustration with being sick, another common male response.[126] In the midst of a war, when masculinity was measured against soldiers in the trenches of Europe, illnesses from influenza felt inexcusable and men routinely expressed their impatience with inactivity and a determination to return quickly to their work. As Thomas L. Sidlo explained in a letter to Secretary of War Baker in November 1918, "I feel it is almost criminal to be getting sick and moping around when you are at your terrific job." Sidlo told Baker, though, that he "ought to be at the office regularly before very long" and that this would be his "first and last illness for this winter season . . . because being ill is the worst form of physical or spiritual punishment that I suffer."[127] Even men who were not sick but were immobilized as a result of quarantine often shared this frustration.[128]

If these divergent private responses by women and men reflected gender norms operating somewhat subtly, in the public sphere the consequences of gender roles were often much more visible. While both men and women volunteered to help out during the epidemic, for instance, Americans often defined voluntarism as a distinctly female activity in 1918. In the late nineteenth and early twentieth century women had gained new access to the American public sphere. Their claims to these new roles, though, were rarely expressed as broad human rights. Rather, women argued for new public responsibilities on the basis of their innate differences from men, suggesting that their feminine traits of purity and domesticity, so valuable within the family, might also produce unique contributions to the community in a kind of "social housekeeping."[129] During the pandemic, while women likely constituted a large part of the volunteer forces, an emphasis on female voluntarism tapped into these notions of women's natural qualities and implied that volunteers *should* be women. As an editorial in early October in the *New York Times* suggested, "The opportunity for young women who want to serve as Red Cross nurses need not be emphasized."[130] Noting the "pressing need" for assistants to help nurses in the homes of the ill a few weeks later, the paper reiterated the chance "for women of goodwill and some natural ability in caring for the sick" to lend assistance.[131] Women were praised for bedside nursing care in homes and in hospitals, and for preparing food, feeding nurses, and delivering meals to the homes of patients, and their feminine behaviors while fulfilling this service brought further applause.[132] The accounts of Red Cross workers' efforts were "veritable documents of sympathy, tenderness and courage," according to one report.[133] It was women's self-sacrifice, their willingness to put others before themselves, which most commonly drew admiration.[134] As a Red Cross report on the contributions of women to its work suggested,

> This is a record of accomplishment. . . . that attempts to set down some of the heroism of the stay-at-homes; a mother, a daughter, perhaps a sister who showed courage of heart in fighting a mysterious foe and a humanity of spirit in aiding the weak and helpless—courage and humanity as richly to be prized as those of a father, a son or a brother overseas.[135]

Making a direct comparison between the contributions of men and women in the crises the United States faced in 1918, the report also distinguished between the kinds of work men and women did: "The work that these women of the Red Cross did in the influenza epidemic was undramatic. There is no drama in scrubbing floors. There is no romance in cooking gruel for the sick. But the very circumstance that their work was undramatic and unromantic gives to these women a reward of praise that needs no Cross of War." If men's proper place in 1918 was in the military fighting the war, women's was, it seemed, in the volunteer forces fighting the epidemic.

The impact of prescribed roles for men and women sometimes played out in much more significant ways as well. With young adults dying in unprecedented numbers, families were decimated by the loss of mothers and fathers. Monmouth County in New Jersey, for example, counted "thirteen motherless children and two fatherless" at the epidemic's conclusion, while the town of Berlin, New Hampshire, with its 3,000 residents, lost thirty-five young homemakers. A small town in Massachusetts found itself with sixteen "motherless children," and Breathitt County, Kentucky, counted at least fifty families in which one or both parents had died.[136] When adult family members died, the consequences were often determined in part by gender norms. Men who lost wives, for instance, might be neither personally prepared nor socially sanctioned to raise surviving children. According to the Associated Charities of Minneapolis, when women died no county aid was provided to families, though the mother might have been an economic contributor in poorer families. Such a circumstance meant "the breaking up of his family" unless the father could afford child care, which was frequently unlikely.[137] When a male adult member of a family died, the problems were often quite different but no less significant. With men the major breadwinners in many families, such a death might leave a family, one Red Cross worker explained, "without any means of support: left really to the mercy of the meager assistance that sympathetic neighbors might give."[138]

Class and the Impact of Poverty

For patients and families alike, the suffering and confusion produced by the epidemic could be made substantially worse by poverty. Shortages of medical and nursing care particularly afflicted the poor. With the well-to-do able to pay for the services of local doctors and nurses, those with limited financial means were often forced to look to local government and charity for assistance.[139] Access to hospital beds for the critically ill was affected by economic status as well. In the two decades immediately preceding the pandemic, hospitals had become increasingly differentiated by their private or public status. While private hospitals came to represent scientific medicine at its most advanced, public hospitals struggled to balance advancements in the quality and cost of care with the continuing mission of care for all. In this context, patients were clearly segregated by their ability to pay for medical services.[140] While all Americans scrambled for access to professional medical care during the pandemic, the poor found themselves at a distinct disadvantage as their numbers overwhelmed the available facilities. (See Figure 2.5.) When death came, too, their poverty sometimes prevented or at least made more difficult adequate burial and funeral services.[141]

For the poorest and most marginalized of Americans, hunger, inadequate sanitation, and preexisting bad health worsened the pandemic's impact. Visiting nurses reported regularly on horrific cases of poverty and emphasized the ways in which "actual want, acute physical suffering and dire distress" tormented patients and their families.[142] In pleas for aid, poor families, too, acknowledged how seriously the epidemic had affected them. "It went badly with my family" 68-year-old J. M. Russell explained in a letter asking for help. "Can you send my husband and myself any clothing of any kind or shoes or even pieces for making quilts?" Russell did not expect handouts, and was willing to send "eggs or chickens" in exchange for aid, and "will be so thankful for anything you can do for us."[143] Others shared this sense of desperation. "I am calling on you for help this winter as I am in need," another supplicant explained. "I have three little children and my husband has been sick.... If anybody needs anything it is us."[144]

For families living with material deprivation before the epidemic hit, the disruption of wage-earning through illness, even for a short time, might mean hunger, cold, and even homelessness.[145] The story of the D. family in Minneapolis reflected how easily the epidemic could derail the fortunes of a family already struggling with poverty. This family first appeared in the records of the Associated Charities of Minneapolis in 1916, when the family sought help with their rent and furniture payments. Though they came to Minnesota from Georgia in 1915 in hopes of both a better climate and employment, by March 1916 Mr. D. had yet to find a steady job, and records suggest the family rarely experienced

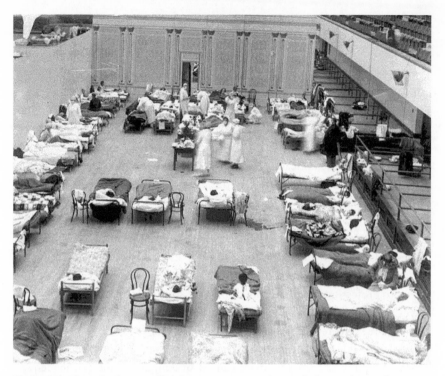

Figure 2.5 The sick often sought refuge in emergency hospitals during the pandemic. In Oakland, California, the Municipal Auditorium was filled with patients suffering through their illnesses. Edward A. "Doc" Rogers, (Photo #277), Joseph R. Knowland Collection, Oakland History Room, Oakland Public Library.

financial stability. In December 1918 influenza struck the family, infecting the father first and later his wife and five children. By December 28, 1918, the father had "been out of work for three weeks" due to his illness and the need to care for his family, and the family needed groceries. For the first two weeks the family had managed on their meager savings and on money sent from a relative. After that, though, the family became frantic, and the Associated Charities of Minneapolis resumed responsibility for the family. Though Mr. D. assured caseworkers that he would return to work, his wife and eldest child's relapses made such a return impossible. At this point, the situation became desperate: "They were absolutely without coal and he had borrowed a pailful from the woman downstairs. The groceries were also gone. He had tried his best to get credit at the grocery but had been unable." Calling his workplace that day, Mr. D. discovered he had lost his position. At that point, "Mr. D. broke down and cried, saying everything was against him."[146] Though the D. family's problems did not originate with the epidemic, their insecure situation was worsened by their bout with influenza, common among Americans already enduring poverty.[147]

The death of an adult family member, in turn, often constituted a serious and long-term economic crisis. A woman widowed in Vermont during the epidemic described a common situation when she lamented, "My husband die [*sic*] from pneumonia at the time of the influenza. . . . It was hard for me to get along after he die [*sic*]." As was frequently the case in working-class families, this woman soon went to work, in this case crocheting altar linens. She recognized her good fortune in having this skill: "How else then could I support myself and three children, except that I scrub floors and do hard work all the time?"[148] For many others, such work was all that kept them from complete destitution. For some families the solution to the loss of an adult breadwinner was the employment of children. Melvin Frank's father contracted influenza during the pandemic, and though he lived almost two more years, in June 1920 he succumbed to the after-effects, in his case cardiac asthma. Like many other youths in that time, Frank found himself prematurely grown, "the man of the family" at the tender age of 12. A week after his father's funeral, Frank lied about his age and went to work as an errand boy, his childhood over.[149]

The problems of poverty were particularly pronounced in Kentucky, a site of special concern for the Red Cross, where "every problem was accentuated."[150] A typical report, this one on work in the community of Pineville, illustrated the severity of conditions there. In the first house the Red Cross worker visited, she found nine people sick, including "the father, mother and seven children ranging in age from 4 months to 15 years, all in two beds and a cot, all in one room without window or door open and hot fire, no one to care for them." The home, in turn, was "perfectly filthy without anything to work with, no medicine, not even a clean rag or towel to sponge them off with, and nothing with which to make them anything nourishing." Such conditions were not unusual in Pineville, it seemed. "The people were starving," this worker concluded, "and had no medicine, and no nourishment."[151] Other reports from Kentucky confirmed similar circumstances.[152] To make matters worse, one nurse reported, patients were often "infested with vermin, and syphilis and trachoma were present."[153] The poverty and rural isolation of many of its communities meant that the shortage of doctors, nurses and hospitals suffered throughout the nation was worse in Kentucky.[154]

Red Cross workers' comments hinted at a deep unease about the people they served in Kentucky, sometimes seeming to blame them for the desperate circumstances they faced. Repeatedly describing those suffering as "desperately poor," "ignorant of the simplest principles of sanitation and hygiene," and "living in crowded quarters," reports intimated that the population's poverty and ignorance, and the resulting living conditions, were actually the cause of the epidemic conditions.[155] Recounting his discovery of a dead woman in a "miserable Shack" and his efforts to get her properly buried and her children appropriately cared for, a Field Supervisor for the Red Cross in this region, Shelly D. Watts, concluded starkly, "I can still smell the terrible odor, and will never forget the nauseating sight. The penalty for filth is death."[156] In a letter written a few days earlier, Watts had offered a particularly scathing assessment of the rural Kentuckians: "The conditions under which the mountain rural people live are so primitive and unsanitary, that the task of properly caring for the patients is impossible absolutely. To make any impression would mean years of intensive social service in most vigorous treatment."[157] MacKenzie R. Todd, Executive Secretary of the Red Cross of the Lake Division, shared this basic view. Describing them as a "primitive people," he worried it would be "a long, tedious job" to educate them to the need for "cleanliness" and "sanitary conditions."[158]

Rural residents of Kentucky were far from alone in facing criticism for their circumstances during the pandemic. The desperate conditions brought on by the epidemic produced unprecedented levels of contact between the Red Cross and working-class homes throughout the country. In turn, the Red Cross was joined by local aid societies, social workers, and visiting nurses in their efforts to offer assistance during the health crisis, providing unmatched opportunities for this range of professionals to observe, and to judge, recipients of their care. As they entered the homes of the poor, aid providers brought their own middle-class assumptions to the interactions, which conditioned their responses.

Especially common in these judgments were distinctions between the "deserving" and "undeserving" poor, between those who were worthy of aid and those who were not. Such categorizing underlay, for instance, the New York Times's presentation of "New York's 100 Neediest Cases" in December 1918, when many of the cases were families recently stricken by influenza. A regular charity effort of the paper during the holiday season, the feature outlined the stories of "some of the Great City's Destitute Families That Are in Desperate Need of Help," families "Selected for The New York Times by Four of the City's Leading Charity Associations," and appealed to Times readers to lend financial assistance. The characterizations of the selected aid recipients illustrated vividly the qualities associated with those who deserved help, and by inference those who did not. Most significantly, the deserving poor were those for whom poverty was the result of misfortune, not misbehavior. As the introduction to the feature explained, "The several hundred individuals whose situation is set forth below . . . are not the victims of their own shortcomings; they are people to whom something has happened."[159] Again and again the feature noted that "it was influenza that brought the problems of the C. family to a crisis," or "it was when the influenza epidemic swept the city that the family became a 'needy' household."[160]

Specific cases illustrated in greater detail that the deserving poor were those who had always been independent and industrious until misfortune struck.

"The N. family has never before needed help," Case 87 began.[161] Reassuring readers that the family would not become a permanent charity case, the story continued, "If they are set on their feet again now there is no fear of dependence in the future. For it is only the father's sudden serious illness that has plunged them into such dire want."[162] Industriousness and thrift were emphasized again and again. As the description of Case 59 noted, "Albert E.'s wife lay ill of pneumonia when he died of influenza during the epidemic. He had been a conscientious worker and a good father, but there are seven children in the E. family and saving was practically impossible."[163]

Though a middle-class definition of men as breadwinners was routinely accepted, indeed celebrated, for the working-class, definitions of womanhood were often more contradictory. On the one hand, women were applauded for being good mothers. Describing a recently widowed mother of five, Case 36 suggested, "She is a wise and capable mother, an excellent housekeeper, a woman whose home is worth protecting."[164] On the other hand, deserving families sent women to work if necessary to regain financial stability. "Mrs. G. intends to undertake the support of the family as soon as that is possible," Case 44 concluded, "but she must have help now."[165] Similarly, Case 74 explained, "Nine people cannot have good food on $12 a week. They need several dollars more than the struggling mother and the good big brother can supply."[166] As this last example suggests, too, a deserving family also sent its children to work.[167] As the description of Case 76 noted, "Leonard's father is dead of influenza and Leonard is bending all his childish energies to doing well in school, so that he can get his working papers the very minute he is 14."[168]

This preoccupation with a family's intentions toward work reflected an underlying tendency among aid workers to suspect the poor of dishonesty and laziness, and of attempting to take advantage of others' generosity. When a family applied for clothing in Minneapolis in late November 1918, the case report noted that in the past the family "had managed some rather clever begging." Subsequent reports questioned the family's need because the parents "were supposed to be working" and had received groceries recently.[169]

Believing some of their applicants for aid exhibited troublesome traits, visiting nurses and social workers sometimes used the opportunity of the epidemic to attempt to reform them. Sometimes aid workers sought only to offer lessons in basic principles of hygiene and health. As an article published by the Visiting Nurse Service of the Henry Street Settlement in New York explained, "One of the best results of the nurse's visit to the average tenement home is the effect of example and precept. Without seeming to teach or preach, the nurse goes about her task— eagerly watched by the patient and by at least some members of the family— emphasizing by actual demonstration the value of cleanliness, of sanitation, of ventilation, of isolation."[170] Other visiting nurses agreed.[171] These commentators imagined themselves as teachers, providing fundamental training in basic hygiene that might promote health among those with limited resources. (See Figure 2.6.).

Yet even these simple interactions might be laden with assumptions about the poor. If visiting nurses sometimes described the people they attempted to help as "intelligent and teachable," such a response also suggested that others might prove ignorant and intractable.[172] As one visiting nurse suggested of a family she visited, "Home conditions were bad, the mother not responsive to teaching, everything untidy and dirty."[173] Implicit, and sometimes explicit, in these educational efforts, then, was an assumption that working-class families might be defective, and sometimes willfully so.

Again and again visitors to the homes of the working poor—both visiting nurses and social workers—critiqued the conditions they found and the people they found living in them, maintaining that their problems derived less from poverty than from their behaviors. A series of recollections from nursing students serving homes in the Boston area during the pandemic illustrate this response vividly. One student nurse visiting a laborer's home critiqued the mother's failures, noting, "Here were three sick children and the mother could not see that it was her duty to stay at home and care for them."[174] Another nursing student described the problem of overcrowding, and, blaming it on large families and small wages wondered, "Why can there not be some way of regulating the size of a man's family to his wages or vice versa?"[175] Another student began

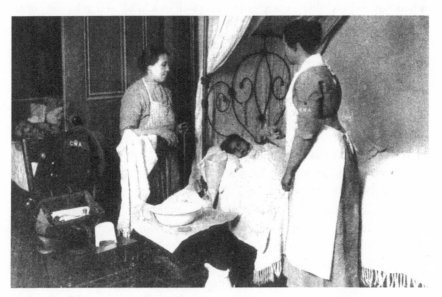

Figure 2.6 Visiting nurses entered homes to assist the ill and often engaged in educational and reform efforts as well. (A102505), Images from the History of Medicine, NLM.

her account with concerns for the patient's situation: "My little patient 8 yrs old [was] lying on an old couch with a filthy ragged comforter for a cover. The child was slightly delirious; flies literally covered her face and she had played and slept in the same soiled clothes for several days. She had no nursing care." Soon, though, her attention turned to the state of the family. "A sister, a mother of an illegitimate child, was sitting by her. It was a hunt to find necessary things for a bath and there was not a thing to be found in the house that could be put on the child as a night gown." And, further, "In this home the usual preparation for bed was unknown. One bed which was without pillows and covers served the purpose of three adults." Describing another visit, this time to a house with three families in it, this student nurse concluded simply, "Dirt and lack of order prevailed."[176] Physical dirtiness was often associated with broader moral problems assumed to exist among the poor—disorderly behavior, sexual promiscuity, and alcohol abuse.[177] As still another student nurse concluded her account of the epidemic, "To nurse in an epidemic was like meeting a creeping foe allied with ignorance, poverty, superstition, immorality, and hopeless fear."[178]

Certain groups of poor citizens were targeted for special criticism. In urban areas aid workers sometimes reported on the particular shortcomings of the foreign poor, whom they depicted as especially ignorant of modern medical care. Such a response was shaped, at least in part, by the unprecedented immigration of the decades preceding the pandemic. Between 1880 and 1924 some 23.5 million people migrated to the United States from other nations. Of note, too, was the source of many of the new residents, who came in unparalleled waves from countries in southern and eastern Europe, as well as in smaller but unprecedented numbers from Mexico, Canada, China, and Japan. Americans had long associated immigrants with epidemics and disease and blamed illnesses ranging from trachoma to cholera, from tuberculosis to typhus, on the arrival of foreigners.[179] During the influenza crisis, though, thanks to immigrants' participation in the war effort, declining immigration numbers, and the unusual morbidity and mortality patterns, there were few broad-based and organized efforts to demonize immigrants. While San Franciscans had been quick to blame the Chinese for earlier epidemics, including the bubonic plague that struck in the late nineteenth century, there was no blanket accusation of them during influenza's attack in 1918.[180] Even without the large-scale suspicion so common in earlier epidemics, individual immigrants nevertheless confronted wariness and criticism as they suffered through influenza in late 1918, reactions fostered by nativism and cultural difference. In Monroe County, Pennsylvania, for instance, the Emergency Service of the Council of National Defense pinpointed "the foreign settlement, where the disease had gained its greatest headway," for "special efforts" while "the relatives of stricken foreigners looked on aghast."[181] Similarly, a visiting nurse in the Boston area described her "continual fight" to get Jewish residents to "have the windows open" because "Jews are so afraid of having fresh air in the house."[182] In this context, leaders in immigrant communities—health care providers, journalists, and social welfare organizations, in particular—came to play a vital role as mediators between public health officials and ethnic communities.[183]

Given their assumptions about the capabilities of the poor, and particular groups among the poor, it is perhaps not surprising that aid workers would set out to reform their clients. The example of a poor immigrant family living in Minneapolis illustrates social workers' preoccupation with the habits of their working-class clients, their assumptions about the immorality of those clients, and their use of the family emergency created by the epidemic as an opportunity to intervene. In this case, initiated by the illness of the mother, the male member of an unmarried couple appealed to the Children's Protective Society in late November 1918 for help during the woman's bout with influenza, seeking to board their 1-year-old child.[184] In mid-December a social worker discovered on a visit to the home that the couple was not married, and from here the case record discusses repeatedly the couple's unmarried status. When the man claimed he was unable to marry because of a wife back in Italy, the caseworker noted that he "does not understand he ought not to continue to visit . . . but says he has a perfect right to see his own child." The woman, too, "does not seem to realize that there is anything morally wrong about living with a man she is not married to."[185] Later entries in the case record further developed the theme of immorality in the home. On January 20, for instance, the social worker noted that the man's "breath smelt strong of liquor."[186] The woman of the household, by this point, had recovered from influenza, but the caseworker noted on January 23 the "very dirty condition" of the room, and the "very careless" appearance of the woman, whom she described further as "dirty" with her "hair uncombed."[187]

Four days later the case appeared in Juvenile Court, where the woman was described as "totally ignorant of any moral laws, altho not what you could term a common prostitute."[188] With the interpreter unable to attend the hearing, the clients' ability to defend themselves was surely compromised, and on February 3 the court ruled that the man would be required to pay the board for the couple's child, the woman's two older children would be temporarily removed to an orphanage, and the woman "would be expected to show improvement and desire to live more cleanly."[189]

Later that month the woman announced that she was now married and began the lengthy process of reclaiming her children.[190] Subsequent reports by caseworkers noted the woman's attempts at "improvement," while nevertheless dismissing her ability to live up to middle-class standards.[191] One suggested that she "is really trying to keep house clean but has not a very high standard of cleanliness," while another explained that she "does not understand modern house keeping and is very primitive about everything in that line." "However," this report acknowledged, "she is making an attempt to keep house clean."[192] Finally, at the end of June 1919, the woman was allowed to recover her children.[193] The children, though, remained in temporary custody of the Children's Protective Society for six months, and the case did not close until 1922 when the woman's new husband adopted all three of her children. Reopened in 1924 on claims that the family was running "a disorderly house," and was "making and selling moonshine," the case would close permanently in June 1925.[194] As this case illustrates, for working-class families contact with charitable organizations could lead not only to "friendly advice" but also to unpleasant interactions with social service agencies and even the local court system.

This case also reveals that the working-class people who were the targets of reform sometimes resisted this interference in their lives. As early as January 1919 the grandfather in the preceding case complained that the intrusion of the Juvenile Court had caused the family to lose the financial support of the youngest child's father; this other male figure was also openly hostile to the social workers and resisted their efforts to shape his behavior.[195] Though the woman in the case attempted to meet the demands of the social workers in order to regain her children, she made clear through a "great deal of weeping and wailing" that she did not agree that her children would be better off in an orphanage.[196] Already living on the edge of desperation, families of lesser means often could not weather the epidemic without aid, but they sometimes discovered this aid came with a high price.

Race and the Epidemic

If the poor sometimes faced the uplift efforts of aid workers determined to reform them, people of color were more commonly stamped by the white majority as beyond redemption. When Edna Hoffer died of Spanish influenza on October 27, 1918, the Bureau of Vital Statistics for the Washington State Board of Health registered her death with some detail. The record included her sex, her age, her marital status, her birthplace, her parents' names, the date of her death, and its cause. It also included her "color or race." Hailing from an "Indian Reservation," Hoffer was listed as "Red." Even in death, it seemed, race marked Americans.[197] People of color frequently experienced the epidemic from positions of economic disadvantage, complicated further by racial prejudice. To make matters worse, dismissive reports by white public health and aid workers routinely charged minority communities with being particularly problematic populations, misdirecting culpability for desperate conditions from widespread and systemic racism to its victims.

The desperate situations faced on many Indian reservations during the epidemic were routinely blamed on residents and their cultural practices, rather than on the poor conditions of reservation life. This tendency was vividly illustrated in the reports of Dr. D. A. Richardson, charged by the Commissioner of Indian Affairs in Denver to investigate the influenza situation at several New Mexico pueblos. First visiting the Isleta pueblo, Richardson discovered the "deplorable condition" there, evidenced in "the death of ten Indians" the day after he arrived. Writing several weeks later, Richardson offered a ready interpretation for the severe situation. While acknowledging a "better portion" of the pueblo, Richardson went on to describe "the southerly portion of the Pueblo which was older and presented a mere mass of low ceilinged adobes, small doors, virtually no windows, one pigeon hole leading into another." The results of living in such quarters were clear. "In these rooms, were, in all stages of the Flu," Richardson noted, "Indians lying dead or dying or advancing well to the conditions which followed the Flu." According to Richardson, the cause of death was as much the Indians' behavior as the illness they faced. The deaths in the epidemic, he maintained, were entirely avoidable if his patients would only adhere to his medical advice. "The Flu itself throughout all the pueblos was a matter of primary importance but where directions were carefully followed out, was seldom followed by pneumonia, pleurisy, nephritis, empyema or aught else of importance," Richardson explained. "Where he [the Indian patient] maintained an earnestness of purpose and remained prone . . . the majority of cases recovered without very much other than symptomatic medication [sic]."[198]

Too often, though, according to Richardson, patients in the pueblos ignored his advice and turned to traditional practices, dooming them to critical illnesses and often death. He described "the combativeness of the Indian," noting that in these cases, "little could be done." Richardson detailed the case of one such patient, Jose Jaramillo, whose early prognosis seemed promising. Though he had been an alcoholic, Jaramillo lived two miles from town and so was "quarantined to the extent that Indians can be quarantined," and his daughter-in-law was "an educated, intelligent woman and did as she was told." The patient remained in bed—"a real bed . . . not lying upon the floor"—taking broth, using a bedpan, and never sitting up, and five days into his illness his recovery seemed certain. With seeming prescience, though, Richardson worried that his patient would disobey the doctor's orders and soon discovered this was the case. Two days later he was diagnosed with double pneumonia and two days after that he was "dying." "This illustrates," Richardson concluded, "the average case with the Indian."[199]

Other Bureau of Indian Affairs employees reached similar conclusions, suggesting that American Indians' illnesses resulted from their intransigence and their continued embrace of traditional healing practices. An agent at the Reno Indian Agency documented the conditions there. In a "shack" he had discovered "four people lying on the dirt floor wrapped in rags apparently all suffering from influenza. . . . The stench which greeted us when we entered was most horrible and could be endured but a short time. An Indian had just been taken from this structure for burial." The reason for such desperation was quickly explained by the agent. Not only had the Indians kept their windows and doors sealed, but "they had refused medicine from the white doctor and Dick Mauwee, a Paiute enrolled at Pyramid Lake Reservation, was the doctor."[200] The agent went on to describe other scenes among the local Native American populations, finding that "the best house in camp" contained similar scenes of horror while another Indian family, "not enrolled on any reservation," was "free from disease" and lived in a "comparatively clean" and "well ventilated" structure.[201] Viewing the struggles of American Indians through the lens of racial hierarchy, aid workers on the reservations sometimes prioritized the long practice of cultural displacement in their efforts during the pandemic.

Though African Americans faced different prejudices and stereotypes, they, too, found their struggles during the pandemic made more brutal by racism. African Americans had long suffered health conditions significantly worse than those of their white contemporaries, the result of racial prejudice and economic and social discrimination. Policies of racial exclusion were fortified by white supremacy, a belief system that assumed the inferiority—physiological, psychological, and cultural—of African Americans. One result of this racial system was the "separate but unequal" provision of health care. Before the epidemic struck, African Americans had pushed municipal administrations to enforce public health reforms in black neighborhoods and sought access to hospitals for the ill. They also developed educational programs for urban residents—many of them new to the city—in sanitation and hygiene, organized cleanup campaigns and a National Negro Health Week, built black-controlled hospitals (118 by 1919), developed training programs for black nurses and physicians, and created professional organizations for these professionals.[202]

Despite these efforts, African American health suffered under the socioeconomic disadvantages of the Jim Crow system. For several diseases African Americans suffered significantly higher rates of mortality. In the southern states in 1917, for instance, mortality rates for tuberculosis, a disease closely linked with poverty, unhealthy living conditions, and physical exhaustion, were generally two to three times higher among African Americans than among whites. Other crucial killers—typhoid fever, whooping cough, and infant diarrheal illnesses—all yielded substantially higher death rates among African Americans as well. While white Americans had achieved a life expectancy of 55.1 years by 1915, African Americans still averaged just 38.9 years.[203] Though scientific racism allowed many in the white community to dismiss the low life expectancy and high death rates among African Americans as symptomatic of their innate weakness rather than their social and economic circumstance, for some it prompted alarm over the dangers posed by neighboring black communities. While such a response sometimes fostered white engagement in public health and medical work that benefited African Americans, it did little to change the stigmatizing of African Americans as diseased and dangerous, and often reinforced demands for punitive controls and segregation.[204]

When influenza struck in the fall of 1918, reports in both the medical and popular press sometimes claimed lower morbidity and mortality rates for African Americans, and many in the black community agreed that they were suffering less severely than whites.[205] The absence of sound data from the epidemic makes it impossible to verify this. What is clear is that, regardless of morbidity or mortality rates, African Americans' experiences during the epidemic were framed by the disadvantages of racial prejudice and the broader poverty and segregated health care system it produced, forcing them to continue relying on their own too limited community resources as they sought to provide sufficient care for their sick neighbors.

Black nurses, who had been barred from service in World War I by the Army Medical Corps with the passive support of the Red Cross, rushed to do battle in the war against influenza, providing care to any American in need without regard for racial identity.[206] Yet beds in hospitals often remained barred to African Americans and their caregivers, and it was only the efforts of the African American community that facilitated the provision of professional care for their stricken. In Richmond, Virginia, though the Red Cross created an emergency hospital at John Marshall High School that served all the city's citizens, African American victims were relegated to the basement until a separate space could be opened at another city school.[207] Such circumstances were not isolated to the south. In Philadelphia, the city's Board of Health eventually provided numerous additional emergency clinics for white residents during the epidemic, but did nothing to help black Philadelphians. Instead, it was Dr. Nathan Francis Mossell, the Medical Director of Frederick Douglass Memorial Hospital, who produced additional beds at a local Catholic school when the city's two black hospitals reached capacity.[208]

Just as many poorer Americans resisted the class assumptions of middle-class aid workers and Native Americans sometimes rejected aid workers' advice and relied on their own traditional health practices, African Americans challenged discriminatory treatment during the pandemic. Newspaper reports represented substantial efforts to defend the African American community against not only influenza but also white supremacy. In Baltimore, the *Afro-American*, a local paper with an increasingly national circulation, detailed the costs in "one of the most pitiful cases." The paper told the story of "an unknown man who was found unconscious" and the struggle "to get him into the already overcrowded Provident Hospital and failing in that to get someone to volunteer to visit him occasionally and administer the necessary medicines."[209] The newspaper did not hesitate to explain the meaning of this story: "This is one of the extremely sad cases that are the pitiable result of the jim crow [sic] policy practiced in white hospitals of the city, and the woeful lack of larger quarters in Provident [a forty-bed hospital]," it argued. "The need for a colored hospital large enough to supply the needs of the city and well equipped for all emergencies has never before been felt so keenly."[210] Publicizing the situation, the *Afro American* determined that the community should remain well aware of the costs racism exacted.

Others took advantage of the crisis to call for the complete dismantling of the racial hierarchy in the United States. The Reverend Francis J. Grimke, an important advocate for African American rights, mused about the meaning of the epidemic in a special sermon in early November at his Fifteenth Street Presbyterian Church in Washington, D.C., and concluded that God was trying to awaken Americans to the sacrilege of the racial caste system.[211] "What ought it to mean to us?" he wondered of the pandemic situation and searched for clues to God's purposes. "Every part of the land has felt its deadly touch—North, South, East and West—in the Army, in the Navy, among civilians, among all classes and conditions, rich and poor, high and low, white and black," he observed. This circumstance surely hinted at God's lesson for Americans. "During these terrible weeks, while the epidemic raged," he argued, "God has been trying in a very pronouncedly conspicuously and vigorous way, to beat a little sense into the white man's head; has been trying to show him the folly of the empty conceit of his vaunted race superiority, by dealing with him just as he dealt with the peoples of darker hue." Stating his case more bluntly, Grimke continued,

> In this terrible epidemic, which has afflicted not only this city but the whole country, there is a great lesson for the white man to learn. It is the folly of his stupid color prejudice. It calls attention to the fact that he is acting on a principle that God utterly repudiates, as He has shown during this epidemic scourge; and, as He will show him when He comes to deal with him in the judgment of the great day of solemn account.

Clear in the workings of the natural world and in the epidemic, racial justice was also obvious in the teachings of Jesus, who commanded people to love God and to love "thy neighbor as thyself." Grimke continued, "Race prejudice, colorphobia, runs directly counter to both of these great commandments. And, therefore, never mind what the white man may think of it, we see clearly what God thinks of it." Certain of the lesson God sought to teach, Grimke was less certain that whites would learn it in time to avoid God's judgment. "Let us hope, therefore," he concluded, "not only for the sake of people of color, but also for the sake of white people themselves that the great lesson as to the folly of race prejudice—of assuming that a white skin entitles one to better treatment than a dark skin, which this epidemic has so strikingly taught, may not be lost upon them."[212] Though Grimke did not hold great hope that white Americans would grasp it, he nevertheless was certain that the epidemic was an event loaded with God's purpose, a powerful mandate for racial justice. If influenza found a ready ally in Americans' social prejudices, such prejudice did not always find cooperative victims as its targets offered alternative interpretations of the epidemic's meaning.

Making Sense of the Epidemic

Grimke was not alone in noting the egalitarian quality of influenza's assault or in finding purpose in its democratizing possibilities. Over the course of the epidemic, Americans went to great lengths to understand what was happening to them, narrating the pandemic in terms that allowed them to regain a sense of control over their lives and to imbue their experiences during the crisis with meaning, even purpose. In this context, it was hard to miss the leveling behavior of the influenza bug. William Pickens, writing in the *Baltimore Afro-American*, suggested, "Whatever other indictments may be brought against the Influenza Germ, it is certainly free from race and color prejudice."[213] For others the epidemic had offered not only the possibility, but also the reality, of democracy, infusing their experience of the crisis with a decidedly positive meaning. While the Red Cross emphasized the shared access to resources for "rich and poor alike" during the epidemic, the Directing Nurse of the Public Health Service suggested that "Caste, color, creed were forgotten, and the desire to render aid seemed paramount."[214] An article published in November 1918 in the social science oriented magazine *The Survey* paid special attention to the epidemic's ability to create a more democratic union. The article, "A Brotherhood of Misericordia," focused on a makeshift hospital that operated in the early days of the epidemic and heralded the social diversity of the staff, which included "army doctors," "army medical students," "trained nurses," and "college professors, teachers, Red Cross aids, volunteers from offices after office hours," and "laboring men, some just over the disease." Noting, "Many were the races represented in that hastily organized hospital," the author concluded with a celebration of the democratic qualities the epidemic had encouraged there:

> I cannot help feeling that in the old building on the river, something more than a fight against influenza had taken place. Another disease was being fought, a disease from which the nurses were suffering as well as the patients, the disease, the plague, of class feeling. Amid the inconveniences

and discomforts of the Lodging House hospital, the kind of democracy toward which we are all working showed a sign of health.[215]

Though the epidemic was tragic, this account maintained, it had nevertheless provided a much-needed opportunity for democratic behavior, and had, in a sense, brought the country closer to real national well-being.

While some Americans found democratic meaning in the crisis, others relied on a religious narrative to provide clues to the pandemic's purpose. For the Reverend Grimke, the pandemic's message of racial equality had distinct secular implications but was also deeply rooted in Christian soil. In addition to racial justice, Grimke pointed to a number of other classically Christian principles Americans might relearn as a result of the epidemic—the power of God and their own complementary powerlessness before Him, the need to focus again on the realities of death and eternity, and ultimately the comfort and security Christianity offered to all willing to accept it. "Let us all draw near to God in simple faith," Grimke concluded.[216] Other Americans, too, viewed the epidemic as God's doing. A report on the epidemic at St. Ann's Infant Asylum in Washington, D.C., thanked God "for his goodness in our regard" as He spared all but three children during the pandemic.[217] Others saw in the epidemic not God's merciful hand but rather His vengeance. Jehovah's Witnesses, for instance, viewed the epidemic as fulfilling Jesus's prophecy on the Mount of Olives of "pestilence and arrows." The evangelist Billy Sunday proposed the use of public prayer to beat the epidemic, and others, too, turned to their faith as the mechanism for their salvation from the scourge.[218]

Not every American was able to find such meaning or purpose in the catastrophe, and many saw it as nothing other than an unimaginable and uncontrollable scourge. One observer tried to describe the wretchedness he had seen in the small town of Simpson, Pennsylvania, noting "the extreme distress of the people there," the "dearth of help," and the "general suffering," but concluded, "It would be very difficult for a person who had not been in the homes of Simpson to imagine how much suffering existed there."[219] Others shared this sense that the epidemic was beyond description, the damage it caused unimaginable to those who had not seen it first-hand.[220] "A blight had fallen," a Red Cross report explained about the situation at Camp Dodge in Iowa. "The Hosts of Death were marshaled—our Camp was invaded, and the enemy, unseen and heretofore undetected, was everywhere in our midst."[221] Everything, it seemed, had changed overnight. As one correspondent lamented simply, "The whole world seems up-side-down. So many people around here have died, and so many are sick."[222]

Even as many described influenza in terms that emphasized the uncontrollable power of the epidemic and their own powerlessness before it, Americans often tried to *explain* the epidemic as well, to suggest what it *was like*. Searching for analogies, they attempted to make the scourge recognizable. For some "it was like a horrible nightmare," or "a horrible dream," something so awful only the imagination could create it.[223] In a subtle critique of modern science, other Americans termed the epidemic a "plague," declaring that "this grippe has been just like a plague of olden times," was "comparable to the historical plagues of the past."[224] For others, comparisons to natural disasters seemed to do justice to both the horror and the power of the epidemic. "It behaved like a storm," or "struck like a cyclone at first."[225] Others viewed the epidemic as a "conflagration" or compared it to a forest fire, while still others described "the tide of the epidemic of Spanish Influenza" and suggested that it had "suddenly swept the country and prostrated communities in its destructive course."[226] Through these metaphorical descriptions many Americans attempted to transform the unprecedented epidemic into terms that made it intelligible.

Americans turned repeatedly to the language of war to describe, discuss, and explain the epidemic. Such efforts to explain disease through metaphor, and particularly military metaphor, were not new with the influenza pandemic of 1918.[227] In 1890 the *New York Times* noted "Grip's Deadly March," while other publications, both popular and professional, referred to influenza as "the enemy" and urged Americans to "fight" that enemy "in his stronghold."[228] Similarly, a 1913 article in the popular magazine *Living Age* recounted the entire history of influenza as a series of attacks by a clever and evolving enemy. In this narrative, the coming of the scientific age allowed humans "to make formidable resistance" against the flu, though in 1889 influenza "began to gather itself together for a mighty effort." Noting the expectation of some that this was influenza's "last concentrated attack upon the human race," the essay reminded readers that influenza was a very clever foe.

> The enemy was only preparing for another campaign. In the parliaments of bacilli it was probably recognized that they must move with the times, adopt modern methods, and abandon the conservative and obsolete policy of existing germ government, which had been living on the reputation of its great success in 1891. So a new campaign was prepared, the army reorganized, and an expedition of pneumo-cocci sent over to England to try to take us by surprise.

Anticipating that this pattern of struggle between humans and influenza would continue, the article reminded readers, "Don't be fooled by the subtle disguises of the enemy."[229]

What made the use of martial imagery unusual in 1918 was the nation's literal involvement in a war at the epidemic's start, which encouraged citizens to view the influenza outbreak through the lens of the war.[230] For some citizens the link between the two was not metaphorical but literal as they imagined the epidemic as an actual battle in the ongoing military conflict, and influenza as the latest weapon of the German enemy.[231] In New York City a rumor circulated that Bayer's Aspirin Tablets contained the organism causing the epidemic.[232] A self-described "Red Cross Woman" wrote to the War Department in September 1918 to share her worry that the Germans had put something in the water to sicken Americans.[233] Similarly, a letter to the Surgeon General's Department wondered whether the epidemic might have been caused by "an enemy submarine or aircraft" spreading germs.[234]

For others, Germany's culpability was not a question but a certainty. A letter to the editor, published in the *New York Times* in October 1918, stated bluntly, "Many thousands of Americans believe that the germs of this plague, which has greatly hindered the Liberty Loan and caused much suffering and many deaths in our army . . . are of German sowing." Suggesting such a tactic was "wholly in accord with previous knowledge . . . of the Germans' barbarous methods of warfare" the letter writer concluded, "Let the curse be called the German plague."[235] Billy Sunday spread the belief that flu was a German plot. As he told an audience during the pandemic, "We can meet here tonight and pray down an epidemic just as well as we can pray down a German victory. The whole thing is part of their propaganda; it started over there in Spain when they scattered germs around."[236] Once tied to the war, influenza became comprehensible as another weapon of the enemy or another battle in the ongoing struggle.[237]

Though most Americans did not accept the rumors of a German plot to infect Americans, they nevertheless relied on the war to help explain the pandemic. References to the war in Europe provided Americans with a shared experience and vocabulary for assessing the new incarnation of influenza. Just as World War I was touted as a truly modern and worldwide war, the epidemic was seen as having a uniquely horrific character. Often, too, influenza was viewed as the more devastating of the two.[238] As a report in a Red Cross publication explained, "The physicians reported the epidemic as 'the worst pestilence they had ever seen,' and Miss Guthrie, a trained nurse, who had returned from work abroad said, it was 'worse than the battlefields.'"[239] Similarly, Hermann Biggs, New York's Health Commissioner, observed, "So far as life and health are concerned, it is apparent that the toll of the epidemic measured in deaths and disabilities will be for the United States four or five times as great as that of the war," and further, "The casualties of the war are in many respects far less serious than the disabilities which will be left from influenza."[240]

Even more common in the narration of the epidemic was the traditional use of martial rhetoric to facilitate a sense that Americans were actively resisting influenza. Describing the onset of influenza as an "attack" and the disease as "the enemy" and "as dangerous as poison gas shells," Americans again and again characterized their situation in the language of a military mobilization.[241] Facing "a flank attack . . . launched by an army of deadly influenza germs," Americans developed strategies "to battle" the epidemic, "to fight Spanish Influenza," to "combat the thing."[242] Influenza became the "invisible foe," and Americans were asked to mobilize for the purpose of "combating the disease."[243] As an article in *Public Health Nurse* argued, "An enemy that attacks city after city in a rapid sweep over the whole country and in a few short weeks takes a toll of a hundred thousand lives needs to be fought by the best mobilization that social forces can provide."[244] Even patent medicine producers adopted the war imagery to sell their products.[245]

Such language also seemed to imply that Americans had the ability to succeed against the epidemic. Specific preventive measures became part of a military campaign; gauze masks became "facial armor for the influenza."[246] Nurses became an "army in nurses' blue," and "led a fight against the dread disease until it was routed," and "hygienists of the world" became the "standing army . . . maintained by society to organize and hold the defenses against such dread invaders."[247] Physicians, too, became soldiers, "the line of first defense," ready to protect Americans and defeat the epidemic.[248] Declaring the Base Hospital at Camp Cody a "Gibralter [*sic*] Against Disease In Any Form," an article in the camp newspaper declared, "Trained physicians and surgeons have their fingers on the health trigger every minute" and every member of the medical detachment "is ready to do more than his full duty."[249] Not just medical practitioners but laypeople had the power to participate in this battle against the epidemic. As a Virginia newspaper exclaimed, "An old enemy is with us again, and whether we fight a German or a germ, we must put up a good fight, and not be afraid."[250] Or as a poster produced by the State Department of Health in Connecticut urged Americans, "HELP FIGHT THE GRIPPE—KAISER WILHELM'S ALLY." (See Figure 2.7.) No longer a mystifying disease, influenza became an enemy to be fought.

This was also an enemy, Americans seemed to say, that they could defeat. Commentators repeatedly noted that Americans had the ability to win this war, just as they expected to win the war in Europe. The Camp Dodge newspaper declared on October 18, "With Germs in Rout, Victorious Hospital Workers Rest a Bit," while an article the next day in the newspaper for Camp Jackson noted that the head of the base hospital was "smiles and smiles since the 'flu' germs have started to 'stack their arms' for complete surrender."[251] An editorial in the *New York Times* entitled "Showing the Courage of Soldiers" celebrated the performance of civilians under the stress of the epidemic, and again drew a direct link to Americans' experiences in the war. Having been trained by the war experience, it seemed, Americans were well prepared for the pandemic, recognizing in it the civilian's equivalent of the soldier's fight. "Probably the general feeling was that the danger here should be borne as bravely as the risks of battle are

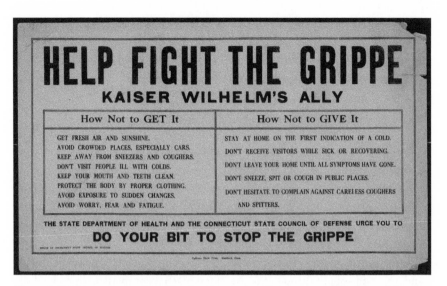

Figure 2.7 This poster produced by the Connecticut Department of Health and the Council of National Defense made it clear that citizens had a patriotic duty to fight influenza. (Broadside 1918 H44), Special Collections Department, University of Virginia Library.

endured by our fighting men abroad," the editors suggested. Perhaps most important, they concluded, Americans were winning both wars. "The danger has been met and conquered, and now we are caring for the wounded just as they do in France after a big encounter with the Germans."[252]

This rhetorical comparison suggested the certainty of American victory over the influenza enemy, while also imbuing the fight itself with meaning.[253] An article from *Literary Digest* illustrated this strategy particularly well. "A war here in the United States, a war that reached into practically every community in the country and took a toll of American lives twice as great as that taken by the war overseas, has raged through the early winter months," the author began. Having established the severity of the epidemic through both metaphor and direct comparison, the article continued, "In the fight against influenza, which is not yet finished, devoted women have served in the front ranks and many of them, uninspired by the interest and honor that helped the dough-boy to act the hero, have gone down to death, if not unwept, at least unsung." Having been "pretty heroic in France," American women had been "none the less so at home," the article concluded.[254] Anxious to garner for nurses the respect and appreciation they deserved, this author compared their service on the home front to their service on the battlefield, a rhetorical strategy that was quite common.[255] In a poem entitled "Your Chance," a student nurse in New York urged other women to join her in the fight against influenza, employing the language of military mobilization in wartime to make her point.

> You who longed for a chance to fight hand to hand
> With the foe, braving death, do ye not understand
> That the worst foe is here? And so here is our chance,—
> For all of the fighting is not done in France.
> Ye women who thrilled with fine purpose before,—
> It is now you are needed, *for this is our war.*[256]

The magazine noted that not long after writing the poem, the author died "from pneumonia during the recent epidemic." An article in a Red Cross publication used a similar tactic to celebrate the service of an emergency hospital superintendent, explaining, "Her service during this time was as unselfish and heroic as the service of nurses at the front, and there is no greater sacrifice than the one she has made."[257]

Again and again Americans celebrated the memory of those who died in the pandemic and sought through the use of the martial comparison to make those deaths meaningful rather than simply tragic. This was perhaps most common in descriptions of the deaths of nurses and doctors who died while serving others. As an account of Red Cross nurses during the war explained, "Nurses were not immune to the disease and many died, as much in line of duty as if they had been nursing the wounded on the Western Front."[258] Or as a tribute to "Our Workers Who Lost Their Lives Fighting the Influenza Epidemic" published by the New York City Department of Health argued, "The supreme sacrifice offered by these workers, quietly and without thought of distinction, ought to rank them with those heroes who have given their lives in France for country and civilization."[259]

Noteworthy is how commonly the language of martyrdom was applied to those who had not performed any service during the epidemic but were simply its victims. The governor of Iowa suggested in a speech honoring troops who had died at Camp Dodge during the epidemic, "We assemble today in the presence of the immortal spirits of these soldiers, who, clothed in the uniforms of their country, were stricken on their way to the battle front. . . . The voice of these will mingle in the mighty chorus of the martyr forces of the past. . . . They ally themselves with the worthy dead from every battlefield where mortal man has fought."[260] Similarly, the University of Virginia yearbook listed many influenza victims among the university's war dead.[261] Or as a chaplain suggested at the funeral of soldiers who died at Camp Sherman in Ohio, "It is sweet to die for one's country. These men are as true martyrs as those who have died in the trenches."[262] One can discern here the almost desperate need to give the deaths from influenza meaning and value.[263] Able to provide literal as well as metaphorical comparisons, to suggest both the enormity of the epidemic as well as Americans' ability to control it, and perhaps most important to infuse the struggles and the losses of the epidemic with meaning, even glory, the war was an ideal explanatory mechanism for interpreting the inexplicable.

As influenza raged through their communities, Americans struggled desperately to make sense of their experiences. For some this took the shape of traditional behaviors and beliefs. Others found meaning in particular interpretations of the pandemic's trials. As they confronted this challenge to their recent gains, health care professionals could only view the influenza crisis through the lens of their efforts to combat it. For public health leaders these struggles would include both the most expansive possibilities and the most troubling defeats.

3

"Let our experience be of value to other communities"

Public Health Experts, the People, and Progressivism

On September 29, 1918, Mr. Sell Litchford, age 41, became the third casualty of the influenza pandemic in Roanoke, Virginia.[1] The week before, W. W. Eastwood and Louise Mapp of neighboring Hollins College had died of "almost identical" symptoms— "pneumonia, following suddenly upon an attack of grippe," but the situation had seemed "well in hand."[2] After Litchford's death, though, the city's health commissioner, W. Brownley Foster, initiated public health precautions; only one member of his family would be allowed to travel with Litchford's body to its burial in Lynchburg.[3] The local paper, the *World News*, immediately joined the fight against the flu. Describing influenza as one of the "spray-borne diseases," it provided detailed instructions on how to avoid infection and, even more significantly, how to avoid spreading it. Including an admonition to "strictly obey" the orders of physicians, the article concluded by reiterating each citizen's responsibility and offering a word of hope. "If all men were religiously to observe these simple rules," the paper maintained, "Spanish grippe ... would be put to rout and its victims would number only hundreds instead of untold thousands."[4]

The reality, of course, was that few communities were to escape influenza, and Roanoke, like so many cities and towns across the nation, soon suffered under the scourge of the epidemic. As concern grew, the political leadership of Roanoke, on the advice of Health Commissioner Foster, upgraded controls on the community's behavior. A ban on meetings in public spaces—from schools and churches to pool halls and motion picture houses—was soon in place. The *World News* applauded citizens' cooperation. Though they had undoubtedly viewed with "grave concern and misgivings" the cancellation of Sunday services, one editorial suggested, "the clergy have borne the enforced abstinence from their godly labors with remarkable fortitude."[5] Similarly, though they had "lost a lot of money during the enforced shutdown," the movie theatre owners showed "a most commendable display of public spirit" by cooperating with the restrictions.[6] Teachers and students, too, were praised for their handling of five weeks of school closure.[7]

From the beginning, Health Commissioner Foster worried that citizens would attempt to return to normal conditions prematurely. He repeatedly urged patients to be conservative during their recovery and asked the community to be cautious about the lifting of restrictions.[8] The newspaper teamed up with Foster to warn citizens, using the case of Gastonia, North Carolina, "where precautions were relaxed in the face of danger" which led to "scores" of deaths and the collapse of local industry, to make their point.[9] As the lifting of the ban approached, the health commissioner urged residents to continue to exercise all precautions and appealed to their sense of responsibility. "Take care of yourself. It's up to the public," he reminded them.[10]

With his admonition, Foster may have been responding to an undercurrent of criticism that had begun to surface in Roanoke. The *World News*, which had been entirely supportive of the public health measures to this point, on October 29 questioned the wisdom of reopening theatres and movie houses only gradually, arguing that limiting the performances would only increase the crowds for the available shows. The editors quickly backed away from any apparent challenge to the health authorities, though, and offered repeated statements of their support. "We offer these remarks in no spirit of captious criticism," they explained. "It is quite likely that they [the health authorities] have considered this matter carefully—indeed we are sure that this is the case—and that they have reasons for the decision as announced which are not plain to us but which nevertheless are eminently sound." Urging readers to avoid any "untoward carelessness or relaxation of vigilance" they acknowledged that the closing orders had been "adjudged to be an effective weapon for combating the spread of the disease."[11] Three days later the editors repeated their hope that the theatres would be able to open fully with the lifting of the ban. Again, too, they backed away from their criticism, though not as far this time. "Of course, the authorities should use their best judgment in this matter and not be guided by newspaper opinion," they opined, "but the foregoing is the way in which the thing looks to us and we pass it on to the public for whatever it may be worth."[12] After churches and theatres reopened on November 3, Health Commissioner Foster again warned citizens against careless behavior. Blaming the "relaxation of precautions by individuals" for an apparent "comeback" of the flu, the Health Department made clear that "parties of all kinds" were "frowned upon." When organizers announced that "a big crowd is coming, with bells on" for a local dance, the newspaper followed up with a report that "the 'bells' were not allowed to ring," and noted that a smaller informal dance was also prohibited by the Health Department. "It is no time to be holding dances and balls," barked Health Commissioner Foster.[13]

Confirming Foster's worst fears, influenza was soon resurgent in Roanoke. On November 23 the newspaper reported on a "rather lively renaissance of the 'flu' epidemic."[14] Two days later there were more cases of influenza in the city than when the restrictions had been lifted two weeks earlier.[15] Believing that a return to the emergency edicts was called for, Foster and the Health Department moved to protect the city a second time. While the newspaper, schools, and theatres remained supportive, other problems quickly arose.[16] One difficulty was the failure by physicians to keep up with the reporting of the disease.[17] A more pressing problem was inattention to the rules of sterilization, a problem that landed a number of soda fountain owners in court.[18] Health authorities also struggled with citizens whose mild cases allowed them to remain mobile and with others wanting to bend or break the quarantine law.[19] As holiday shopping made it impossible to prevent crowds in town, the World News reported that people seemed to be ignoring the Health Department postings and reminded readers that "the doctors say, and statistics support them, that death is borne to the breezes from coughs and sneezes" and called on the public to "do its part."[20] "It isn't right for the individual to put on the city all the responsibility for protecting him," Foster railed as influenza continued to tighten its grip on the city in early December.[21]

By December 9 Roanoke was facing a "secondary epidemic."[22] That evening the City Council met and released a "Notice to Public on Influenza Situation," prompted by the failure of the public to respond to the warnings of the Health Department.[23] The next day estimates suggested the city had suffered 1,000 cases in the first ten days of December, and Roanoke's Board of Health and City Council decided to put the "'flu' lid" back on the city, again banning public meetings and calling for the closure of "schools, churches, theatres, pool rooms, bowling alleys, dances and other public gatherings" in two days.[24] Noting that "preventive measures were apparently cast to the winds by the individual" in the wake of the earlier ban's lifting, the newspaper's editors again supported the officials, admitting that "under the circumstances it is just as well, perhaps, that Roanokers should be forced—and not merely asked—to keep out of crowds and away from places where the influenza germs are apt to be prevalent."[25]

Challenges to the new ordinance were immediate, prompting both the city council and the city solicitor to state their intentions of punishing those resisting the ban, including an initial group of "seven pool room proprietors and a theatre."[26] In open defiance, some of the pool-room operators whose cases had been set aside by a technicality "flung open their doors and proceeded to operate as if nothing had ever happened."[27] In turn, two defendants, once brought to court, openly admitted they had opened their business and announced their intention to test the "legality of the ordinance."[28] The city maintained that its "policing powers" permitted such an ordinance and pointed to both the state and federal supreme courts for support.[29] An account of the debate before the judge made clear that feelings surrounding the case were strong and the atmosphere in the courtroom charged.[30] This second ban was in place only a few days. The closing order was soon rescinded, replaced by another, looser ordinance.[31] At this point even the editors of the *World News* wondered about the machinations of the Health Department and expressed hope that the return of Health Commissioner Foster, who had been away at the American Public Health Association meetings, would improve the situation.[32]

The arrival of the Christmas season did not make Foster's job any easier, though the latest ordinance gave him the power to control holiday festivities. Christmas celebrations or any parties involving "two or more families" were "a violation both of the spirit and letter of the law," and weddings, too, were to be kept as small as possible.[33] Foster pleaded with citizens to follow the regulations, suggesting that prosecutions in court would be a less effective approach to community health than simple cooperation.[34] Then, as the holidays approached, the city faced a nursing shortage.[35] Stunned that citizens had not responded to Red Cross calls for aid, the paper chastised the community for its failure. "In addition to the lives that may be lost unless help comes now," the paper lamented, "the fact will remain that Roanoke has fallen down on a big job."[36] The situation was likely complicated by the rising number of influenza cases. Though there had been a slow decline in influenza figures the preceding week, by Christmas Eve the numbers were again on the rise. Reminding the public of their experience in November, when the decline had been followed by a slow, and then rapid, increase, the day before Christmas Foster again cautioned the public to practice restraint in their holiday celebrations.[37]

Finally, though, relief came. In the wake of the holiday, conditions grew steadily better. The day after Christmas the nursing shortage had "improved considerably," and the next day the number of new cases was the lowest since the epidemic's beginning.[38] Public health authorities celebrated the apparent success of their actions, and while continuing to encourage citizens to take all possible measures to avoid infection, they again loosened the restrictions. When schools reopened on December 30 students had been away from their desks for the previous three weeks.[39] A week into January, three months after Mr. Litchford's death, the city could finally imagine an end to the epidemic.[40]

As the city's leaders orchestrated a public health response to the emergency, and as the people of the town reacted to the new edicts controlling their communal activities, the city of Roanoke acted out a drama repeated in cities and towns across the United States. When the epidemic threatened their communities, public health leaders shouldered responsibility for protecting the well-being of their citizens. As the example of Roanoke suggests, this required massive mobilization—of government power, of financial resources, of local health care providers, and perhaps most significantly, of public cooperation.

As with patients, there was no single public health experience of the pandemic, and each community suffered and survived in its own way. The story of Roanoke, though, was typical in many ways. As Health Commissioner Foster's early pronouncements suggest, public health authorities' decisions were informed by their recent successes in improving community health and by their resultant confidence in their ability to protect the citizenry. Though they initially hoped that simple precautious would suffice, the realities of the epidemic soon led them to take more dramatic actions. Some of the measures they employed were simple and required little change in the public's habits, but others required significant sacrifice as well as substantial organization, education, and mobilization of the public. Though health leaders needed to convince their constituents that the emergency called for drastic measures, only rarely did they detail the horrors of the pandemic or the misery of influenza patients. Instead, they relied on arguments that drew on citizens' sense of duty and patriotism.

As was the case in Roanoke, local health officials initially found the public supportive. From providing emergency budgets to organizing their communities, Americans cooperated with many of their requests, looking to experts to guide them through the epidemic and working together to help their communities. And yet this early cooperation was not always enough to halt the epidemic, which too often returned to communities in a renewed wave. As the crisis persisted, the public sometimes became restive. Resisting the continued impositions in their lives, individuals began to defy the authorities and to duck their communal responsibilities. As public health authorities attempted to shape American behaviors, they adopted the strategies of Progressivism, seeking to use government power to control the epidemic while educating and mobilizing the public to support these actions. Similarly, citizens' reactions—their initial support for and eventual weariness with the actions of officials—reflected the broader ascendance and collapse of Progressivism. In this sense the epidemic ended just in time, preventing what might have been a much broader rebellion against the authority of the state in the realm of public health.

Public Health in 1918

Public health leaders faced the emerging epidemic in the fall of 1918 with notable optimism.[41] As the second wave struck, some public health figures, largely unaware of the spring incursion, expressed the simple hope that this particular manifestation of influenza would be a mild one, lacking the "many serious complications and sequelae" of the 1890 outbreak.[42] Others hoped the epidemic would pass naturally, that it would "gradually subside" if weather conditions cooperated.[43] Most significantly, though, public health leaders' hopes were buoyed by their confidence in their expertise and the efficacy of their work.[44] As one public health leader suggested simply, "We ought to be in time to prevent the epidemic from assuming severe proportions if there is anything to public health education at all."[45] This confidence was encouraged to some extent by public health leaders' sense that they understood influenza and could employ their expertise in controlling the epidemic. As a special Editorial Committee formed by the American Public Health Association stated simply in a lead article in the *American Journal of Public Health (AJPH)*, "Something is known concerning the nature of influenza."[46] In particular, experts agreed, the epidemic was caused by a germ, it was extremely communicable, and it spread very quickly.[47]

While broadly dismissing criticism of germ theory itself, public health leaders were forced to admit that influenza's precise causative agent was a mystery, as was its explosion into worldwide pandemics.[48] As the APHA's special Editorial Committee rejoined, "Much remains to be determined."[49] This sense that their knowledge was easily balanced by their ignorance, that what they knew was fully matched by what they did not know, was shared by public health leaders around the country. In New York, for instance, the governor's Commission on Epidemic Influenza agreed on ten "Accepted Points" regarding the disease, including its origins in an "infectious agent," its acute communicability, the role of coughing and sneezing in spreading the infection, the consequent importance of hygiene and quarantine in preventing infection, and the need for legislation to control public behaviors.[50] Yet these shared insights remained frightfully limited. Recognizing that there was "no specific cure for the disease," with "rest in bed with careful nursing" as "the most essential factor in promoting recovery and preventing unfavorable complications," the commission complemented its ten "Accepted Points" with fourteen additional "Points in Regard to Which Information Is Desired" as well as "Proposed Investigations," the majority of which had to do with issues of communicability, patient care, and preventive measures. As they approached the epidemic, these public health leaders, and others like them across the nation, recognized in influenza both a disease about which they understood some important essentials and an epidemic incarnation of that disease about which they knew very little.

Even these challenges, though, could be recast as possibilities. From the beginning, public health officials recognized that the pandemic would create unique opportunities to develop their work. Data collection, for instance, could help to answer their myriad questions about the epidemic and would facilitate future understanding.[51] On November 23, 1918, two representatives of the

American Public Health Association wrote to Charles E. A. Winslow, the chairman of the recently founded Department of Public Health at the Yale School of Medicine, to announce the formation of a Committee on the Statistical Study of the Influenza Epidemic. "An unprecedented opportunity for collecting the facts of the epidemic of influenza is presented to the American public health movement," the letter began. It urged Winslow to participate in what could prove a "statistical contribution of the highest importance to American epidemiology."[52] At the first meeting of the committee a few weeks later, the chairman announced the "opportunity to show what statistics, especially vital statistics, and its methods can do for preventive medicine."[53] The Surgeon General, in turn, recognized that, because influenza was not on the list of "reportable diseases" in most locales, it was difficult, if not impossible, to measure the extent of the disease in the general population. He called for both state health officers and the officers of the United States Public Health Service (USPHS) to give regular reports, which he published in the agency's weekly *Public Health Reports* to allow for the epidemic's course to be tracked.[54] Even without this additional information, though, public health authorities felt ready to act, and to act quickly, to control the rapid spread of influenza.[55] Though lacking specific etiological information, they maintained that they could, indeed should, proceed with their efforts to mobilize and organize the nation to face the flu.

Organizing the Public Health Forces

The first hope was to limit the severity of the epidemic by hindering its entry from overseas, an effort likely doomed from the start.[56] On August 16 Surgeon General Rupert Blue sent a circular to Medical Officers at all United States Quarantine Stations, asking for particular alertness in the inspection of vessels coming from Europe.[57] Though infected ships were to be held in quarantine to halt Spanish influenza's spread, he did not call for a broader quarantine of all incoming ships.[58] Almost a month later *Public Health Reports* detailed measures necessary to block influenza's entry into the country.[59] Even as the journal went to print, though, influenza was gaining ground in the northeastern United States, making clear that influenza could not be kept out.

As this initial attempt suggests, public health efforts to fight the flu would be grounded in preventive work, the primary agenda of the public health profession. This work required substantial preparation, including the coordination of public health forces, the organization of local resources, and the mobilization of the public. The *AJPH* addressed the issue of preparedness directly, acknowledging that in this case preparation for actual cases would be an important part of the work. "What should health officers do in those communities where the disease has not yet struck? Shall they build fences to try to keep people from falling off the cliff or shall they invest in ambulances to take care of those who will have fallen?" For the *AJPH* editorialist the answer was clear: "Regrettable and discouraging as it is, we must nevertheless admit that in this specific catastrophe, the ambulance possibly will help more than the fence." And further, "With one in two hundred persons of the stricken populations dying, no community will criticise the health officer who may have prepared too thoroughly." What did such preparation entail? "The health officer should . . . put into effect with great vigor all of the preventive measures at his disposal. Let him not neglect, however, to plan for those who are sure to become sick . . . or those who will die."[60] Organizing available resources, particularly those sure to prove scarce during the epidemic, was a vital first step in preparing for the epidemic.

Doctors and nurses were the most valuable of those resources. At the national level, the USPHS shouldered responsibility for organizing medical and nursing personnel for the country as a whole during the pandemic. As influenza erupted in the Boston area, the Surgeon General recognized that the need for health care professionals would far exceed those immediately available, particularly given the depletion of their ranks due to the war.[61] While the USPHS quickly deployed both its regular officers and additional nurses to communities hit by the epidemic, it also asked for aid from the "American Medical Association, the Volunteer Medical Service Corps, the Red Cross, the medical and nursing professions as a whole" as well as the broader public in its search to supply additional staff to serve.[62]

Though additional physicians were soon employed by the USPHS, the problem of the nursing shortage struck the agency as a more difficult one. The Red Cross would lead efforts to mitigate this crisis, while also playing several other important roles.[63] Over the course of the epidemic the Red Cross organized nursing resources and supplied nurses to those communities in the greatest need of emergency assistance. They also took on responsibility for establishing and supplying emergency hospitals and kitchens; providing transportation for patients, medical professionals, and supplies; offering aid to families stricken by the scourge; and participating in the broad-based educational efforts necessary to mobilize the public.[64] To help coordinate the local work, a Red Cross representative was appointed for each state.[65]

Even as the Red Cross played a leadership role, the USPHS retained substantial control over its work. The Health Service appointed a field director for every state, often the state's health officer.[66] These officials were to work alongside the Red Cross representative to bring "the best results possible" and prevent "duplication of effort," but this partnership was never an entirely equal one.[67] The USPHS would "conduct all necessary dealings with the state and local boards of health," and the Red Cross would provide nurses and supplies "only upon the request of the Federal Public Health Service."[68] Thus while the Red Cross would play a very significant role in providing personnel, supplies, and avenues of com-munication, its efforts would be orchestrated by the Public Health Service.

The Red Cross, in turn, hoped to command the local nursing groups with which it worked but knew it would need to navigate relationships with local health officials with some care.[69] Who would decide whether gauze masks were needed? Who would distribute them? The Red Cross expected to intervene as necessary to provide health care for the poor during the epidemic, but who would pay for these services?[70] In addition to its preoccupation with the proper division of responsibilities, the Red Cross recognized the potential tensions that could arise with local authorities. As the Director of the Bureau of Nursing for the New England Division, Elizabeth Ross, reminded her colleagues, "Your organization should cooperate in every way with the local Boards of Health, but should take great pains not to force its opinions or services or criticize in any way their actions. You must remember that the Red Cross is not an officially recog-nized medical organization."[71]

The USPHS attempted to be clear about the lines of authority, deferring to state and local health officers while maintaining its own central role in the work nationwide.[72] To ensure this, "requests for medical, nursing and other emer-gency aid in dealing with the epidemic" were to originate with state health officers, who would forward them to the USPHS.[73] Public Health Service officers would oversee all of the medical and nursing personnel under the USPHS umbrella, including those that were organized by both the Volunteer Medical Service and the Red Cross.

The power of local public health agencies varied widely. In many states, cities, and towns public health administrators had the authority to act in the face of a health crisis, closing public places such as schools, prohibiting crowds and public gatherings, imposing quarantines, and enforcing other sanitary measures deemed necessary.[74] As important, these health leaders had long employed educational efforts to mobilize citizens and encourage their voluntary compli-ance with health measures. Though they would benefit from the strategies and support of the USPHS and the Red Cross, these local administrators would serve on the front lines of the epidemic, working directly with the public both to prevent and control the invading illness.

Finally, other national organizations, including professional organizations like the American Public Health Association (APHA), the American Medical Association (AMA), and the National Medical Association (the NMA, which served African American physicians who were barred from AMA membership), joined the effort to combat the epidemic, mobilizing their membership for ser-vice, designing programs for combating influenza, promoting educational efforts among laypeople, and collecting and publishing data related to the epi-demic and influenza.

For public health officials and activists, the epidemic had clearly cast them in a leadership role, placing on their shoulders responsibility for "safeguarding the health of the nation," a responsibility of unquestionable importance, but also one full of great "opportunities . . . to help."[75]

Educating the Public

Given the importance of their work, the public health forces understood from the beginning the significance of "spreading the gospel" of public health, of motivating the public to "stand squarely" behind their recommendations.[76] As a result, their efforts were always multi-pronged: they designed programs to educate and mobilize the public, and they planned mechanisms to prevent and control influenza. National leadership relied, in part, on local public health agencies for the implementation of their plans, and so needed to provide information and support to these officials to encourage cooperation. These local officials, in turn, often looked to political leaders for both funding and authority. But it was the public that would play the largest role in shaping their community's experience of the epidemic. Citizens needed to be either convinced or policed to accept control over their public and private behaviors.

Education, then, was a top priority for public health leaders, who targeted both local health officials and the populace in their efforts to spread the messages of prevention, relief, and research. The campaign was led by the USPHS and spearheaded by the Surgeon General, who argued that the best way to "check the spread of the epidemic and to minimize the ravages of the disease lay in an aroused and educated public opinion."[77] The APHA, immediately on board, detailed the education needed. Physicians would need reporting guidelines as well as information on resource availability and treatment standards. Doctors, school superintendents, and factory-floor managers required instruction on the importance of "immediate home and bed treatment at the first sign of respiratory disease." Families should be provided with information regarding "where aid may be secured," guidance on "what to do till the doctor comes" and "the problems of care during the physician's absence" and warnings about "the danger of returning to work too soon, etc."[78] With this range of educational materials, national public health leaders hoped, communities and individuals might face the epidemic armed with the best public health information experts had to offer.

Early in the epidemic the USPHS published a circular, *"Spanish Influenza" "Three-Day Fever" "The Flu,"* that provided "the known facts regarding the nature of influenza and the precautions to be observed in dealing with the disease."[79] By epidemic's end, the USPHS had published six million copies of this essential text. In addition, it produced countless posters and articles for publication in the popular press as well as a "daily bulletin" for "the large news-gathering associations" that included both "a summary of the situation from day to day" and a "brief comment on new features regarding preventive measures."[80]

The USPHS recognized the need to appeal to different citizens in different ways and prided itself on its accessibility to the average citizen. An article describing the intentions of a "striking" new poster drawn by a "well-known Washington cartoonist" in the November 15, 1918, *Public Health Reports* explained, "This shows at a glance and in language understood by everybody just how influenza and other respiratory diseases may be guarded against." The poster depicted an elderly gentleman wearing a hat labeled "THE PUBLIC," who, upon seeing a young boy about to sneeze, offers the youth a handkerchief and exclaims, "USE THE HANDKERCHIEF AND DO YOUR BIT TO PROTECT ME!" Celebrating the "modern method of health education" represented by this new poster, the article compared it to the "official, dry, but scientifically accurate" messages of the past, burdened with "technical phraseology," which would have been useless to the "man in the street, the plain citizen, and the many millions who toil for their living."[81]

The USPHS was joined by the Red Cross in its educational efforts. One Red Cross pamphlet, "Spanish Influenza," included a single-page discussion of "How to Protect Yourself from Spanish Influenza," which it made available in eight different languages—Hungarian, Italian, Bohemian, Spanish, Polish, Russian, Yiddish, and, of course, English.[82] As the historian Alfred Crosby noted of the educational effort by public health forces, "If influenza could have been smothered by paper, many lives would have been saved in 1918."[83]

In these educational efforts, prevention took center stage. "Prevention in this disease is worth many pounds of cure," a message from the USPHS to the men in uniform explained.[84] Most important, public health advocates urged Americans to be active in protecting their own health and that of others. The first step in safeguarding themselves was to shore up what was assumed to be their existing good health.[85] A local representative of the USPHS told soldiers at Camp Bowie, "If soldiers and civilians alike will just use common sense in keeping themselves in fighting trim much will be accomplished in the conservation of man-power and in stamping out this disease in the various sections of our country."[86] According to the APHA, Americans needed to avoid "physical and nervous exhaustion" by "paying due regard to rest, exercise, physical and mental labor and hours of sleep."[87] The Red Cross urged citizens to "keep in good condition, eat regular meals, drink plenty of water, keep the bowels open, stay out in the open air . . . as much as you possibly can. . . . Get enough sleep and sleep with the windows open so that you breathe the open air, but keep out of drafts."[88]

Experts acknowledged, though, that "youth and bodily vigor" alone would not ensure immunity.[89] They urged individuals and communities to pay close attention to personal and public hygiene. Washing their hands frequently, keeping their hands and any objects they touched out of their mouths, sterilizing eating utensils, and avoiding the common drinking cup were all basic precautions.[90] Americans were implored to avoid overcrowding in their homes and to keep them clean and ventilated.[91] Such guidelines applied beyond the walls of the household as well. Rupert Blue advised, "One should keep out of crowds and stuffy places as much as possible, keep homes, offices, and workshops well aired, spend some time out of doors each day, walk to work if at all practicable—in short make every possible effort to breathe as much pure air as possible."[92] One could not always avoid crowds, of course, but even in these circumstances individuals had the opportunity to protect themselves, avoiding, as the Red Cross warned, "ignorant or careless persons who sneeze or cough without covering the nose or mouth with a handkerchief."[93]

As this last bit of advice implied, public health guidelines also urged Americans to recognize their role in helping others stay healthy. Public health leaders exhorted against "carelessness."[94] The Surgeon General was direct in his instructions: "*Cover up each cough and sneeze, if you don't you'll spread disease.*"[95] The Acting Army Surgeon General agreed, urging soldiers to "smother your coughs and sneezes—others do not want the germs which you would throw away."[96] Making a similar declaration, the Red Cross proclaimed, "Do not spit on the floor or the sidewalk anywhere. Do not let other people do it."[97] (See Figure 3.1.) With this last admonition, the Red Cross reminded Americans that they might police their own behaviors in public as well as in private, and they might also demand the same vigilance of others.

As influenza spread, public health leaders called for more significant preventive measures to contain the epidemic and limit its impact, measures that required Americans to change the patterns of their public lives. Some of these recommendations were fairly basic and required only minimal disruption. The banning of common drinking cups, for instance, was widely encouraged by public health advocates and understood to be an easy way to stop the spread of the disease. Other measures required both greater inconveniences for citizens and greater action by civic leaders. Preventing overcrowding on public transportation, for example, often meant staggering the schedules of workers and shoppers.[98] Still other measures—such as requiring public masking, closing public places, and prohibiting public meetings—while similarly disruptive to regular practices, also required still greater efforts on behalf of public leaders and were largely inconceivable without enforcement mechanisms.

Not coincidentally, these measures prompted both more discussion, and ultimately more disagreement, as public health leaders discussed the best approach to the epidemic crisis. For example, public health experts generally advised the use of masks by doctors and nurses and others who would be in close contact

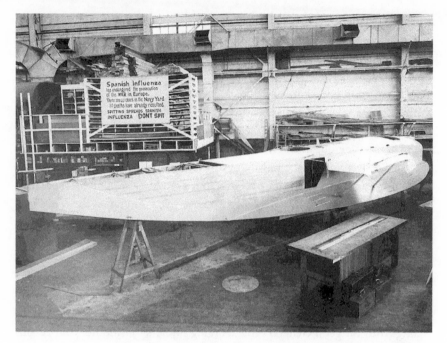

Figure 3.1 Public health signage at the naval aircraft factory in Philadelphia warned workers that their behaviors affected others, urging, "SPITTING SPREADS SPANISH INFLUENZA—DON'T SPIT." (Photo NH 41731), Department of the Navy—Naval History and Heritage Command.

with the ill.[99] Even as they made these recommendations, though, some public health leaders, including the Surgeon General, recognized that they were not based on any definitive information. Since the masks were only useful if they were "properly made," officials debated their use by the general public.[100] In San Francisco, the Board of Health succeeded in getting a masking ordinance passed through the Board of Supervisors, effective November 1. Others feared such rules would backfire if the public used masks improperly and gained a false sense of security as a result.[101] As Heman Spalding of Chicago declared of the mask, "As it is worn by most people, it is worse than useless."[102] (See Figures 3.2 and 3.3.)

If masking caused minor disagreements among public health officials, debates over the banning of public gatherings and the closing of public spaces caused much greater conflict among the professionals. The general logic behind bans and closures was simple and broadly accepted. As the USPHS maintained, because influenza was an infectious disease spread from person to person through droplet infection, keeping individuals away from one another, and especially away from crowded situations, was the key to slowing infection rates.[103] The APHA agreed and called for a blanket prohibition on all "non-essential gatherings."[104] At the same time, it recognized that while closures

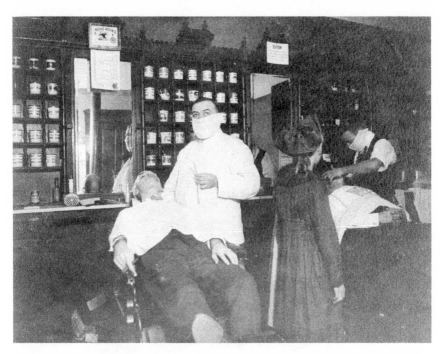

Figure 3.2 These barbers in Cincinnati donned masks, though their clients did not. (165-WW-269B-14), Still Picture Branch, NA.

might be effective in smaller communities that could function without interpersonal contact, in major urban areas people would be forced nevertheless to interact in crowded conditions at work and on streetcars.[105] Others shared the APHA's assessment that closures might be impractical in certain contexts, given the impossibility of halting all public business during the epidemic. Most public health leaders, though, continued to argue that at least limited bans and closures were necessary.

Even when such a position was broadly accepted, the devil was in the details. If some places such as dance halls and saloons were easily categorized as unnecessary, indeed hazardous, during an epidemic, decisions about certain other institutions such as churches and schools were hotly contested. For some, religious services were a necessity during such a difficult time. Dr. John Dill Robertson, the Commissioner of Health in Chicago, argued that closing churches would eliminate opportunities for health education in addition to robbing citizens of the "spiritual uplift which they should have at such a time."[106] Alternatively, the APHA imagined that churches might sometimes remain open but only with restrictions designed to limit services and minimize contact.[107] Others continued to argue that church services, like most public gatherings, were simply too dangerous during the worst of the epidemic.[108]

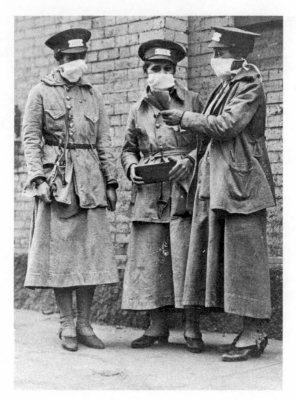

Figure 3.3 Like many in the urban work force, these "Conductorettes" on New York City's public transportation wore masks. (165-WW-269B-17), Still Picture Branch, NA.

It was the closing of schools, though, that generated the greatest conflict among public health forces. The USPHS recommended the closure of schools.[109] At the same time, the Health Service also acknowledged that all closures and prohibitions were local matters to be handled "after consideration of circumstances."[110] The APHA, in turn, noted the particular intricacy of understanding the impact of school closures. Such questions ranged from whether children would be "exposed to inclement weather or long rides in overcrowded cars" if they attended school to whether an "outbreak" would simply be stalled by school closure and would resurface when schools reopened. Perhaps most important, the APHA recognized as a central issue whether school closures would increase or decrease contacts among children.[111]

Others agreed that local conditions were relevant and suggested that, with careful sanitary controls, keeping the schools open could prove safer than closing them. When New York City's Commissioner of Health, Royal S. Copeland, asked Victor Vaughan, a recent President of the American Medical Association, to assess the city's response to the epidemic, Vaughan reassured him that keeping the schools open seemed a reasonable response. While noting that the city might want to reevaluate their decision if the epidemic among children worsened, Vaughan argued, "At present I believe that under the proper sanitary supervision the majority of children are better off in the schools than they would be in their homes or on the streets." As Vaughan's comment illustrated, many public health experts worried that school closures placed a heavy responsibility on an unready public, even as they eliminated valuable opportunities for public health education.[112] In Chicago, Health Commissioner Robertson offered a similar line of reasoning, suggesting that closing the schools "would be to send the children into the streets and alleys without supervision," while in school they would be "under the scrutiny of a doctor and a nurse and the corps of teachers."[113]

Even while deferring to local handling of the epidemic, the Surgeon General continued to maintain the importance of school closures. When the Chief of the Bureau of Communicable Diseases for Maryland, C. Hampson Jones, looked to him for help in preventing the future closure of schools during epidemics, Blue reiterated his belief in the tactic's efficacy. While acknowledging that prohibitions on public gatherings and the gating of schools could not halt the disease altogether, Blue nevertheless maintained that closures slowed the pace of the epidemic and bought communities time to prepare for influenza's full onslaught.[114]

The issue of the use of vaccines also prompted substantial disagreement among the public health forces, often pitting national against local leaders. Throughout the crisis the Surgeon General reminded Americans that without the identity of the causative agent, vaccines could be little more than exploratory and were simply "not reliable."[115] The APHA agreed.[116] Despite the clarity of national public health voices on the issue, local public health leaders sometimes advocated the use of vaccines.[117] In Illinois, for instance, the State Department of Public Health disseminated a vaccine to the populace.[118] In New York City, vaccines developed by William H. Park at the city's renowned public health laboratory were distributed with much fanfare and reassurances by the city's Health Commissioner.[119] In San Francisco roughly 31,000 residents received inoculations, and in Seattle city health workers produced vaccines for local use.[120] (See Figure 3.4.) Though often employing them as a prophylaxis against fear rather than influenza, or in order to facilitate research on prevention and cure, public health leaders who advocated the deployment of vaccines ensured that the public received mixed messages about their importance in a plan of prevention.

At least some local health officials recognized vaccines' limited medical value. In Philadelphia, for instance, the Health Department distributed doses of a vaccine, one developed by their own C. Y. White, a bacteriologist at Philadelphia

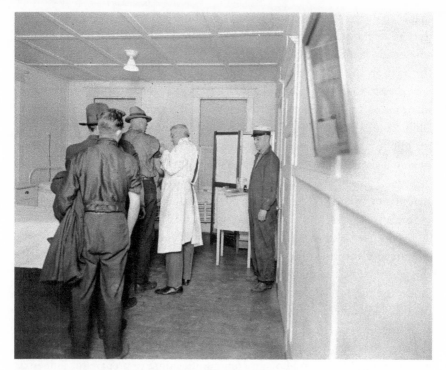

Figure 3.4 In Seattle, health authorities distributed flu vaccines according to a priority list that included military personnel. (165-WW-269B-9), Still Picture Branch, NA.

General Hospital and a member of the city's Bureau of Health, though White himself acknowledged some uncertainty about the vaccine's dangers and bene-fits.[121] Recognizing its purposes would be strictly preventive, White noted, "Vac-cines for prophylaxis use at least do no harm, and from the general application of vaccines in other diseases they possibly do good."[122] Such admissions about the unknown and likely limited value of vaccines were common among public health forces nationwide.[123] It may be that public health authorities recognized above all the psychological value of the vaccine—its ability to make people feel safe and its contribution to the appearance of an alert and active government working to protect its citizens.[124]

For some public health officials, including Chicago's Health Commissioner Robertson, this was clearly the case, at least as he explained his decision at a meeting of the Public Health Section of the Illinois Medical Society in May 1919. "Anyone who has studied psychology knows that when you get a fear you want to run," he explained. "Every animal runs but man. He does not run because he is too proud. The other animals run. You cannot control your heart. Fear does control the sympathetic system. You are apt to get cold feet. If you get cold feet you are apt to get pneumonia, and if you get pneumonia, you are likely to die."[125]

He explained further, "If you had been in charge of the great city of Chicago when the fear was getting aroused so that you could not keep the policemen on the wagons, what would you have done?" For Robertson the answer was clear: "Give them a vaccine. I said it was good because when I injected vaccine into those policemen they stayed on the job." For some public health authorities the dangers posed by a frightened public outweighed the benefits to be gained by an alarmist approach.[126]

Although most public health leaders did not go as far as Robertson, it is clear that the effort to minimize public fear was a central feature of public health work during the epidemic. In their educational work, health leaders balanced the need to alert citizens with a determination to avoid frightening them. This strategy is very clear in the USPHS pamphlet *"Spanish Influenza" "Three-Day Fever" "The Flu."* The pamphlet began by asking simply, *"What is Spanish Influenza?"* The answer was at once familiar and direct: "The disease now occurring ... resembles a very contagious kind of 'cold' accompanied by fever, pains in the head, eyes, ears, back or other parts of the body, and a feeling of severe sickness."[127] Having compared the epidemic disease to the common cold, the pamphlet went on to describe a sickness little different from the yearly flu. "He [the patient] feels weak, has pains in the eyes, ears, head or back, and may be sore all over," it noted. "Many patients feel dizzy, some vomit. Most of the patients complain of feeling chilly, and with this comes a fever in which the temperature rises to 100 to 104." Put simply, "The patient looks and feels very sick." The USPHS conceded, too, "in some places the outbreak has been severe and deaths have been numerous." At the same time, the pamphlet carefully introduced such potentially frightening information alongside descriptions of a more pedestrian outcome. "Ordinarily," it suggested, "the fever lasts from three to four days and the patient recovers." And further, "When death occurs it is usually the result of a complication." The pamphlet reassured readers that epidemic influenza was nothing new and had "visited this country since 1647," in "numerous epidemics of the disease." While these descriptions made clear that this was a potentially dangerous disease and epidemic, they also adopted the traditional strategy of domesticating influenza.

Having introduced Spanish influenza in familiar terms, the pamphlet went on to suggest how readers could participate in the fight to prevent and control it. "It is very important that every person who becomes sick with influenza should go home at once and go to bed," the Surgeon General explained. "This will help keep away dangerous complications and will, at the same time, keep the patient from scattering the disease far and wide." Reinforcing the importance of isolating the patient from the uninfected, the pamphlet provided clear guidelines on how to care for patients. There were advisable and inadvisable ways to take care of the sick and caregivers need only follow the advice of the experts to help control the disease.

What is remarkable about this pamphlet is how carefully it balanced the need to inform the public with a complementary determination not to frighten them. The Surgeon General did not exploit what might seem the most obvious message for motivating the public—the direct expression of the danger posed by influenza and the seriousness of the burgeoning epidemic. Nowhere did he describe the horrible scenes witnessed as the epidemic struck or depict in detail the appalling symptoms that had frightened even the most experienced physicians. Instead, he kept his references vague and his language muted.

This approach was common throughout public health leaders' communications with the American public. Certainly some worried early in the epidemic that the public did not understand the seriousness of the situation. As the *AJPH* editors suggested, "Very few health officers, and no communities, appreciate the terrific devastation of the epidemic until it strikes them."[128] In this context, public health advocates recognized the power fear might play as a motivator. As Heman Spalding of Chicago explained, "In the face of danger, even the indifferent will listen to the words of the health officer."[129] The Director of the Bureau of Nursing for the Red Cross in New England agreed and implored her colleagues to "impress upon your community the gravity of the situation."[130]

Yet direct expressions of the degree of danger the epidemic posed were unusual in public health communications. Instead, these officials attempted to mobilize the public without reliance on the rhetoric of alarm. A public health worker attempting to control influenza at the Groton Iron Works urged supervisors to be careful how they approached the subject of the flu with employees. Beginning by explaining the certainty of influenza's arrival, he went on to outline the symptoms and the important role supervisors could play. "Ask you to help by watching men under you and sending any men with symptoms to yard hospital immediately," he pleaded. Even as he urged them to be on alert, though, he also cautioned the foremen to avoid causing undue anxiety among the workers. "Work quietly," the message concluded, and "do not alarm [the] men."[131]

Others in the world of public health went still further, overstating their ability to prevent the disease and control the epidemic. The mayor of Tacoma, Washington, announced in early October, "Public health officials feel sure that the epidemic will be short-lived if we all help to head it off."[132] In order to facilitate such a success, the mayor closed all theatres and dance halls and placed a ban on public gatherings. Two days later the City Health Officer, Dr. Robert D. Wilson, reassured the public that such measures were purely preventive: "There is no immediate need for all this," the doctor explained, "but I believe that Tacoma should be prepared as far as possible to meet any emergency likely to arise whether we expect it or not." Wilson seemingly did not expect a crisis to develop. "With the precautions we've taken," he reassured residents, "I doubt if this city will be hit by the influenza as may other cities."[133] A circular from the

Boston Health Department took a similar tack, downplaying the danger of infection and the risks posed by the disease. Following instructions on "How to Avoid Infection Generally," the circular concluded, "If one takes these precautions, the chance of being infected is not great."[134] The circular was similarly comforting about the consequences of infection. Outlining "What to Do Until The Doctor Comes," it reassured, "If you take these steps—the chief of which is to remain in bed—you will probably not be seriously sick."

It may have been New York City's Health Commissioner, Royal S. Copeland, who most thoroughly employed these reassuring narratives. On August 14, 1918, before readers had confronted the emerging disease themselves, the *New York Times* reported the possibility that passengers on a recently arrived Norwegian liner were suffering from Spanish influenza.[135] While the next day's paper confirmed that several passengers had indeed arrived ill with influenza, "Spanish or some other kind," the overall tone of the report was reassuring, noting that neither Copeland nor the Port Health Officer believed there was "the slightest danger of an epidemic of Spanish Influenza in New York."[136] New Yorkers were safe, the paper reported, because "it seldom attacks any but persons who are badly nourished." Further reassurance was offered by Health Commissioner Copeland, who contrasted the safety of Americans with the reality of the disease in Europe. "You haven't heard of our doughboys getting it, have you?" he queried. "You bet you haven't, and you won't. But you have heard of cases in the German Army. . . . No need for our people to worry over the matter."[137] Over the next few days, health authorities in New York contradicted themselves on the need for a quarantine of incoming ships but never ceased their campaign to calm the public.[138]

When influenza reached New York in late September, Copeland continued to downplay the danger and overstate the authorities' ability to control the disease. On October 1, well before the worst of the epidemic had hit the city, the *New York Times* reported Copeland's claim that the disease and the epidemic "had been checked."[139] The very next day the newspaper reported Copeland's announcement of the "important" discovery of "a vaccine that would be a preventive against Spanish Influenza."[140] Making his announcement on a day with 836 new cases of influenza, Copeland "warned the public against undue alarm," suggesting the figures reflected not a developing problem but only the tardy reporting of backlogged cases.[141] The health commissioner would continue to provide reassuring accounts over the next several days. On October 3, a day that posted 903 new cases in the preceding 24 hours, he noted he was "gratified that the increase is no greater than it is," and assured New Yorkers that if the increases remained gradual they would not "swamp" the city's health care resources. "We have every reason to feel encouraged and to believe that there will be no serious impairment in the health

of the community," he concluded.[142] The next day, with 999 new cases, Copeland continued to mouth reassurances, suggesting, "There are no alarming
symptoms about the spread of influenza in New York."[143] Even as the city
implemented new restrictions on October 5, and as infection figures rose ever
higher—2,070 new cases in 24 hours reported on October 6—Copeland continued to deny the seriousness of the situation. "Considering the population
here," he told New Yorkers, "I do not consider that the city is stricken."[144]
While Copeland sought to keep the city calm, his caution was sufficient to
alarm the New York Times.[145] The next week Copeland would finally establish
an Emergency Advisory Committee, but he continued to call for "calmness"
and "coolness."[146] Though Copeland was clearly an extreme case in his efforts
to reassure the public, this commitment to keeping the public calm was widespread.

Mobilizing the Public

Having rejected fear tactics as a mobilizing mechanism, public health advocates
were forced to rely on other rhetorical choices to encourage the citizenry's cooperation. Given the wartime context, it is not surprising that leadership would
turn to appeals to duty, patriotism, and the war effort to convince Americans to
join the fight against influenza. Public health leaders attempted to engender a
sense of responsibility among the citizenry, suggesting that each individual's
behavior mattered and the best way to protect oneself from influenza was to act
according to guidelines offered by public health authorities. As one Red Cross
pamphlet stated directly, "You owe it to yourself and to your fellow man to do
everything you can to stay the progress of this crippling and all too swiftly fatal
disease."[147] Appeals to individuals, then, were complemented by the suggestion
that citizens also had a responsibility to others. In Chicago, a public health poster
designed for theatres let patrons know the theatre was "cooperating with the Department of Health," and commanded citizens to do the same in order to "keep
Chicago the healthiest city in the World."[148] A similar tactic appeared in a USPHS
posting in West Point, Mississippi. "IT'S UP TO YOU," the circular opened.
Suggesting that the timing on the lifting of the local quarantine was dependent
on citizens' continued "strict observance of all the precautions" recommended
by the health service, the circular criticized those who had failed to carry their
share of the public health burden. "Impatience, carelessness, and a premature
assumption that the epidemic has passed has caused a rather general **Relapse in
This Part of the State**," the poster chided, concluding, "This means that continued restrictions must be imposed upon some places, the duration of which will
be a **Direct Result of Your Conduct**."[149]

This invoking of individual responsibility was often framed as a responsibility to the broader community of the nation, allowing public health advocates to link efforts to fight the flu with a broader commitment to the well-being of the nation. As the USPHS opened its "Health Almanac for 1919," "It is the patriotic duty of every loyal American to keep well. Our country needs every bit of assistance from every individual."[150] These directives applied to all citizens, not only "the fighting man" but also "the farmer, the industrial operative, the transportation employee, and all the rest of the general public upon whom the soldier must rely for food, clothing, and weapons."[151] While the Almanac framed all public health efforts as patriotic, other public health materials spoke directly to the needs of the country as it faced the epidemic. Introducing the dangers of the influenza epidemic to soldiers at Camp Bowie, for instance, Captain J. G. Townsend of the USPHS intoned, "It is . . . the patriotic duty of each one, soldier and civilian alike, to do all in their power to keep from being incapacitated from this disease."[152] The Red Cross called on "all patriotic available nurses" to help in the fight against influenza and hoped representatives could recruit their local "patriotic newspaper" to help with publicity.[153]

Not surprisingly given the wartime context, public health advocates often raised the rhetorical power of patriotism by linking efforts to fight the flu with the broader fight to win the war. Germs and Germans were allies against the United States, and Americans needed to join the cause against influenza if they hoped to win the fight against the Hun.[154] A message in the *Illinois Health News* declared, "TALK ABOUT BULLETS SPRAYED FROM MACHINE GUNS—THEY ARE NOT MORE DEADLY THAN THE MUCUS SPRAYED IN MILLIONS OF DISEASE-BEARING DROPLETS FROM PEOPLE'S MOUTHS! DON'T COUGH OR SNEEZE INTO ANYTHING BUT YOUR HANDKERCHIEF! DON'T TALK OR LAUGH INTO ANYONE'S FACE!"[155] Comparing germs to dangerous weapons, this illustration suggested that individuals carried significant responsibility for combating influenza. Others noted parallels between this responsibility and those of military duty. As the mayor of San Diego suggested as he voiced his support for a quarantine in the city, "There is a class of people blind and indifferent to the death and sick rate. . . . If we cannot put life and health above dollars and pleasure for a few days, we had better abolish the Bible and the Constitution. I cannot see a particle of difference between the invasion of France by the heartless, lustful Huns and the invasion of our homes by some epidemic permitted by greed and politics."[156] A USPHS representative at Camp Bowie used the same essential appeal. "The more cases of influenza we have in this country so much more will the German Kaiser be pleased," it suggested.[157] The messages here were clear. Each American had a role to play in fighting the epidemic, such a role was a patriotic duty in this time of crisis, and defeating influenza was both similar to, and integral to, winning the war in Europe.

Popular Support for Public Health

How did the public respond to these requests and demands for compliance? The reactions were as diverse as the country itself. In some cases local public health authorities were resoundingly successful in implementing programs of prevention and treatment that matched precisely the plans outlined by national leadership. In other cases, the mobilization of community members proved more difficult, sometimes reflecting chaos and disorganization, other times a blatant rejection of public health education, advice, and strictures.

One way to measure popular support for public health directives was the degree to which governments provided the financial resources necessary to implement their agenda during the pandemic. On October 1 Congress approved a $1 million appropriation for the USPHS "to combat and suppress 'Spanish Influenza' and other communicable diseases," a decision the Surgeon General found "as encouraging as it was gratifying."[158] The APHA also encouraged local health officials to organize local fund-raising, hopeful that the epidemic's presence would ease such efforts.[159] In many cases these hopes seem to have been met. Massachusetts was the first state hit, and it suffered not only from the scourge of influenza but also from surprise at its rapid spread and its unusually high morbidity and mortality rates. As the state's situation worsened, its governor, Calvin Coolidge, established a State Emergency Health Committee with a budget of $100,000, a figure increased to $500,000 by late October, with the expectation that it might climb still further.[160]

In addition to financing, national authorities had also hoped the epidemic might prompt significant infrastructural development for public health forces. Already an important part of the public health agenda, organizing the state and local public health communities and their resources quickly became a vital component in the struggle against the epidemic. Again, the local populace often responded to these needs, creating new bodies or enhancing the authority of those already in existence in order to allow them to manage the epidemic crisis effectively. One common mechanism was the establishment of an emergency committee—sometimes at the state level, other times at the level of the county or city—to deal with the overwhelming need for organization, communication, and cooperation among individuals, agencies, and organizations. In Illinois, for instance, the Council of National Defense organized the Illinois Influenza Commission, which included representatives from the state and city health departments, the USPHS, the Red Cross, the military, and others. They met regularly, indeed nearly every day, until the worst of the epidemic was over.[161] In Pennsylvania the State Department of Health created nineteen Epidemic Emergency Districts in the state and mobilized and coordinated the actions of countless "Health, Patriotic, Civic, Religious, Business and Social organizations" as well as the State

Guard.[162] In Washington, D.C., the USPHS Medical Officer in Charge was appointed to oversee the work of a Central Office and four Medical Districts, each with its own Medical Officer, Assistant Directing Nurse, Supervising Nurse, and nursing staff. Cooperating agencies included the District Health Department, the Board of Education, the Visiting Nurse Society, the Washington Diet Kitchen Association, the National Organization for Public Health Nursing, the Children's Bureau, the Red Cross, other governmental departments, and local churches.[163]

One purpose for the enhancement of public health structures during the crisis was the collection of data related to the epidemic, a need fulfilled in part by establishing influenza as a reportable disease.[164] Requiring the reporting of influenza cases and actually succeeding in acquiring accurate statistics on its prevalence proved to be two entirely different things, particularly as the epidemic boomed. In New York City, for instance, Health Commissioner Copeland criticized irresponsible doctors who had failed to report cases of influenza and blamed them for thousands of unnecessary illnesses and countless deaths.[165] Though Copeland was clearly outraged by physicians' neglect of their record keeping, others acknowledged that the turmoil of the epidemic made failure to report cases understandable.[166] Such behavior, though troubling to some public health leaders, was not necessarily an intentional challenge to the efforts of the public health establishment.

In the end, it was the response of the general public that mattered most to public health leaders during the pandemic. They would measure their success to a large degree by the behavior of the populace—by communities' willingness to establish controls based on public health leaders' guidelines and by individuals' willingness to comply with the new regulations. With education the first step in mobilizing the citizenry, getting the message out through popular channels was one important goal. In this arena the public health forces were notably successful. National circulation magazines joined the effort from the beginning. The *Literary Digest,* a weekly magazine that focused on current events and excerpted other print media to represent the broad range of public opinion, regularly printed articles such as "Spanish Influenza," "How to Fight Spanish Influenza," "How Influenza Got In," "How the 'Flu' Mask Traps the Germ," "Expert Medical Advice on Influenza," and "How the Hand Spreads Influenza."[167] The *Survey* followed suit with "Plagues in Europe and America," "Spanish Influenza and Its Control," "The Effects and Cost of Influenza," and "A Program to Combat Influenza."[168]

Health authorities often found the local press compliant, even supportive. From coast to coast local papers published editorials echoing the specific messages of the public health leaders and calling on citizens to follow the precautions offered by health authorities. The *Press-Times* of Wallace, Idaho, illustrated just how closely some newspapers mirrored the efforts of public health leaders. Early in the national epidemic, before influenza reached Wallace, the paper reassured the citizenry and worked to maintain the public calm. "Wallace has had no serious epidemic to contend with," the paper reported on October 11. It argued that the situation could be maintained with proper observance of the public health directives. "Do your part and Wallace will be a healthy community in the future, as it has been in the past," the paper claimed.[169] The paper took a similar position eleven days later, relying on familiar public health rhetoric.[170] The editors began by domesticating the epidemic, comparing it favorably to earlier epidemics. "Each year these epidemics run through the country," the editorial explained. "They travel under one name or another. Usually they are worse than they are at this time, due to the fact that many people take no precautions." From here the paper suggested the strength of the public health forces, reminded readers of their authority, and offered further reassurances. "The thing to do," the paper concluded, "is not to be alarmed but to take the precautions advised by those in authority and to strictly observe the rules against public gatherings. Wallace and vicinity are shown to be extremely healthy now. The epidemic has gained no foothold here and if people will only keep their heads, observe the rules laid down and guard their health with more than usual care there will be no spread of it here."

As the health department implemented restrictions to protect the city, too, the newspaper employed public health rhetoric to praise their actions. "Expressions of complete confidence in the officers responsible for the closing orders were heard on every hand in the city yesterday," the paper reported on October 11, and "the inconveniences and real financial loss to some lines of business are being accepted without complaint."[171] On November 2, the paper reiterated its support for the health authorities' actions, acknowledging, "The health authorities here are taking the proper precautions and their prompt measures in putting a ban on public gatherings of all kinds show that they are awake to the situation."[172] The paper reinforced its support for the health officials by providing information designed to facilitate the public's proper behavior. Immediately below an editorial entitled "Stop Spread of Influenza," for instance, it ran an article entitled "Make Your Own Mask; It Is a Simple Task."[173]

As they urged the public to cooperate with the health authorities, the Wallace paper's editors also demonstrated the profound influence of those authorities as they adopted arguments of duty and responsibility in their efforts to encourage readers to obey local precautions against the flu. In an editorial entitled "Keep Healthy" the paper suggested, "Each and every person should do his part in preventing the spread of Spanish influenza. The time is here for all to act. The responsibility rests upon you."[174] Such messages were repeated a number of times by the paper over the next several weeks. "The community itself can take certain precautions, but the individual must realize his or her responsibility," another editorial declared on November 2. "This is a time for cooperation. Let each one assume his or her full responsibility. Then the epidemic will soon pass away. Do not be selfish. Think of the others."[175]

The *Wallace Press-Times* was not alone in adopting the words of the public health leaders or praising them in their pages. Across the country, in small towns and major cities, at military camps and college campuses, editors and writers of local newspapers supported the efforts of the public health forces, lending their columns to the cause. In Tacoma, Washington, the *News Tribune* noted that the mayor had "very properly" closed schools, wrote approvingly of the prohibition on public meetings and the closure of theatres, and urged citizens to follow basic "precautions" to avoid the flu.[176] A leading African American newspaper, the *Chicago Defender*, which had a nationwide distribution, used its regular public health column by Dr. A. Wilberforce Williams to spread the word of the public health forces to their readers.[177] Even student editors joined the chorus of commentators supporting the work of public health officials. At the University of California, Berkeley, the *Daily Californian* was a strong proponent of public health efforts on campus.[178]

Again, the importance of this editorial support lay in its ability to mobilize individuals to accept the emergency regulations. The ready support of the popular press suggests some level of possibility here, and indeed, the success of public health leaders was extraordinary in some communities. In Quitman, Georgia, for instance, the mayor and city council established a new Board of Health and granted it "full power and authority to adopt such rules and regulations as may seem to them proper and necessary" in order "to check the spread of the disease and save human life."[179] The board soon enacted twenty-seven directives that reached into every aspect of public life.[180] According to the new regulations, physicians were responsible for reporting influenza cases, the clerk of the Board of Health for recording and reporting the physicians' news. "All cases of influenza" were to be quarantined, with the chief of police responsible for enforcement. Individuals were required to "sneeze and cough in their handkerchiefs," and spitting "on streets, sidewalks, or in stores, offices or other places of business" was expressly forbidden. Crowds were not allowed to gather "on the streets, in stores, offices or private homes," and the police were charged with the dispersal of any gatherings that arose. Businesses were required to be "thoroughly ventilated at all times during business hours." "Clerks, salesmen, bookkeepers, porters, barbers, waiters in restaurants and hotels and all other employers and employees engaged in serving the public" were required to wear masks. Some of the restrictions on businesses were quite specific. Rule 7, for instance, concerned the serving of ice cream, which was to be served only in cones or "individual receptacles for that purpose," while Rule 6 detailed the special circumstances in which drinks could be served. "The picture show" was closed. Other regulations mandated public actions of private individuals. Indoor funerals were prohibited, as were all "social gatherings," and "private classes." With these twenty-seven detailed directives, the Board of Health brought to fruition the plans articulated by public health leaders, creating almost total control over the public behavior of the local population.

Milwaukee, Wisconsin, was a larger community that found significant success not only in creating rules to govern the public but also in broad-based support for those measures. Influenza reached Milwaukee in late September, as in so many cases carried by two sailors training nearby. In this case it struck a city with strong public health leadership and a well-established public health system already in place. Having anticipated the disease's arrival, Milwaukee Health Commissioner George C. Ruhland was ready to act and soon initiated the prohibition of further visits from sailors at the nearby Great Lakes Naval Training Station, the reporting of influenza cases, and the creation of a special advisory committee that broadened his connection to the community. Ruhland followed these initial responses with further efforts to fight the flu. Isolation of the infected and education of the population were top priorities, but as the city continued to suffer, Ruhland called for more dramatic actions, including the always-unpopular closure of public spaces. Despite some resistance among business owners and religious leaders, the response was remarkably supportive. The community's cooperative attitude persisted, even when a new wave of the disease forced a second round of closures in December, and resulted in one of the lowest mortality rates reported for a major city (see Figure 3.5). Milwaukee's experience illustrated the success of the public health forces in both mobilizing the public and limiting the damage wrought by the pandemic.[181]

Public Resistance

Though the public frequently responded to the pleas of the public health leadership, in some communities chaos and fear combined to disrupt even the best of intentions. Philadelphia, for instance, exemplified the case of a city whose commitment to fighting the epidemic was simply overwhelmed by the circumstances of the catastrophe. Though among the hardest hit of American cities, Philadelphia's "travail," as the historian Alfred Crosby suggests, had much in common with other American cities.[182] Despite having some warning that the epidemic was coming, Philadelphia did little to prepare for influenza's onset. Though Boston was under siege, by late September few in the country had really recognized the extent of the catastrophe headed their way. Philadelphia continued to conduct business as usual throughout the month, proceeding, for

Deaths from influenza and pneumonia.(all forms) in certain large cities of the United States, Sept. 8, 1918, to Mar. 1, 1919, inclusive (25 weeks); also excess deaths from all causes as compared with 1917.

City.	Population July 1, 1918, estimated.	Deaths from–		Deaths from influenza and pneumonia (all forms.)		Excess deaths[1] from all causes.		For comparison. [2]1917 deaths.
		Influenza.	Pneumonia (all forms).	Number.	Number per 1,000 population.	Number.	Number per 1,000 population.	
Albany, N. Y	112,565	570	178	748	6.6	534	4.7	119
Baltimore, Md	[3]669,981	1,956	3,006	4,962	7.4	4,118	6.1	853
Boston, Mass	785,245	4,711	1,472	6,133	7.9	5,107	6.5	942
Buffalo, N. Y	473,229	2,172	903	3,075	6.5	2,766	5.8	465
Cambridge, Mass	111,432	501	197	698	6.3	661	5.9	103
Chicago, Ill	2,596,681	7,878	5,298	13,176	5.1	9,956	3.8	2,557
Cincinnati, Ohio	418,022	1,897	366	2,263	5.4	1,670	4.0	418
Cleveland, Ohio	810,306	3,054	1,351	4,405	5.4	3,254	4.0	787
Columbus, Ohio	225,296	726	212	938	4.2	710	3.2	237
Dayton, Ohio	130,655	527	221	748	5.7	460	3.5	142
Fall River, Mass	128,392	766	136	902	7.0	749	5.8	167
Grand Rapids, Mich	135,450	96	248	344	2.5	206	1.5	62
Los Angeles, Calif	568,495	2,636	557	3,193	5.6	2,968	5.2	304
Louisville, Ky	242,707	150	1,056	1,206	5.0	869	3.6	290
Lowell, Mass	109,081	174	521	695	6.4	554	5.1	117
Milwaukee, Wis	453,481	339	1,247	1,586	3.5	1,333	2.9	403
Minneapolis, Minn	383,442	1,099	194	1,293	3.4	1,023	2.7	206
Nashville, Tenn	119,215	640	254	894	7.5	928	7.8	144
New Haven, Conn	154,865	914	227	1,141	7.4	860	5.6	206
New Orleans, La	382,273	2,199	1,114	3,313	8.7	2,767	7.2	431
New York, N. Y	5,215,879	15,449	16,511	31,960	6.1	24,329	4.7	6,505
Oakland, Calif	214,206	975	250	1,234	5.8	1,268	5.9	119
Philadelphia, Pa	1,761,371	8,807	6,750	15,566	8.8	12,790	7.3	2,394
Pittsburgh, Pa	593,303	2,545	3,153	5,698	9.6	4,743	8.0	1,333
Providence, R. I	263,613	1,091	531	1,622	6.2	1,389	5.3	288
Rochester, N. Y	264,856	1,002	272	1,274	4.8	703	2.7	226
St. Louis, Mo	779,951	2,188	1,425	3,613	4.6	2,323	3.0	961
St. Paul, Minn	257,699	894	197	1,091	4.2	852	3.3	158
San Francisco, Calif	478,530	3,192	593	3,785	7.9	3,586	7.5	360
Toledo, Ohio	262,234	567	318	885	3.4	561	2.1	170
Washington, D. C	401,681	2,294	822	3,116	7.8	2,637	6.6	422
Total	19,503,836	72,009	49,598	121,607	6.2	96,674	5.0	21,949

[1] Excess deaths means the number of deaths from all causes in excess of the number which would have occurred had the 1917 death rates for the corresponding months prevailed.

[2] Number of deaths from influenza and pneumonia (all forms) in January, February, September, October, November, and December, 1917.

[3] Large annexation Jan. 1, 1919; population estimated as of July 1, 1919.

Figure 3.5 These statistics from *Public Health Reports* provide information on influenza and pneumonia death rates for major American cities during twenty-five weeks of the pandemic (September 8, 1918–March 1, 1919). "Deaths from influenza and pneumonia (all forms) in certain large cities of the United States, September 8, 1918, to March 1, 1919, inclusive (25 weeks). . . ." *PHR* 34 (March 14, 1919): 505.

instance, with an ill-advised opening parade for the Fourth Liberty Loan on September 28. The pandemic exploded in its wake. The city reported 635 new cases on October 1 alone, and this figure was likely an underestimate.[183]

The city council moved quickly to support the needs of the Health Department, providing an "emergency appropriation" of $25,000 to provide for the hiring of physicians and whatever preventive measures the director thought necessary.[184] According to accounts by the city's Department of Public Health and Charities, the population of Philadelphia—health care professionals and laity alike—cooperated fully with the authorities and responded admirably to the needs of the community during the crisis. In an editorial comment in its monthly bulletin the department recounted both the "scourge" the epidemic had represented and the support the department received as it fought back.[185] Noting the shortage of physicians and nurses brought on by the war, the essay acknowledged the "suffering, the frightfulness and the pitiful sights in the homes of the afflicted" witnessed by the doctors. Quickly, though, the editorial shifted from this negative focus to emphasize the heroic work of health care professionals and the superb support of the public. "Too much praise cannot be given to the civilians who offered their services, their homes, their cars and themselves to curb the dreaded pestilence." Special praise was reserved for "the Red Cross, with its admirable corps of motor messengers, its nurses and its ambulances," as well as "the Emergency Aid, the Department of Public Safety, the fraternal societies, the industrial plants, the Philadelphia Rapid Transit Company, and many others," all of whom "gave the health officials every service within their command."[186] According to the Health Department, then, the public had done all that was asked of them as the city fought the epidemic.

Even with this broad-based cooperation, however, the city was overwhelmed by the epidemic. Part of the problem may have been the Health Department's failure to prepare adequately.[187] The epidemic struck quickly and ferociously, and the sick overwhelmed available health care resources. The shortage of doctors and nurses spread overwork and exhaustion, and city services struggled to function as well. From keeping the phone lines running to collecting garbage, from firefighting to interring the dead, the city could not keep up with the demands of its residents once the epidemic took hold. A leadership vacuum caused by political corruption produced a disorganized and chaotic response.[188] Gradually, with the help of the Council of National Defense and the remarkable cooperation of the city's residents, Philadelphia succeeded in marshalling its forces "to keep the living alive," and soon after conquered its problem of laying the dead to rest.[189] Nevertheless, the city suffered an extraordinarily high death rate during the epidemic.[190]

If in some cities, such as Philadelphia, even widespread cooperation by the citizenry was not enough to allow for an entirely effective struggle against the epidemic, in other cases public health leaders contended with a less pliable public and found their efforts disrupted, if not entirely corrupted, by citizens' resistance to their emergency measures. Sometimes public health authorities seemed to bring the problem of noncompliance on themselves as their efforts at reassurance produced not only calm but indifference. As late as October 3, for instance, the editors of the *New York Times* were still suggesting that citizens "should not worry too much about the Spanish influenza" and describing the outbreak with surprising nonchalance. "At the worst it is no more, in many cases it is considerably less, than the old grippe, without the Iberian adjective, which we all endured, mostly had, say, in 1893," the paper concluded, reflecting the costs of Commissioner Copeland's campaign to calm the public.[191]

Before long, any illusions about the dangers of the encroaching influenza were destroyed by the stories unfolding across the nation. As the realities of the pandemic became obvious, even in communities still unscathed by Spanish influenza, resistance to public health authorities became more notable. Under these circumstances, refusal to adhere to the guidelines and restrictions produced by local leaders represented much more purposeful intentions. Those who pushed back against the behavioral restrictions were not unified in their motivations, but were prompted variously by disagreement with the approach chosen by local authorities, by growing frustration with government control over their lives as days turned into weeks and then months, or by utter disregard for the importance of the public health efforts. An exploration of the efforts of local officials to implement some of the essential measures called for by the public health profession—the preventive use of vaccines, the masking of the general public, the prohibition of public gatherings, and the closures of public spaces—illustrates the range of responses authorities confronted.

For reasons often quite different from those professionals who awaited a viable vaccine, many Americans found little comfort in the widespread employment of vaccines. An anti-vaccination movement had emerged years earlier, leading to the founding of the Anti-Vaccination Society of America in 1879 and the Anti-Vaccination League of America in 1908. Opponents of vaccine programs were a diverse group, and individuals criticized the safety and efficacy of vaccinations, sometimes on the basis of religious beliefs, other times on what they viewed as the governmental tyranny implied by coercive programs. During the Progressive era, the rising power of both the "expert" and the state, including health authorities, encouraged a corresponding rise in anti-vaccine activism.[192] A letter from a citizen, John H. Faulkner, to the Secretary of War illustrates both the arguments and the emotions attached to this position. He explained, "Vaccination has no place in the Twentieth Century. Modern Sanitation has taken its place. It is obsolete."[193] The problem, according to Faulkner, was that "the injection of germ matter and the scum of disease in the blood of a healthy person" led to resistance against that particular germ or disease, but made the body vulnerable to "attacks of other bacteria" and the overtaxing of the system as a whole. In the context of war, such damage was unconscionable, endangering the entire nation with a weakened army. Though Faulkner and others expressed their opposition with vehemence, their correspondence was easily ignored by public health authorities at both the federal and local levels.[194] Vaccines never garnered unified support among public health leaders during the epidemic, nor were they ever a required action on the part of citizens, and so opposition to them did not pose a meaningful challenge to the authority of public health leaders.

Other protests were not so easily dismissed, as the uproar over the closure of public spaces, the banning of public gatherings, and the wearing of masks demonstrated. In each case, public health authorities tested the boundaries of public obedience. The Surgeon General had recommended the closing of "all public gathering places" if a community was "threatened with the epidemic," and authorities in small towns and major cities moved to prohibit public meetings and prevent public crowding of every possible sort.[195] Leading this work, the State Emergency Committee in Massachusetts on September 25 called for the cancellation of public events and the closure of public amusements and schools.[196] Other states, counties, cities, and towns soon followed.[197]

The tone of the objections as well as the nature of the defiance varied to some extent according to the particular public space being closed. In the case of schools, for instance, the arguments did not necessarily challenge the importance of combating influenza or the essential authority of public health officials but questioned instead the closure of schools as the best tactic for the community to employ. Given that Progressive-era reforms had brought routine medical inspections and hygienic training for students and nursing care to some schools, communities sometimes saw in their schools a site for waging the fight against the epidemic.[198] In Illinois, for instance, the Influenza Commission allowed schools to continue to operate if they offered appropriate medical inspections of their students.[199] In Chicago, Health Commissioner Robertson took a strong stand against closures and focused on school inspections and home visits by school nurses to control influenza among children.[200] With approximately a million young people in its school system, New York was the largest city to keep schools open, and public health officials carried out medical inspections there.[201]

In other cases, community leaders agreed to close their schools and follow the restrictions, but they did so under vocal protest. In Seattle, for instance, Superintendent of Schools Frank B. Cooper was outspoken in his opposition to the closing of the city's public schools. Claiming the closure was a result of the mayor's "hysterical" reaction to the crisis, Cooper argued, "I consider it more dangerous to have children running around the streets loose than to have them in school where they will be under strict medical supervision."[202]

Other communities attempted to minimize the closing of their schools, either shutting the doors slowly or seeking to reopen them as quickly as possible. In Massachusetts, when the State Emergency Committee asked schools to close only "in so far as the proper authorities considered it advisable," some school boards, including Boston's, moved slowly in ordering closures.[203] In Deer Creek, Minnesota, school officials wavered repeatedly about closing their schools and were later blamed by the local paper for the community's influenza plight.[204] In South Carolina school officials acted quickly to request permission to reopen as soon as new case figures showed a decline.[205]

The closure of churches led to similar dynamics. In some communities public health officials allowed churches to remain open. The Illinois Influenza Commission countered the general acceptance of closures and suggested that the potential values of churches, like schools, outweighed the benefits of their closure. Certainly the commission asked churches to act responsibly if they remained open, keeping meetings to a minimum while preventing crowds, ensuring ventilation, and barring any cold sufferers from attendance, but also maintained that churches had a valuable role to play in the pandemic. As a report on the work of the commission explained, "It was felt that there was definite need for an outlet for the public emotion which was clearly manifesting itself in connection with the epidemic."[206]

In cases where they did close churches, citizens often expressed both disappointment and opposition. When Philadelphia's Director of the Department of Public Health and Charities Wilmer Krusen included churches in the general closing order, significant opposition surfaced "among clergymen of the various denominations," opposition that apparently met a unified front in the medical community.[207] In Washington, D.C., the local African American newspaper chastised local preachers for their resistance to closures suggesting, "These preachers ought to be ashamed of themselves. Their attitude suggests superstition or mediaevalism [sic] or pure selfishness; certainly not a regard for the public good."[208] Or as a local newspaper in Rathdrum, Idaho, suggested simply regarding the response to closures among the clergy there, "The churches and lodges are chafing under the ban."[209] Despite such "chafing," however, churches—their leadership and their congregations—generally conformed to the requirements of any restrictions once they had made their protests (see Figure 3.6).

Such was not always the case as public health authorities attempted to close a number of other public spaces, in particular those associated with popular amusements. In this context both customers and business owners engaged in protest that reached beyond words and into actions. The simplest and most common expression of resistance to public health restrictions was the steady stream of citizens rushing to catch one last performance or attend one last party before bans went into effect. In Minneapolis, for instance, the local paper reported

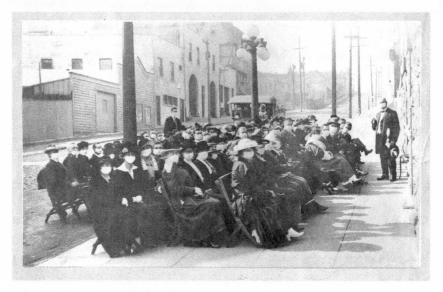

Figure 3.6 Church services sometimes escaped public health closures. Here, congregants in San Francisco meet outdoors and comply with public masking requirements. (FN-30852), Photography Collection, California Historical Society.

the "packed" theatres and "long lines" of people rushing to see the final performance.[210] Similarly, when authorities announced the upcoming quarantine of Camp Lewis outside Tacoma, Washington, soldiers "made a bee line for the bus stations," according to the *News Tribune*, "bound to get away until the last minute, if only to stand on the streets of Tacoma, or to spend a brief time with friends."[211]

Once public entertainments were closed, the public began clamoring almost immediately for their reopening. In some cases the protest was mild, as citizens simply complained about the limits on their recreation. On military bases, for instance, camp newspapers often recounted the frustration of soldiers confined to the base, and in some cases quarantined in their quarters. The *Camp Dodger*, for instance, described the "relief" soldiers felt when recreation inside Camp Dodge was restored in late October, noting that for soldiers who had escaped the flu "the quarantine has been growing more irksome every day."[212] Local businessmen complained bitterly about the loss of profits they faced due to the camp quarantine. "In fact," the *Camp Dodger* explained, "practically every owner of a movie show, restaurant, temp bar, dance hall, taxicab or other place of business which has catered to the boys in khaki claims that the 'flu' has hit him hard" and taxicab and bus drivers described business as "rotten."[213] Similarly, in West Point, Mississippi, the USPHS representative there faced significant problems with a continued ban. "We had some local negotiations to prevent a resumption of public gatherings," he suggested, as a result of "certain vested interests . . . having become somewhat impatient."[214] The motion picture industry's trade journal, *Moving Picture World,* covered the epidemic closely and noted not only the closures and the resultant loss of revenue but also the growing resistance of theatre owners to emergency restrictions and the growing number of lawsuits challenging the government controls late in the pandemic.[215] It was never businesses alone that fought to remove bans on public gatherings, however. In cities and towns across the country citizens organizing Liberty Loan parades and the United War Work Campaign sought exemptions to the rules to allow their "patriotic" activities to take place.

In most cases citizens ultimately accepted the decisions of local authorities, but on rare occasions protests rose to a more brazen disregard of health officials' authority over public life. In Globe, Arizona, both the school district and private citizens pursued legal challenges to the restrictions they faced. Upset by the requirement that schools close during the epidemic, the Globe School District took health officials to court to block the order. In the end, the Supreme Court of Arizona ruled against the schools, suggesting that in the context of a health emergency the power of state, county, and city health boards to act to protect the public health trumped that of the school trustees and educational administrative officers to "govern and regulate" the schools.[216] Even in this extreme case citizens worked within the established legal system to challenge the restrictions and accepted the authority of the courts to determine the outcome.

The response to the closure of public amusements in Globe was not so tempered. According to the *Journal of the American Medical Association,* a theatre owner was arrested for the crime of "wilfully [*sic*], maliciously and unlawfully conducting and carrying on a moving picture show" despite restrictions in place as a result of the pandemic. Taking his protest one step further, this businessman, like the school district, appealed his case all the way to the Arizona Supreme Court. Arguing that the local public health officials did not have "constitutional authority to . . . compel him to close his place of business," the theatre owner believed he was within his rights to open his movie theatre.[217] The Arizona Supreme Court again disagreed. Pointing to its earlier decision in the *Globe School Board* case, the court maintained that the actions of the Health Board were legitimate.[218] Legal challenges were repeated in other cities, including Wichita, Kansas; Terra Haute, Indiana; and Roanoke, Virginia.[219]

While the closure of public spaces and the prohibition of public gatherings brought some vehement resistance, such protest was always limited to a small number of individuals willing to challenge the authorities. It was the wearing of masks that produced the most broad-based and visible challenges to the emergency measures. In the early days of the crisis most citizens followed the health authorities' rules, including orders to don masks. As the epidemic retreated, however, resistance rose. Even the renewed strength of influenza, returning in new waves to threaten communities, did little to restore authorities' earlier control over the population. With massive noncompliance, local public health leaders were ultimately unsuccessful in exerting full control (see Figure 3.7).

Events in San Francisco offer a classic example of the waxing and waning of popular support for public masking.[220] Thanks to its West Coast location, San Francisco's epidemic hit late, with the first case announced on September 24, 1918. Three days later the state's Board of Health acknowledged the coming crisis and added influenza to the list of reportable diseases. Despite the awareness of

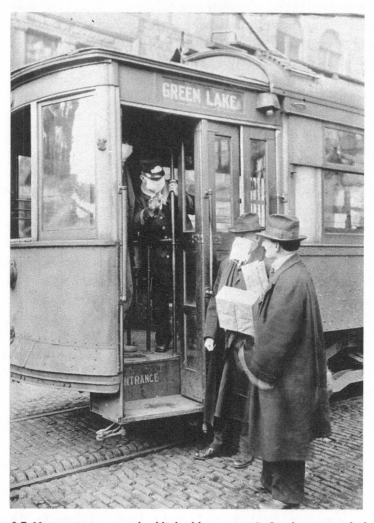

Figure 3.7 Not everyone accepted public health measures. In Seattle, an unmasked passenger was denied passage by a streetcar conductor. (165-WW-269B-11), Still Picture Branch, NA.

the looming epidemic gained by the experience of communities nationwide, San Francisco, like so many other cities and towns, kicked off its Fourth Liberty Loan drive with a parade on September 28, an event soon followed by two weeks of public occasions designed to secure the loan and demonstrate the city's patriotism. Not until October 18 did the city finally begin taking direct action against the epidemic, closing the doors of schools and popular amusements and prohibiting public gatherings. The city also employed vaccines with some enthusiasm, as the Board of Health provided them free of charge to local physicians and inoculated residents who turned up by the thousands.

Though the city relied on the range of preventive techniques encouraged by public health authorities nationwide, it was the masking of the public that many locals credited with slowing the epidemic. Health care workers had worn masks from the beginning, and early in the crisis the Chief of the Board of Health William Hassler had urged others in close contact with the public to do so, in particular those working in stores and barbershops. Soon Hassler called for the entire city to wear masks, and the Board of Supervisors passed an ordinance unanimously that required all citizens to wear masks when on public streets, in any place where more than two people assembled, and even in their own homes if more than two people were present. Further, anyone who handled or distributed either food or clothing was also required to don a mask. To educate the public and assert the measure's importance, local leaders as well as several organizations joined together to publish a full-page ad in the *San Francisco Chronicle* that announced the near-foolproof protection offered by masks and maintaining that their use would save lives.[221] San Franciscans responded enthusiastically, exhausting the supply of masks as quickly as they were offered. "It will soon be impolite to acknowledge an introduction without a mask," the *Chronicle* commented, "and the man who wears none will be likely to become isolated, suspected and regarded as a slacker. Like a man of means without a Liberty Loan button he'll be shy of friends."[222] According to the Board of Health, the vast majority of residents were complying with the ordinance even before it became law on November 1. Within days the epidemic began to recede, and as Hassler and his constituents celebrated their success, observers nationwide took notice.

Hassler had hoped to continue to control the disease by keeping the city in masks until the epidemic had fully passed, indeed until one week *after* the last case was discovered. Such a strategy proved impossible. Gradually, San Franciscans abandoned the masks. At first the police responded with arrests, including 400 during one raid on hotel lobbies. Soon, though, authorities from the mayor to the chief of the Bureau of Health were discovered maskless. On November 21 citizens were finally allowed to shed their masks. By this point, though, the masks had become not only unpopular, but an object of humor, and even ridicule.

During the first week of December influenza returned. Hassler, reminding the city of the earlier success, urged citizens to once again wear masks. During this new wave the city suffered roughly half the infections and deaths it had faced during its first encounter with the epidemic.[223] Left to a voluntary code of conduct, 90 percent of the population failed to return to using masks. Businesses, worried about Christmas shoppers, announced their opposition, as did the Associated Culinary Workers. A letter to the *Chronicle*, signed "What's the Use," recounted the illness of a man who had followed the public health recommendations to the letter and yet had suffered not only influenza but pneumonia. The newspaper itself warned of the fear that accompanied masking, while providing only the most tepid support for the authorities. By mid-December neither the Board of Supervisors nor the Public Health Committee sought responsibility for decision making on the issue. Citizens arrived by the hundreds to join the public debate at a meeting on December 16, and on December 19 the Board of Supervisors voted down the proposed order by a close margin. But influenza continued to plague the city, and on January 10 the Board of Supervisors revisited the issue. Again citizens came in droves to oppose the order. This time the supervisors were swayed by the persistent crisis, deciding 15–1 to resume masking in one week's time.[224] Despite countless arrests, citizens wore their masks haphazardly, and the strongest opponents joined together in a new Anti-Mask League. As influenza declined, opposition increased apace. By the time the order was reversed on February 1, enforcement had become impossible. While the retreat of the epidemic allowed public health leaders to reverse this order without humiliation, by the time they took this action they had lost control of San Francisco's population. In this case it was not just a few individuals intentionally challenging the constitutionality of one of the emergency measures but rather large numbers of the populace simply disregarding them altogether.

Such circumstances posed a dilemma for public health officials—how to preserve the public's health even as the public grew tired of restrictions and more suspicious of health officials' authority and power. As early as mid-December the USPHS worried that the public was relaxing its attitude toward the epidemic despite the resurgence of influenza in many communities. As the Surgeon General reminded the people:

> I may have been misunderstood, but I thought I had emphasized the fact that not only was the epidemic still present in many parts of the country, but in a number of places it is even more prevalent than it was in the early part of the epidemic. Any statement at the present time that the epidemic has "come and gone for good" can only do harm, for it will lull people into a false sense of security, and cause them to relax the precautions they should take to avoid the infection.[225]

Such a plea on the part of the Surgeon General reflected the growing resistance public health authorities faced in the waning weeks of the epidemic, not only in San Francisco but throughout the nation.

Public Health and Progressivism

Long before the epidemic concluded, public health leaders began assessing their work. As they struggled against the skyrocketing infection and death rates in the early weeks of the pandemic, some public health professionals expressed their surprise and their chagrin that such circumstances had befallen the nation. State Health Commissioner Hermann M. Biggs of New York, for instance, admitted to colleagues in October that he "felt that it was rather a serious reflection upon public health administration and work, and medical science in a way, that we should be in the situation we now are."[226] An editorial in *Scientific American* in November lamented the same situation. "It is certainly a disconcerting fact that, at the very time when the country had organized itself . . . to fight disease and prevent suffering, we should be smitten with a visitation which caused more casualties and deaths in the homeland than occurred among our troops in the great world-war."[227] In January 1919 Biggs acknowledged in the popular press that despite recent progress made in bacteriology and the resulting successes against infectious disease, "The question naturally arises as to how such a pandemic of disease should be possible at the present time."[228] Because scientists understood the transmission of the disease, influenza, "theoretically at least, should be preventable."[229]

For many in the public health profession, though, success was never measured only by death rates. As they shouldered their responsibility and wielded their power during the epidemic, they sought to investigate, educate, mobilize, and legislate to control the problems the health crisis presented. In the process, they hoped both to assert their authority as experts and to establish their role in protecting the public. From simple victories in inter-agency organizing to the conquest of influenza itself, their comments emphasized especially their successes in demonstrating their value *as a profession*. Even as they began their struggle against the pandemic, public health leaders believed the meaning of their work should be assessed at least in part according to educational developments, by opportunities for learning exposed by the epidemic and met, and here health leadership was nearly unanimous about their successes. In Philadelphia, they dedicated an entire issue of the *Department of Public Health and Charities' Monthly Bulletin* to "What the Health Department Has Done to Curb the Epidemic of Influenza." "The epidemic has passed, only to be renewed in other sections of the country," the editors explained. "Let our experience be of value to other communities that they may be even better prepared to handle the situation and reduce their morbidity and mortality to a minimum."[230] Though the city had faced an horrific death rate, Philadelphia's public health leadership remained convinced that the knowledge they had acquired constituted a valuable chapter in the story of the nation's developing public health system.

Perhaps the most important measure of their success, according to health authorities, was the support they gained from the general public. Reporting on their efforts in the early weeks of the epidemic, health leaders congratulated themselves on mobilizing the public to accept the regulations they established to handle the crisis, and the broader support for public health this response reflected. As one nurse serving outside Camp Lewis reported, "Our patients see Uncle Sam in a guise they have never seen him before; they may have been good citizens before, but these experiences have not impaired their citizenship at all."[231] The *Journal of the American Medical Association* (*JAMA*) was even more effusive. In mid-October *JAMA* acknowledged the danger of making claims about the incidence of the disease "without great fear that it will have completely changed by the date of publication."[232] At the same time, *JAMA* did not hesitate to celebrate the changed relationship between public health officials and the public. Crediting the war for preparing the public to "accept freely orders and suggestions as to their mode of living," the journal explained, "When health authorities place a ban on public gatherings, when they insist that the windows of public conveyances be kept open, when they insist on absolute quarantine in order to stop the spread of the disease, the public is ready to obey, and does obey to the fullest measure."[233] It was not only a willingness to obey that encouraged public health leaders but also the public's new belief in the power of public health and its leaders.[234] The citizenry, according to *JAMA*, had expressed their support through their ready acceptance of the restrictions the epidemic demanded.

These comments did not anticipate the resistance that emerged late in the epidemic. Implicit in the public health plan for the epidemic was a willingness to coerce the public if necessary to ensure behavior that comported with the vision of public health authorities. Progressivism always held the potential to employ coercive measures to accomplish its goals, a potential public health leaders had made real during earlier health emergencies. Public health authorities assumed that their authority should include the power to control Americans' behaviors, both public and private, when such behaviors threatened the "welfare of the community," the "well-being of the body politic."[235] The pandemic constituted just such a crisis and warranted not only their wielding of power but also the embracing of that authority by the lay public, even when that authority included repressive measures. During the epidemic and in its most immediate aftermath, some argued that this was precisely what was occurring. Yet the reality of public

resistance, particularly as the epidemic wore on, suggests that the relationship was not so simple. While early in the epidemic citizens rallied to the public health cause, relying on experts for guidance and entrusting their health to the authorities, such a reaction did not outlast the epidemic.

Like public health authorities who measured their successes by the changed relationship with the citizenry, physicians and nurses, too, would judge their experiences during the pandemic in terms of their interactions with the broader public. And though they worked together closely and shared the heavy burdens of patient care in the midst of the disaster, their perceptions of their work, of their successes and their failures, would prove markedly different.

4

"The experience was one I shall never forget"

Doctors, Nurses, and the Challenges of the Epidemic

In the fall of 1918 student nurses at Fort Des Moines answered a call to service, joining the fight against the epidemic that was sweeping through the American Midwest. Recording the experiences of her classmates for the school yearbook, Mabel Chilson recalled the resolve with which she and her classmates faced the dreaded disease. "We wondered, 'were we helpless or could we fight?' With eager determination we entered the ranks." Once at work, according to Chilson, the nurses "soon became the happiest family, and when off duty we had jolly good times. The greatest comfort we possessed was the knowledge that each girl was doing her best and making good as a nurse."[1] Mabel Chilson was not alone in her positive reaction to her experiences during the epidemic. Her sense that nurses had performed well in providing much-needed care to a country in crisis was mirrored in the responses nurses recorded in diaries, letters, and published accounts as they fought the influenza outbreak. While acknowledging the horror of the disease and the wretched state of its victims, these women described the pride they felt in doing their duty and the satisfaction, even joy, they found in serving others.

The narratives of physicians reflected no similar sense of satisfaction. "Give us another war with Germany, Mexico and all the other heathenish countries in preference to another blast of this distressing flu," a physician from Tennessee grumbled in an article published in December 1918.[2] Describing the devastation wrought by the unchecked epidemic, he continued, "The family of orphans, the lone widow, the cattle at the barn, with no one to feed them; the plow standing in the field, rusting, the corn not gathered, and the general panorama of desolation viewed through tear-dimmed eyes, usher to our senses and observation that a great, merciless juggernaut has rolled over the land and left weeping and wailing in its path." Before such a scourge, this physician acknowledged, he had stood powerless. "Like a hideous monster, he went his way, and none could hinder," he concluded. Conceding his own sense of failure in combating the epidemic, another medical man summed up the mood of many when he declared years after the epidemic, "You can't do anything for influenza."[3] Such responses were not uncommon among American physicians. Ignorant of the disease's etiology, uncertain of the best methods of treatment, and unable to ease the suffering of their patients, physicians often expressed a sense of helplessness as individuals and humility as members of a profession as they narrated their experiences during the epidemic.

That doctors and nurses could react so differently to their shared service during the epidemic seems surprising, given how closely they worked together during the crisis. (See Figure 4.1.) By 1918, though, these health care professionals understood their roles and their responsibilities quite distinctly, and measured themselves against sharply divergent standards. With the medical profession an almost exclusively male preserve and nursing the acceptable alternative for women working in health care, profession-specific standards had also become gender-specific. Men working as physicians gauged their work against the masculine standards of skill and expertise and embraced an understanding of their profession as one that healed patients and cured disease, standards difficult to meet during the pandemic. Though there were exceptions to their self-critical reaction, most notably among African American physicians, far more prominent were expressions of masculine failure. In contrast, women working as nurses aspired to what they viewed as the uniquely feminine qualities of domesticity, compassion, and selflessness. To measure up to these standards nurses needed only to care for their patients, not cure them, and this they proved able to do. Believing they had met the highest standards of both womanhood and nursing, these women found in their work in the epidemic both personal and professional satisfaction.

The American public, too, looked at the work of nurses and doctors during the pandemic through a gendered lens. While physicians were celebrated for their skill and bravery, nurses were hailed as angels who had manifested the womanly qualities of selflessness and caring. Yet doctors also saw their cultural authority subverted as their patients turned to other medical practices—to folk remedies, patent medicines, or alternative medical systems—for aid against influenza, and as alternative practitioners openly criticized the inadequacy of "regular" or "orthodox" medicine. For doctors and nurses, as for their patients, contemporary thinking about social identity shaped their experiences in profound ways.

Doctors and the Challenge of Spanish Influenza

When influenza exploded in September and October, physicians faced a disease that was, in theory, a familiar one. And yet as they began to see cases of Spanish influenza and recognized the reach of the outbreak, physicians struggled to place

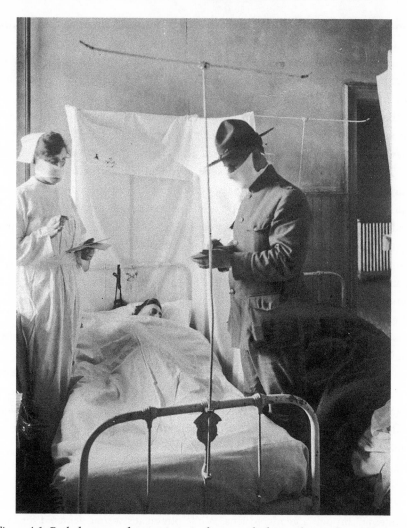

Figure 4.1 Both doctors and nurses were in short supply during the pandemic. Here a nurse and doctor attend to a patient at U.S. Army Hospital No. 4 at Fort Porter in New York. (165-WW-269B-4), Still Picture Branch, NA.

the new epidemic in the context of their existing understanding of the disease. In the pages of their professional journals physicians retraced the steps their predecessors had traveled in the pandemic of 1890. Their articles on the epidemic frequently opened with an overview of the long history of influenza. One physician began in "prehistoric times" before tracking influenza through the centuries.[4] Similarly, a piece in the *Journal of the American Medical Association* (*JAMA*) explained, "Under various names, epidemics corresponding to epidemic influenza have occurred at irregular intervals since accurate descriptions have been made of disease."[5] Others went on to confirm that the disease wreaking havoc in

1918 was not a new foe.[6] "Although its name suggests to the laity some new out-landish disease," one doctor wrote, "we find Spanish influenza to be distin-guished only by the greater virulence of its infection from the ordinary grippe."[7] Physicians often emphasized a link between the 1918 flu and its epidemic and pandemic predecessors, especially that of 1889–1890, and affirmed that it was another episode and represented "nothing new."[8]

Even as many physicians maintained the essential familiarity of the disease, increasingly they admitted that they were also confronting something unusual that fall. Indeed, influenza's shocking presentation jolted some physicians into the recognition that there was nothing customary about this disease. Shortly after the fall wave began, Victor Vaughan, William Welch, and Rufus Cole, men accomplished in the field of scientific medicine and all serving as medical officers in the army, traveled to Camp Devens on behalf of the Army Surgeon General, William G. Gorgas, to survey the situation there. Cole, whose expertise on respi-ratory disease was already well established in 1918, still evoked his sense of awe when he described that visit almost thirty years later. "We were at once struck by the cyanosis which most of the patients exhibited. One could pick out the infected men among those standing about, by the color of their faces. We went to the morgue and saw a large number of bodies piled up waiting to be exam-ined. In one after another of them, when the chests were opened we saw large amounts of bloody fluid in the pleural cavities, and on cutting open the lungs there were large areas of wet, hemorrhagic consolidation." Suggesting just how unprecedented these conditions were, Cole noted, "Even Dr. Welch was startled and alarmed. It was the first and only time I ever saw him lose his customary calmness and self possession."[9]

Though the disease they confronted was influenza, physicians suggested, it was a more dangerous form than that to which they were accustomed. As one of the earliest articles to appear in *JAMA* explained in September 1918, "The disease is similar to the familiar endemic influenza, except that it is often more severe, the complications are more frequent and serious, and it shows an extraordinary degree of contagiousness."[10] Others stressed that this one was in a class all its own, "a new disease and a new influenza, namely the 'Spanish' influenza," an ill-ness that "has had no parallel of its kind."[11] As one physician noted simply but definitively in October 1919, "No book I have ever read has properly or correctly described the disease as I saw it in the late epidemic."[12] In the end many physi-cians abandoned the notion that they were on tested ground.

Questions about the etiology and treatment of this new scourge replaced the comfortable familiarity that had once surrounded the yearly influenza visit. An editorial in *JAMA* suggested in early November 1918, "It is of great interest that there is no unanimity of opinion whatever as to the nature of the primary infecting agent."[13] No consensus was reached throughout the epidemic, despite substantial and ongoing research among bacteriologists and clinicians, and debate filled the pages of the professional medical journals, as it did public health journals.

Not surprisingly, the role of Pfeiffer's bacillus in causing the disease was debated as the pandemic intensified the challenges to its importance.[14] Some physicians continued to identify Pfeiffer's bacillus as the infective agent in influenza, while others maintained that the influenza bacillus was responsible for the epidemic but suggested that there was something unusual about its presentation.[15] Anna Williams conducted extensive research at New York City's Health Department Laboratory, and discovered the bacillus in the vast majority of samples she tested, leading to efforts to develop an influenza vaccine. The lab's head, bacteriologist William H. Park, acknowledged throughout this work that though Pfeiffer's bacillus seemed a possible "starting point of the disease," there was also "the possibility that some unknown filterable virus may be the starting point."[16] The caution displayed by Pfeiffer's advocates is not surprising, given the rising chorus of detractors they confronted in the medical press.[17] Recapping a recent meeting of the American Public Health Association in their pages in December 1918, the editors of *JAMA* announced, "The discussions relative to the etiology of the present epidemic resolve themselves into the belief that the bacillus of influenza is not the primary etiological factor, and that the actual cause is as yet unknown."[18] Others were a bit harsher in their conclusions. "There seems to be no justification for the belief that the epidemic was due to the influenza bacillus," three physicians announced in January, 1919.[19] The sense of certainty that had accompanied Pfeiffer's discovery evaporated in the epidemic with the heat of new research.

Throughout the months of the scourge, medical authorities ranging from the United States Surgeon General to those physicians publishing in *JAMA* were forced to concede that the "causative agent" for influenza remained unknown.[20] As the epidemic progressed, medical commentators acknowledged repeatedly how little they understood about the disease.[21] As one diagnostician lamented in December 1918, "The real cause, I am afraid, we must admit to be some vagary of plant life beyond our ken up to the present time. In these modern days, we are not permitted to invoke sun spots or world girdling volcanic dust."[22] "It is certain that the cause of influenza remains a mystery," responded *JAMA*'s editors in January 1919.[23] "Epidemic influenza is a disease of unknown origin," and "nothing is definitely known as to its [influenza's] causative agent," acknowledged others in March.[24] Commentators noted, too, that this ignorance persisted despite the significant efforts to isolate and identify the infective cause that were underway in laboratories across the country.[25] Such uncertainty did little to assuage the anxiety of medical practitioners.

Doctors were similarly unable to explain some of the secondary infections that soon accompanied influenza and were frequently the actual cause of death.[26]

Physicians were quick to acknowledge the important role of these sequelae. As an article in the "Current Comment" section of *JAMA* suggested in mid-October, 1918, "The great danger is not from influenza, but from secondary complications."[27] "The complications of influenza," a physician from South Carolina, J. Heyward Gibbes, observed, "are without limit."[28] Gibbes listed "the most common ones" as pneumonia, empyema, sinusitis, laryngitis, psychoses, complications with pregnancy, peritonitis, and subcutaneous emphysema.[29]

Though other physicians would share Gibbes's view that there were several important sequelae evident during the epidemic, it was pneumonia, appropriately, that dominated discussions in the medical community. "The large number of deaths incident to an epidemic of influenza is not due to the influenza," an article in the *Journal of the National Medical Association* (*JNMA*) explained in late 1919, "but almost entirely to a virulent type of pneumonia which accompanies it."[30] Although the relationship between the two diseases was unclear, "There seems to be no doubt that there is some unexplained or peculiar relation between these two diseases."[31] In a context in which it was often not influenza itself but its sequelae, particularly pneumonia, which brought death, doctors admitted that these, too, remained beyond contemporary wisdom.[32]

Nonetheless, physicians attempted to treat their patients throughout the epidemic, using a wide range of therapies. Perhaps the most common treatment plan was a simple one, emphasizing basic pain relief, isolation, bed rest, ventilation of the sick room, and protection from chills.[33] A preoccupation with the bowels was also common, with calls for "the free ingestion of water and hot drinks" or other methods of "purgation" to ensure a cleansing process a fairly standard prescription.[34] Beyond this common course of treatment, clinicians employed a dizzying array of strategies to fight the flu. An account of the treatment employed at the Camp Brooks Open Air Hospital near Boston suggests the multiple approaches potentially employed by even a single practitioner. In addition to the general emphasis on "open air and sunshine," keeping the patient warm, "four-hour feeding throughout the entire course of the fever," and "free catharsis by calomel," the hospital also deployed a number of other treatments:

> In the way of special medication were sponging for fever, coal tar preparations, acetylsalicylic acid, quinin, salicylates; for cough, brown mixture, Dover's powder, codein and expectorant mixture; for throat, mentholated throat tablets, Dobell's spray, red gum lozenges; for kidney irritation, hexamethylenamin, spirit of nitrous ether, milk; for nosebleed, plugging with cotton saturated with epinephrin solution; for heart, digipuratum, digifolin, camphor in oil, strychnin; for pneumonia, cotton or paper jackets, forced feeding, calcium iodid, codein, morphin, atropin, bromids, expectorant mixture and oxygen

inhalation; for delirium, bromids, codein, ipecac; for meningitis, Flexner's serum; for arthritis, sodium salicylate; for convalescence, tonics of iron, arsenic and strychnin.[35]

Clearly there was no scarcity of treatments to be tried during the epidemic. As had often been the case in the past, doctors advocated treatments in direct contradiction with those of other practitioners. For instance, while some prescribed coal tar drugs as a central feature of treatment, others believed they "undoubtedly did an immense amount of harm."[36] Similarly, while some advocated the use of alcohol or narcotics, others stood steadfastly against their use.[37] Some emphasized the importance of regular food intake; others argued for restricted diets.[38]

Despite this therapeutic chaos, an occasional physician nevertheless expressed confidence in the efficacy of a particular approach and claimed success in treating his patients. For instance, in a "Letter to the Editor" in *JAMA*, Dr. Thomas C. Ely of Philadelphia maintained his own "very successful experience in the epidemic with the saturation of the system with harmless alkalis," which he used to produce "poor soil for bacterial growth."[39] Another letter writer noted that his use of injections of "quinin hydrochlorid," coupled with the ingestion of "quinin bisulphate" and "sodium salicylate" and "a brisk flushing of the bowels" had proven "a treatment from which my results have been most satisfactory."[40] Other practitioners would express a similar certainty about a variety of treatments, for instance the use of calomel to stimulate the liver, turpentine enemas to ensure "elimination," and "the transfusion of total citrated immune blood" to create "an acquired immunity" as a "corrective to influenza and its complications."[41]

Doctors repeatedly acknowledged that their treatment was aimed at controlling symptoms, not the disease itself.[42] "In our hands no specific treatment seemed to have greater value than the induction of symptomatic relief, which we believe should be the hub of the treatment," two physicians at the Michael Reese Hospital in Chicago conceded in November 1918.[43] By the end of 1918, this was also the position staked out by the Assistant Surgeon General. Given the absence of "accurate knowledge of the cause and transmission of the disease," it was not possible to create protection from the disease or to cure it.[44]

Like their public health colleagues, some medical practitioners found relief from this sense of uncertainty by investing hope in the promise of future research, suggesting that ongoing investigations would decipher the mysteries surrounding the disease. Though noting that it was "too early to consider in detail the outcome of the etiologic investigations of the present outbreak," *JAMA*'s editors suggested hopefully in October 1918, "We may anticipate, however, highly valuable and interesting contributions" when that research was completed and its results published.[45] Other physicians expressed the same hopes that the current outbreak might hold the key to unlocking the secrets of influenza. As

Mazyck Ravenel suggested at a meeting of the Advisory Board of the United States Public Health Service (USPHS) Hygienic Laboratory on January 8, 1919, "We medical men and scientific workers throughout the country cannot but take off our hats to what the laboratory has done, and it is the place we are looking to for comfort and to be set right on things."[46]

Many physicians staked their hopes on vaccination. Throughout the pandemic medical researchers applied themselves diligently to work in the laboratory with this goal. In mid-October, for instance, two naval physicians in Massachusetts published what they conceded were still incomplete results because their findings suggested "the possibility in the use of convalescent serum."[47] A few months later these physicians followed up with more conclusive results, based on further experimentation and suggested confidently, "Pooled serum from convalescent influenza bronchopneumonia patients at this hospital has greatly reduced mortality, has shortened the course of the disease, and has proved almost a specific, not only during a waning epidemic but also during the more recent recrudescence."[48] Both William H. Park of the New York City Health Department's laboratory and the highly respected scientist Paul Lewis in Philadelphia put significant effort into developing both preventive and curative vaccines.[49]

The reality, though, was that none of the developed vaccines proved effective against influenza as either prophylaxis or treatment. In mid-October, *JAMA* reported on the work of two state committees appointed in Massachusetts to investigate the potential of vaccines in the treatment of influenza. Recognizing the failure of the research, the state chose not to endorse or supply a treatment vaccine.[50] In an editorial in late October the *JAMA* editors acknowledged their own skepticism. "The main point to keep always in sight is that unfortunately we as yet have no specific serum or other specific means for the cure of influenza," they began. "Such is the fact," they continued, "all claims and propagandist statements in the newspapers and elsewhere to the contrary notwithstanding."[51]

Confounded by both the disease and the epidemic, doctors increasingly conceded their confusion and uncertainty as practitioners. "It was freely confessed by all that we are at sea as to the proper methods of treatment, cure and prevention; that we do not know as yet how to prevent and control the spread of the disease, and that most of the methods employed in fighting it, though pronounced efficacious by some of their adherents, have been held of little value by others," one physician admitted.[52] Incapable of stopping either the disease or the epidemic, and uncertain about the best treatments, doctors often conceded there was little they could really offer their patients. As another practitioner recalled, "There wasn't much a doctor could do. The patient would be dead before he could get back to see him. He could diagnose you and give you some medicine and the next day you'd be dead." And further, "The main thing of visiting every day was to find out who was dead and then bury them."[53] Another doctor experienced a similar fatalism, as he remembered, "It got to the place where I would only see patients twice—once when they came in and again when I signed their death certificate. It was horrible."[54] Still another physician noted how ghastly he found his experience of watching his patients, too many in number, progress too rapidly toward death.

> These men start with what appears to be an ordinary attack of La Grippe or Influenza, and when brought to the hospital they very rapidly develop the most viscous type of pneumonia that has ever been seen. Two hours after admission they have the mahogany spots over the cheek bones, and a few hours later you can begin to see the cyanosis extending from their ears and spreading all over the face, until it is hard to distinguish the coloured men from the white. It is only a matter of a few hours then until death comes, and it is simply a struggle for air until they suffocate. It is horrible. One can stand it to see one, two, or twenty men die, but to see these poor devils dropping like flies sort of gets on your nerves.[55]

The editors of the *New York Medical Journal* tried to caution readers in November 1918, "Probably nothing serves so well to add emphasis to the warning of the great fathers of medicine that the first duty of the physician is expressed in the Latin phrase, *non nocere*—to be sure to do no harm—as the history of therapeutics for influenza." They reminded doctors, "There is much more likelihood that jumping to conclusions in the midst of an epidemic shall prove wrong rather than right and much more than a possibility that biological remedies of various kinds, except when employed under the most rigid control, may do ever so much more harm than good."[56] In this context, some doctors concluded, "The best thing that the physician can do for the patient is to leave the patient alone."[57]

Unable to cure their patients or to check the epidemic, many physicians experienced an unfamiliar, and unexpected, sense of helplessness. One physician suggested that after 400 years of the disease one might expect that "the medical profession would be unfailing in its [influenza's] recognition and somewhat proficient in its control," but suggested that "the records of our army camps and our bureaus of vital statistics too plainly establish the futility of our efforts at control."[58] Another practitioner concluded, "There was just nothing you could do."[59]

For many this sense of powerlessness was completely unanticipated. Certain about the utility of germ theory, confident in their scientific methods, and proud of recent successes with infectious diseases, many doctors had embraced a belief in their ability to handle any health crisis. Their failure to control the epidemic or help their patients came as a terrible surprise and a blow to their professional identity. As an article in the *JNMA* stated simply, "In the future we will look back on this epidemic of influenza with wonder and surprise; yes, in spite of our vaunted advancement, we have utterly failed in the recent crisis."[60] Confronted with the reality that this epidemic was beyond their command, many physicians experienced a new sense of the limitations of their profession. Aware of each generation's tendency to see its own time as "enlightened" in comparison to the "benighted" eras that preceded them, one practitioner intimated, "I fear that even before two generations have passed, some of our therapeutics of this latest epidemic of influenza will seem to be absurd."[61]

For many physicians the epidemic constituted a professional low point as the epidemic challenged their former confidence in the promise of modern medicine. Mystified by the disease and unable to slow the epidemic or save their patients, doctors experienced it as a time of distress and humility.[62] A group of physicians, writing in *JAMA* in 1919, described the crisis they witnessed at Camp Upton and noted how haunting their experiences had been. "The impression received in going through our pneumonia wards . . . was one of horror at the frightfulness of the sight of the hopelessly sick and dying and at the magnitude of the catastrophe that had stricken wholesale the young soldiers prepared to fight another enemy but helpless before this insidious one," they explained, concluding, "The memory of this sight will haunt for life the minds of those who saw it."[63] Or as another doctor exclaimed with notable directness, "I shall never forget that experience!"[64]

Nurses and the Experience of Success

Working alongside doctors, nurses agreed that these images of destruction were ones they would never forget. One leader in American nursing, Anna C. Jamme, recounted her first visit to a military flu ward: "From the moment I left the train I saw that terrible look of horror in the face of everyone whom I met. . . . At the nurses' quarters there were 67 nurses in the throes of the disease . . . and the stricken horror in the eyes above the masks was something never to be forgotten. The wards were quiet with the stillness of death. . . . It was a spectacle never to be forgotten."[65] While acknowledging the unforgettably appalling reality of the epidemic, Jamme's reaction to what she saw, and the impact it had on her understanding of her profession, were quite different from those expressed by doctors. Describing nurses who "stood to their tasks like brave soldiers" and detailing the appreciation her nurses received from commanding officers, Jamme articulated her admiration for the "splendid work" of nurses during the epidemic.

Jamme's reaction to the epidemic was not uncommon among nurses. "The happy memories of the epidemic are many," wrote Eunice H. Dyke. "The list of treasured experiences," she concluded, "is long."[66] Or as Miss Condell, a nursing student in Boston, remembered, "We enjoyed the work and as it was considered a war measure to nurse the civilian population we were very glad we were nurses and able to do 'our bit.'" In short, she concluded, "The nursing experience was wonderful and we have learned many valuable lessons. The self control, the endurance, and the splendid willing spirit of all the nurses were marvelous."[67] Though few were as effusive as Dyke and Condell, nurses' memories of the epidemic, at least those they recorded, were rarely as wholeheartedly negative as those of physicians. While most shared the doctors' sadness, and even revulsion, at the suffering and dying they witnessed, this dismay was often coupled with more positive associations with this period in their lives.[68] "All of us who had any part in helping in the epidemic," a report on visiting nurses in Boston explained, "must look back upon it as one of the most immediately satisfactory experiences of our lives, and this is true even though we were borne down with the knowledge that, do all we might, the pressing, tragic need for nursing was much greater than could possibly be met."[69] Or as another account maintained, "Terrible as was the influenza epidemic, with its frightful toll, there was a certain tremendous exhilaration to be felt as well as many lessons to be learned from such a terrific test."[70]

That nurses were able to narrate their work during those months so much more positively reflects their assessment that they had been able to do a great deal of good during the emergency. One nurse recounted how much others had appreciated the assistance she and her colleagues had been able to lend. "So we had that," she concluded, expressing how much it had meant to her to be able to offer significant help to others.[71] The Annual Report of the Visiting Nurse Society of Philadelphia shared this perspective, reporting, "It was the high privilege of the Visiting Nurse Society to be able to give that which was most needed—skilled nursing care."[72]

For some their success was as simple as providing basic comfort to their patients. One Red Cross account detailed the aid two nurses brought to a family suffering in the tenement district of a major city, making clear the simple but important work they completed: "In two dirty, unaired and unheated rooms, lighted by one oil lamp, with no one to prepare food or give any attention, they found thirteen suffering people—nine of whom were children. Immediately several were sent to a hospital; bedding was sent for, fires were built, the rooms were aired and cleaned, in almost less time than it takes to tell of it."[73] Another story in this account highlighted how meaningful for the patient this basic caregiving could prove. Describing the work of a Red Cross nurse in the mountains of Virginia, it queried, "Can you imagine what it meant to those people, isolated as they were from all possibility of help, to have a capable, willing woman appear suddenly in their midst, and without any preliminaries set to work and make them comfortable—a veritable angel of mercy in a cap and apron."[74] For nurses, providing comfort in the context of the crisis was an accomplishment, one worthy of angels.

Other accounts celebrated even greater achievements. A nurse who served in the Boston area felt her spirits restored by her sense that her actions mattered: "It was a great help to flagging spirit and weary back to find that by bringing trained hands and minds into these places [patients' homes], one could bring also hope, cheer, and a decided improvement in the patient's surroundings and conditions."[75] Another elaborated, "Through the confusion and terror spread by the epidemic the visiting nurses, who had but little time to nurse, rushed on, instructing and leaving behind them a world of comfort, of reassurance, of encouragement, forming inseparable ties of trust, unity, and confidence between the patients and themselves."[76] Others expressed the certainty that "due to the unselfish work of these women, a great many lives in this vicinity have assuredly been saved."[77] Nurses did not claim that they had cured influenza or stopped the epidemic. They did, however, feel that their ministrations had contributed in a meaningful way to patients' well-being.

Not unlike the reaction of public health workers during the epidemic, nurses suggested that these successes had demonstrated both the importance of their profession and the quality of its practitioners. As the president of a local nursing association explained in a letter during the epidemic, "The situation is critical, the hospitals are filled, the doctors are ill, and the District Nursing Association and the few nurses and doctors worked in relays. No call went unheeded. . . . We were taken quite unawares. But I feel we were not found wanting."[78] Another woman noted the "great pride" she felt regarding the performance of her local Red Cross branch.[79] Nurses' satisfaction in their work often reflected their sense that they had brought honor to themselves and their profession. "The name of every nurse at this hospital should be placed high on the nation's *Roll of Honor*," one head nurse proclaimed. And further, "The wonderful team work and spirit shown was beyond expression. . . . No soldier went over the top with more will to do or die."[80] Another woman, the Superintendent of the Army Nurse Corps, shared this perspective about her own nursing staff: "They were untiring in their efforts and met the situation in a manner which cannot be praised too highly, taking no heed for their own comfort or the number of hours they served. The heroic self-sacrifice and fidelity to duty shown by the nurses is without parallel."[81] Or as a letter published in *Public Health Nurse* suggested in the wake of the epidemic, "We nurses who tried to do our best do not want any Distinguished Service Medals, but we *do* want to be considered by God and men what most of us tried to be: Good and faithful servants."[82]

Proud of their profession and of the work of their colleagues, nurses' personal reactions to the epidemic were often markedly positive. "I am so glad to find that I can help," one volunteer nurse proclaimed simply.[83] One report recounted the story of a volunteer nurse who died after just eight days of service. "In the last moments she stated she had obtained more joy from her work in the past eight

[days] than she had in the twenty five years of her life," the report claimed.[84] Over-
worked to a state of exhaustion and witness to devastating disease and death,
nurses nevertheless embraced their experience in the epidemic. "I feel thankful to
have been able to help out a little and to keep up during it all, yet I shall never want
to go through the same thing again. The sight of so much suffering, death and
sadness, and the leaving behind of so many little orphans, in some cases both
parents taken, was very depressing indeed," one student lamented. "However,"
she concluded, "it was all a very wonderful experience, and one which will never
fade from my memory."[85] Another nurse agreed. "It was a most horrible and yet
most beautiful experience," she explained, elaborating, "Our supply of nurses was
entirely inadequate to the sudden need. The constant tragic appeal for nurses
which could not be satisfactorily met were [sic] heartrending, and the experience
of the nurses in the homes was overwhelmingly sad. It was distressing to watch
the nurses working long over time, and to see them gradually becoming more run
down, and finally succumbing to the disease." And yet, she concluded, "They
would not have spared themselves even if they had been told to do so. Too many
lives depended upon them for them to think of themselves. They rendered as
noble service as any soldiers in battle."[86] Certainly saddened, these nurses nevertheless also found value and nobility in their experiences during the epidemic.

For African American nurses this response was especially pronounced as they
found in their work in the epidemic confirmation of their place in the nursing
profession, a position long contested by white Americans uneasy with black success. African American nurses recognized an opening in the epidemic, a chance
to prove their value to a nation too busy with the epidemic to enforce racial restrictions. Nursing had long offered a unique opportunity for African American
women, who faced circumscribed possibilities in a society that excluded women,
and especially women of color, from most professions.[87] African American
nurses had found their offers to serve during the war largely refused. Though the
Army Nurse Corps and the Red Cross engaged roughly 33,000 nurses during
the war, they accepted only about thirty African American nurses into their
ranks, forcing them to develop their own opportunities for service, for instance
through the Circle for Negro War Relief.[88] African American women's work in
the epidemic, then, was meaningful not only for the valuable contributions they
made to their patients' well-being but also for the opportunity it offered for
showcasing their professional competence. It was the epidemic, for instance,
which finally forced the army to accept their help.[89]

African American nurses joined the chorus of nurses celebrating their profession's accomplishments in the epidemic. Bessie Hawse, a 1918 nursing school
graduate, recounted her own work in the epidemic.[90] Like many other nurses,
Hawse acknowledged the harsh conditions she had confronted during the
epidemic but found herself nevertheless feeling very positive about this time in

her life. "Eight miles from Talladega in the back woods, a colored family of ten were in bed and dying for the want of attention," she began. "No one would come near. I was asked by the health officer if I would go. I was glad of the opportunity," she explained. Venturing into the countryside to aid the family she discovered that the dead mother's body was still in the family's midst, and other family members were suffering from either influenza or pneumonia. Friends and relatives had abandoned the family to its fate, but this nurse felt compelled to help them. "I saw at a glance," she declared, "I had work to do. . . . I worked day and night trying to save them for seven days." Hawse emphasized her commitment to her work, and the joy she found in the opportunity to serve others. "I didn't realize till it was over just how brave I was. I did feel happy when they were out of danger. I only wished I could have reached them earlier and been able to have done something for the poor mother."[91] Like other nurses, Hawse felt joy and pride in the service she was able to offer and articulated a narrative of success in stark contrast to the preoccupation with failure voiced by physicians.

In the aftermath of the epidemic, Dr. John A. Kenney celebrated the accomplishments of African American nurses during the crisis in the pages of the *Journal of the National Medical Association*, a journal established by black doctors in the face of their exclusion from the American Medical Association. "The Negro woman has long been recognized and accorded the place of an experienced nurse," he argued, "and as such she has done untold good in caring for the sick and relieving the suffering." And further, "In point of devotion, endurance, sympathy, tactile delicacy, unselfishness, tact, resourcefulness, willingness to undergo hardships—yea, in all that goes to make a good nurse, she has been found not one whit behind her white sister."[92] Describing the work of nurses from the St. Agnes Hospital and Training School for Nurses in Raleigh, North Carolina, Kenney applauded their efforts, suggesting, "The nurses from this school carried on the work for four weeks untiringly and diligently, and as a result many were saved that would have died for want of care."[93] For Kenney and others, African American nurses' successes contributed to the broader struggle for racial justice even as they eschewed the racism evident among their white counterparts.[94] Despite the awful costs of the epidemic, then, for some African Americans the accomplishments of black nurses during the crisis warranted notice, and perhaps even celebration.

The Gendering of Health Care

That most doctors and nurses should react so differently to the same epidemic seems surprising at first glance. The two groups of professionals worked together with unusual closeness during the epidemic, sharing the same risks to their personal health, as well as the experiences of understaffing, overwork, and the desperate need for their services. The obvious explanation for their divergent reactions would hold that medicine and nursing had different responsibilities during the epidemic—medicine to cure, nursing to comfort—and that doctors failed in their charge, while nurses succeeded. Yet this explanation ignores the deeper question of why doctors and nurses had come to understand their roles in these ways. By the early twentieth century, health care in the United States was the province of two distinct professions, defined, at least in part, by the presumed gender identity of its practitioners.[95]

This gendering of the health professions had evolved over the course of the previous century. In the early years of the American colonies, care of the ill was shared by men and women. The label "doctor" encompassed both a clergyman and a midwife, both a pharmacist and a surgeon. Much "health care" was handled within the household, largely by female family members. By the late eighteenth century, though, a growing number of physicians began to imagine themselves members of a more exclusive profession, basing this identity in formal education.[96] It was in this context that male practitioners of medicine moved largely to exclude women from the profession. During the nineteenth century the struggle over professional identity persisted, as "regular" physicians, those associated with allopathic medicine, faced enduring competition from a variety of directions, from lay providers to adherents of "irregular" medicine.[97]

By 1918, the "regulars" had consolidated their power in the medical profession and had established for themselves a position of prestige in American life. The recipe for success called for several ingredients—the establishment of an exclusive professional organization, the American Medical Association; "rapprochement" between the regulars and the most significant of the medical sects; the restoration of medical licensing; comprehensive restricting and reform of medical education; and increasing control over drugs at the expense of patent medicine producers.[98] With these moves, medical men had succeeded in eliminating all but a few women from their profession. Though women had trained for careers as doctors in ever-increasing numbers in the late nineteenth century, this rise was followed by a rapid drop in the early twentieth century. Tightening admission standards, declining spaces in medical schools, and rising costs for medical education affected all potential practitioners; in turn, restrictive policies in admissions and training appointments worked to eliminate women specifically from medicine.[99] By 1915 women constituted only 3.6 percent of physicians, a number that would grow to 5 percent by 1920 but fall again in the following decades.[100] As male practitioners developed a professional identity, then, this identity was increasingly associated with doctors' male identity.[101]

Parallel developments affected the field of nursing. Up until the late nineteenth century, most medical care took place in the home, with nursing largely the province of female family members, but this field too began professionalization in the latter years of the nineteenth century. In the 1870s the first nurses' training schools opened. Other vestiges of a developing profession—the establishment of professional organizations, the publishing of professional journals, and the requiring of professional examinations—soon followed.[102] Nursing's emergence from a domestic responsibility to a paid profession did nothing, though, to change its gender identity. Nurses were expected to embody traditional "feminine" characteristics—to be caring, self-sacrificing, domestic, and submissive—even as their work shifted out of the home and into paid labor.[103] Professionalization did not change this ideology but reinforced it.[104] Though African American women's relationship to dominant American gender norms was complicated by their families' economic needs and by the white community's racialized gender stereotyping, within their own communities African American women continued to be viewed as particularly suited to nursing because they were women. Professionalization, though, only increased white resistance to black nurses.[105]

By the time of the flu epidemic, these gendered and racialized notions of American health care were firmly established and helped shape the standards by which doctors, nurses, and laypeople alike measured the success of health care professionals during the epidemic.[106] A poem in the *American Journal of Public Health* in 1914 sang the praises of "The Health Department Nurse" and concluded, "So we'll doff our caps and help her when we can, /As she goes about among the sick—and worse, /For she's doing what can not be done by man / She's a woman—and a Health Department Nurse."[107] Or as one male physician explained in 1925, "A hospital is a home for the sick, and there can be no home unless there is a woman at the head of it."[108]

If nursing required womanly qualities, the work of the doctor was best done by men. Describing the role of the physician in the aftermath of the epidemic, one practitioner demonstrated how completely his understanding of their responsibilities was tied up with masculine notions of action and efficacy. While some doctors felt there was little use for treatment, he believed this reaction contradicted the central responsibility of the physician. He explained, "I believe that the only real claim that a man may have to the title of doctor is to do something for somebody who is distressingly sick."[109] The trauma of their helplessness and its impact on their sense of themselves and their profession was especially evident among medical officers in the armed forces.[110] As doctors described their failure during the epidemic, then, it was a failure to fulfill the male responsibilities with which they had imbued the role of doctor.

The response of African American physicians may be particularly instructive here. In the years preceding the epidemic the number of black physicians had risen dramatically, one part of the African American community's commitment to its members' health. Numbering only 900 in 1890, by 1920 the forces of

African American doctors had risen to roughly 3,500.[111] They continued, though, to face institutionalized racism throughout the system of American medicine as they sought medical and post-graduate educational opportunities, attempted to gain membership in the American Medical Association, and pursued professional positions at white-controlled hospitals.[112] Their sometimes upbeat and hopeful responses to the epidemic experience as they found opportunities for both service and advancement constituted a dramatic contrast to the sense of failure exhibited by so many doctors. "The Negro physician played a most prominent part in treating and relieving victims of every race in all parts of this country," an essay in *JNMA* proclaimed.[113] Though the situation had arisen from the prejudice that had kept African American physicians out of the armed forces while producing a shortage of white physicians among civilians, the experiences of the epidemic produced a unique opportunity for African American doctors, like nurses, to prove their capabilities as medical practitioners. Describing the changes he had seen during the epidemic, the author continued, "A new brand of professional democracy was born. No one stopped to inquire into the racial identity of the doctor. The one and sole purpose was to get medical assistance for the stricken member of the family."[114] "The Negro doctor will possibly never be cited in the history to be written of the 1918 epidemic," he realized. "However we want to call to the attention of the medical profession of America the unselfish devotion to duty that impelled three thousand legal practitioners of medicine of African descent to work night and day to aid in checking the monster scourge." The upbeat and laudatory tone of this piece stood in marked contrast to the more common lamentations by physicians about their failure during the epidemic.

Such a response is easily explained by the unique role of African American physicians in 1918. Leaders in their communities thanks to their educational and professional status, African American men serving as doctors during the epidemic had alternative community standards by which they could judge themselves. As the *JNMA* essayist described the role his black colleagues had played in the epidemic, "We are pleased to state the Negro physicians of this country have made new and excellent history for the race, because of their recent experiences."[115] While this single example can only offer a glimpse of African American physicians' experiences, it seems to suggest that African American physicians sometimes found it possible to locate their work during the epidemic within the realm of the masculine, as their efforts to save lives cast them in the role of "race men" fighting for the reputation of their people against the forces of prejudice. Redefining masculinity to reflect their community's circumstances, African American physicians could view themselves as successful men during the epidemic in a way many of their white colleagues could not. Though their reactions during the epidemic were thus more positive, they were nevertheless intimately connected with their view of themselves, and their profession, as masculine.

The Public and Health Care Professionals

Americans lavished significant praise on both doctors and nurses for their efforts during the crisis. Much of the praise caregivers received was gender-neutral, heralding qualities shared by doctors and nurses alike. For instance, contemporaries commended the devotion to duty and heroism exhibited by both doctors and nurses during the epidemic.[116] It was a widely held assumption that their dedication often weakened the resistance of physicians and nurses to influenza, and that many lost their lives trying to protect the health of others.[117] Such behavior earned accolades as observers acknowledged the courage and nobility of doctors and nurses who endangered their own health as they cared for others, "risking their lives for the cause of humanity."[118] Both doctors and nurses were also praised for efficiency, a quality highly regarded in early twentieth-century American culture.[119]

While both men and women earned the appellation of hero for their care-giving efforts during the epidemic, in many accounts the nature of their heroism, as described by their contemporaries, hinted at gender norms, illustrating that it was never only health care professionals who envisioned their work according to gender-inflected standards. The broader American populace, too, expected doctors to perform *as men* and nurses *as women* as they battled the epidemic. Doctors, for instance, were often praised for the expertise with which they fulfilled their responsibilities. Describing the contribution of doctors from Camp Crane in Pennsylvania to their neighboring communities, one account highlighted the proficiency evident in the physicians' apparent success in saving lives: "Only by hard and skillful work were they able to save the large percentage of lives which they did. In all places where these men have been stationed the disease has been wonderfully checked."[120] That the characteristic of expertise or skill was associated with doctors but not nurses was highlighted still more obviously in an editorial published during the epidemic in a small town newspaper in the Pacific Northwest. Describing an epidemic "becoming worse instead of better," the newspaper noted the shared devotion of doctors and nurses. When it came time to herald the skill of practitioners, though, only doctors warranted this praise. "The doctors and nurses are working overtime," it explained, "and to the physicians too much credit cannot be given for the able manner in which they are combatting the situation."[121]

An occasional source complimented the skill of nurses.[122] Others, though, seemed to suggest that nursing did not require skill, only a woman's dedication. As one woman suggested regarding her own volunteer work during the epidemic, "I am so glad I can help. I have not had a nurse's aide course, nor, in fact, any training. I probably have no qualifications for nursing except for my desire to relieve some of the suffering."[123] Still others simply suggested that influenza itself did not require "technical nursing" but rather only "intelligent care, diet,

ventilation and cleanliness," qualities that "volunteer workers" succeeded in supplying "with remarkable aptitude and unselfish courage."[124]

It was not skill, then, but innately feminine qualities that marked nurses as
successful during the pandemic. This viewpoint was made especially clear in a
graduation message for student nurses in 1919 by a professor of medicine at the
University of Pennsylvania Training School for nurses. "You are about to enter
upon a career full of trials," he reminded them,

> but equally full of that joy which comes from giving comfort, and often
> returning to health those committed to your care. It is not given to us to
> cure all of our patients, but do not forget that, even if the battle with
> disease goes against us, the fact that we have been able to assuage the
> sufferings of those in affliction, may be as great a triumph as saving life
> itself.... Do not forget that the greatest triumphs are sometimes those
> of the vanquished, and that if material victory does not perch on our
> banners, the feeling that we have been kind, gentle, sympathetic, and
> untiring in our efforts to relieve, as well as cure, will more than counter-
> balance the regret at failure to achieve that which, perhaps, was impos-
> sible from the very beginning.[125]

For nurses, then, their "greatest triumph" need not include a recovery but rather
only "kind, gentle, sympathetic, and untiring" care. Understood to be driven not
by a desire for glory but by an unselfish dedication to service, too, nurses were
commended for their quiet and self-sacrificing commitment to duty.[126]

Celebrating nurses for their feminine touch, Americans sometimes acknowledged directly their belief that it was its female qualities that distinguished
nursing. The *Monthly Bulletin for the Department of Health* in New York City
made this point, heralding volunteer nurses for "ministering as only a woman
can."[127] Poems seemed to be a favored genre for singing the praises of nurses. A
poem published in the *American Journal of Nursing* was very direct about the
importance of women's gender in suiting them for the nursing role. "Let the
khaki be worn by the men who must fight," it suggested, "Your work can be done
in the gingham and white."[128] Accounts of nursing during the pandemic often
employed familiar female imagery—for instance, referring to the nurses as
"ministering angels" or referencing the motherly quality of their care— reinforcing the idea that women succeeded as nurses *because* they were women. Another
poetic paean began by describing the nurses who, "like angel guides . . . so still
and white," attended the sick, and went on to describe the impact of their care:

A fair-haired boy
With bandaged eyes

> Starts from his slumber
> And faintly cries—
> *"Mother, mother/I see!"*[129]

Or as a tribute to nurses at a military hospital explained, "The hospital was started in the early days without nurses, but now includes this necessary and helpful and pleasant part of hospital life—the white gowned sister of mercy, who bring[s] not only healing and practical assistance to the sick, but an indefinable spirit of cheer that only womanhood can give."[130](See Figure 4.2.)

Challenges to Orthodox Medicine

Though very few commentators questioned doctors' dedication or hard work during the catastrophe, the epidemic nevertheless produced challenges to their cultural dominance in the health care field. Sometimes the challenges were fairly muted, as Americans shook their heads at the apparent disarray of medical thinking. Faced with vastly divergent reports on the causes and cures of influenza, Americans began to accept the reality that the epidemic remained, in many ways, a mystery even to those dedicated to understanding it.[131] Counter to the image of physicians as medical, and thereby social, authorities, this realization soon encouraged criticism of the medical profession, criticism that emphasized the failure of physicians to fulfill their roles as skilled and able practitioners of medicine. As an editorial comment in the local paper in Roanoke, Virginia, suggested, "There seems to be no question but that the 'flu' got the best of the doctors for a while. They fought it indefatigably and they fought in intelligently but it can hardly be said, all things considered, that they fought it effectively."[132] In the pages of the *New York Times*, a pair of editorials in October 1918 articulated a more hostile version of these sentiments. The first, entitled rather boldly "Science Has Failed to Guard Us," opened with an attack on both science and its practitioners. "When the history of this influenza epidemic comes to be written," the editorial argued, "it will not reflect much glory on medical science, or, to be more explicit and to recognize the great truth that responsibility is always personal, on the doctors in whom medical science is embodied."[133] The editorial did not suggest that doctors had not cared about their work, or even that they had proven entirely incapable. "That the doctors have been either idle or helpless nobody imagines," the editorial continued. "Widespread as the malady is, and serious as are its effects, it can be claimed without the possibility of contradiction that it would have been worse, the fatalities more numerous, except for the wisdom of our physicians and the labors of the nurses trained by them." "That, however, is poor consolation," he concluded.[134] A week later the same newspaper

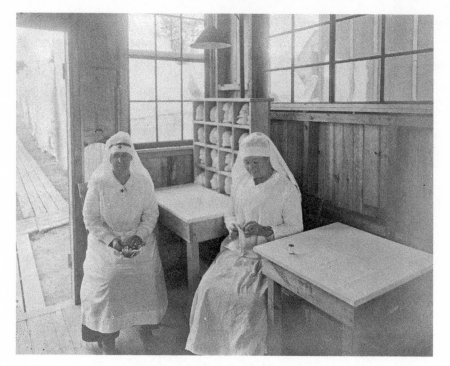

Figure 4.2 Popular imagery of nurses often emphasized their feminine qualities, including their selfless dedication to others. Here Red Cross nurses produce masks in Lawrence, Massachusetts. (165-WW-269B-38), Still Picture Branch, NA.

returned to this topic, again criticizing the medical profession for its arrogance and its failure to prevent the epidemic, suggesting that the cost of medicine's failure would be long in payment.[135]

Similar concerns emerged in more direct challenges to mainstream medicine. An ad in St. Louis for "Dr. Allen's Number 7," a patent medicine, blamed physicians for the high death rates during the pandemic and offered a ready alternative. "It is estimated that over 5,000 have died in this city, and nearly 100,000 in the United States," it began, "but not one has died as far as we know who took this remedy and they did not have to call a Doctor." Continuing, the ad made clearer its position that medical practitioners were not to be trusted. "WAS THIS ENORMOUS DEATH-RATE CAUSED BY THESE DISEASES?" it queried, "or was it caused by drugs, anti-toxins, stimulants and whiskey given or recommended by the doctors who treated them. . . . It is a fact that less than half that number would have died, if they had taken no drugs at all." And further, "It is not enough to have faith in your doctor, there should be a certain amount of knowledge and common sense [to] go with that FAITH." Denouncing germ theory, the ad described the futility of following doctors' prescriptions. "Drugs have proven a failure, injections of anti-toxins much worse, and those doctors who believe GERMS the cause of disease and have to give drugs to KILL the GERMS are butting their heads against a stone wall and will have to start a new theory of disease." Describing the cost of medicine's mistakes, the ad concluded, "The saddest thought is not that all these things are so' / 'But sadder is the fact, the people do not think, or know."[136] Though this ad clearly had as its intent the sale of its alternative therapy, it pitched the sale by detailing the failure of doctors, their theories, and the resultant practices.

Losing confidence in physicians' expertise, citizens sometimes dismissed both their authority and their advice. "There is more than a mere grain of truth in the statement of a Boston paper that there is nothing in the current epidemic that can be twisted into a compliment for the medical profession," one diatribe began. Tracing its dissatisfaction to the willingness of physicians to act with authority without the expertise to back it up, the critique continued, "The doctors know little or nothing about the causes of the disease, according to their own admissions. . . . The unprofessional mind might conclude that doctors who know nothing of a disease's cause, effective methods of checking it, and little about how to treat it, might be less profuse in prophecies about what is to come."[137]

If editorials sometimes contested the counsel of medical doctors, others took the critique a step further, offering different approaches to the treatment and cure of influenza. From folk practitioners to patent medicine producers, from the "irregulars" of the medical sects to Christian Scientists, challengers offered Americans other ways of thinking about influenza and alternative therapies for its treatment.

Even Americans who subscribed to the basic belief in a scientific approach to health and disease often turned to folk remedies offered by relatives or neighbors. In New Orleans some locals turned to voodoo, buying charms—"anything from a white chicken's feather to an ace of diamonds for the left shoe"—or performing an incantation, "repeated three times a day when rubbing vinegar over the face and palms: 'Sour, sour, vinegar—V /Keep the sickness off'n me.'"[138] On a farm near Lawrence, Massachusetts, a young boy's parents attempted to protect him from the flu with "white chips of camphor in an old sock around his neck," while a nurse in nearby Boston also found patients relying on what she viewed as "old superstitions."[139] One "lover of our Boys" in Michigan recommended powdered lobelia, sprinkled on chests readied with olive oil for "fine results."[140] In Nevada, many tried "sagebrush tea," brewed of boiled sagebrush root, while reporters noted the longstanding employment of Indian root by the local Washoe.[141] In South Chicago Ann Olds Woodson offered "the old woman's (octigenarian's [sic]) remedy," that involved two or three large, ripe red peppers, stewed at a boil for an hour or two with the windows and doors secured.[142] And in Louisiana the superintendent of a Methodist hospital recommended a quilt made of wormwood, sandwiched between layers of flannel, dipped in hot vinegar and placed on the chest of flu sufferers.[143] Other folk remedies ranged from the burning of "Coal Tar" to "destroy any germs" or the consumption of pine pitch to asafetida necklaces, from onion plasters or an onion diet to heavy doses of whiskey.[144]

Private citizens and businesses intent on selling "cures" to make a profit off the epidemic promised surprising relief through their products. Sherwin-Williams marketed Phenolene as a household disinfectant, sure to "prevent contagion and stop the spread of influenza," and suggested that it might also be used as "gargle, snuff up the nose . . . on handkerchiefs and gauze breathing masks."[145] Lysol promised that "no germ, no matter how great its strength, can live for an instant, in its presence."[146] Businesses often attempted to lay claim to the scientific mantle usually reserved for doctors to sell their products, while hoping to make a buck in the bargain. "In this Time of Danger of Infection from Influenza" the Kolynos Company suggested, its dental cream "was evolved under the influence of bacteriology" and had gained "approval among dentists and physicians."[147] Patent medicine producers, in particular, promised relief from the symptoms of influenza and its aftereffects. According to Charles V. Chapin, Health Officer for Providence, Rhode Island, and a leader in the field of public health, his local papers were flooded with ads for thirty-two different products promising to control or cure influenza. As the epidemic exploded, "compounds previously advertised as remedies for indigestion, rheumatism, constipation, headaches, as general tonics, etc., suddenly became specifics for influenza," he observed.[148] The claims for such cures ranged widely. The producers of Eatonic, for instance, maintained that their product could help those "suffering from the after effects of the deadly flu . . . by giving attention to the stomach—that is removing acidity and toxic poisons," while Loudon's Catarrhal Jelly could ease the discomfort of a sufferers' nose and head, Dr. Kilmer's Swamp-Root promised to heal kidneys damaged by a bout with influenza, Hypo-Cod guaranteed to help those recovering from illnesses, including influenza, to "avoid constipation, headaches, lassitude, weariness and long convalescence," and Dr. Pierce's various medicaments would "assist nature" both "before or after the influenza."[149] Other patent medicine companies made more grandiose promises, pledging their products could prevent the dreaded disease.[150] Demonstrating these companies' attempt to share the mantle of medical authority, many of the products bore the name of a doctor or offered "scientific" evidence of their efficacy as part of the sales pitch.

If folk medicine practitioners and patent medicine producers challenged only the success of the allopaths, rather than their way of thinking about health and disease, alternative systems of medicine offered a more comprehensive challenge. Some of these challengers operated from far outside the medical establishment, positing theories that never gained either popular or professional followings. For instance, Professor Albert F. Porta, a civil engineer and architect from San Francisco, penned a letter to the Surgeon General that included his "study on certain peculiar connections . . . between the various positions of the planet Jupiter and the progress of the successive waves of the influenza epidemic."[151] Even this marginal figure attempted to pose as an alternative authority, using the language and methods of science to establish himself as an expert worthy of attention, though his theory would never escape obscurity.

Other critiques of mainstream medicine, particularly those posed by the "irregulars," offered a more comprehensive and meaningful challenge. During the epidemic, practitioners from these other schools of medical thought openly criticized "regular" medicine and offered their own practices as viable, indeed preferable, alternatives.[152] Though they often shared with the allopaths a gendered vision of the meaning of success and a commitment to the scientific method, these practitioners rejected entirely the superiority of allopathy as a medical system.[153]

Though they shared with the allopaths the sense that the pandemic constituted a serious crisis, homeopaths rarely expressed the sense of helplessness and defeat so common among mainstream physicians.[154] Rather, in the pages of their professional journals, homeopathic practitioners celebrated their achievements in combating influenza and in controlling the epidemic. Articles described the "remarkable success of the homeopathic school" and "the phenomenal success attained by homoeopathic practitioners during the epidemics of influenza" and highlighted the "unqualified testimony of the low mortality following treatment."[155] "Many people are alive today," one practitioner maintained, "because of the curative action of homeopathic remedies, carefully prescribed and conscientiously given."[156]

Homeopaths also noted that their accomplishments stood in marked contrast to the failures of other practitioners. As the editors of the *North American Journal of Homeopathy* proclaimed in their October 1918 edition, "The impartial observer who is familiar with all therapies must admit that the homeopathic treatment of Influenza is superior to all others."[157] The editors of the *Hahnemannian Monthly*, the monthly journal of the Homeopathic Medical Society of Pennsylvania, agreed. "It is a great satisfaction . . . that the homoeopathic method of prescribing has proven eminently more successful than the empirical method of treatment in vogue among the members of the dominant school of medicine," they suggested.[158] Mortality rates, they believed, confirmed this conclusion, showing the superiority of homeopathy to other approaches.[159]

If allopaths expressed shock over their inability to contain influenza, homeopaths articulated no such surprise—about either their own successes or the failures of the allopaths—and instead used the occasion of the epidemic as an opportunity to chastise orthodox medicine for its discrimination against homeopathy. In the context of their disastrous performance in the epidemic, homeopaths argued, regular physicians should reconsider their exclusionary approach to medical practice. As one editorialist, W. D. Bayley, suggested in the *Hahnemannian Monthly* in August 1919, "If our allopathic brethren were disposed to accept friendly criticism we would gently remind them of their self-confessed helplessness in influenza and pneumonia, and show them that at least, until some new therapeutic miracle is wrought, the adoption of the homoeopathic methods would have vastly lowered the mortality in these diseases."[160] Such criticism was necessary, according to Bayley, because of the close-minded approach of the orthodox practitioners to their medical brethren.[161] While Bayley remained optimistic about the possibility of "complete friendliness and mutual understanding," other homeopaths were less certain about the goodwill of their allopathic colleagues and much harsher in their criticisms. An editorialist who signed his or her essay with only the initials "J.W.W." launched a scathing critique of "dominant medicine" and its "control of all medical treatment" in the American army and navy in the aftermath of the war and the epidemic.[162] *"It is unbelievable,"* the editorial maintained, *"that we are forced to admit the positive dictatorship of allopathic control."*[163] Noting the discrimination that had kept homeopaths from offering soldiers and sailors treatment, the editorial did not hesitate to suggest the costs of such prejudice evident in the "thousands of bereaved homes."[164] In this context, the continued control of medicine by the regulars was inconceivable. *"The indictment stands!"* the editorial exclaimed. *"Dominant medicine has bamboozled American life long enough. Dominant therapy has been 'weighed in the balance and found wanting.'"*[165] *"The silent voices of the unnecessary dead"* demanded that homeopaths receive such recognition.[166]

Osteopaths, relative newcomers to the field of medicine in 1918, also challenged allopathic practice in the throes of the epidemic. Osteopathy's founder, Andrew T. Still, began his medical career in the United States in the 1850s when methods such as bloodletting and often harmful pharmaceuticals were still the standard of mainstream medical care. Still lost confidence in allopathy after three members of his family died from spinal meningitis. Disturbed by what he came to see as the immorality and harmfulness of medication in the treatment of patients, Still looked to the medical sects for methods free of drug use. Strongly influenced by the magnetic healers and the bonesetters, his creation of a new approach to illness—osteopathy—borrowed from both schools. Still came to believe that the manipulation of the vertebrae might be used to repair the maldistribution or blockage of the body's fluids and to treat a wide range of problems from heart trouble to rheumatism. In 1892 Still founded the American School of Osteopathy. In 1896 the first state, Vermont, began to license osteopaths; by 1901 osteopaths were licensed practitioners in fifteen states, and by the time of the epidemic that number was nearing forty.[167]

Though today osteopaths (DOs) practice alongside MDs with only minor differences in their approaches—osteopaths still view themselves as more holistic in their approach to treatment—in 1918 the differences between the approaches were sizable. Most osteopaths, like most allopaths, had accepted germ theory and shared with their mainstream counterparts a belief that influenza was an infectious disease, but they rejected all drug therapy and relied instead on traditional osteopathic therapy—manipulations of the spine and ribs designed to "normalize visceral functions and specifically build up resistance to and disperse fluid in pneumonia, which was a common sequela."[168]

Like homeopaths, osteopaths saw in the epidemic both a powerful critique of the practices of the orthodox physicians and a stunning recommendation for their own alternative practices. Occasional critics softened their blows by acknowledging the "education and devotion to duty" allopaths brought to their work. Such praise, though, served only to highlight the failure of the allopaths' medical system.[169] Similarly, while some critics granted that a small number of allopaths brought real talent to the practice of medicine, this praise for the few only reinforced the criticism of the many.[170] Other critics were even harsher. Describing the "scourge," the "great plague" that "has swept, and is still sweeping, our land," an osteopath from New York exclaimed that "modern medical practice availed but little to check its ravages." And further, "Whole families were wiped out. Medicine failed."[171] Another critic suggested that he was "convinced that as many patients have been killed by physicians as have been cured."[172] Casting this failure in a particularly gendered way, one set of authors in the *Journal of the American Osteopathic Association* concluded that "organized medicine" had proven "impotent" during the epidemic.[173] The editors of the journal agreed, concluding that "the system practiced renders it impotent in many of the most serious diseases," including influenza.[174]

The use of vaccines and drugs drew especially harsh criticism from osteopaths. Describing vaccines as a "dangerous diabolical conglomeration of germs," one critic emphasized the backwardness of allopathic treatments: "One million five hundred thousand dead bugs injected into some poor body at a squirt. . . . It reads like the practices of the physicians in the dark ages when pulverized chickens' entrails were given to patients afflicted with dysentery, and live toads were bound on the throats of sufferers from goiter."[175] Osteopaths found the use of medications similarly appalling, as well as both immoral and harmful.[176] As one journal article explained, "The toxemia of influenza is quite enough for the patient to overcome without the additional handicap of promiscuous drugging."[177] In the end, according to the osteopaths, allopaths did very little to aid their patients and instead inflicted a great deal of harm.

Also similar to homeopaths, osteopaths contrasted the failure of the allopaths with their own successes in articles such as "Influenza Deaths Unnecessary" and

"Making the World Safe for Osteopathy."[178] From the early days of the epidemic, osteopaths suspected their patients were faring better than those of the allopaths, and two of their professional journals—the *Osteopathic Physician* and the *Journal of the American Osteopathic Association*—set out to test this hypothesis, with 2,445 practitioners contributing information on their efforts and their outcomes. According to this research, osteopaths achieved a low 2-percent death rate for influenza and a 10-percent rate for pneumonia, impressive accomplishments next to the rate they claimed for allopaths.[179] Such results led osteopaths to expressions of pride in their profession.[180] Noting the successes osteopaths were having in treating pneumonia in particular, one practitioner announced,

> We turn from all drug therapy and we look with unstinted pride and we acknowledge our most profound gratitude, and we hail with honor and unspeakable admiration that modern Moses who in 1874 with his magic wand, that inseparable staff, smote the rock of scientific research and caused to flow therefrom a rational system of therapeutics that has not only revealed an effective and rational treatment for pneumonia but has also given to the therapeutic world a rational and efficient method for the treatment of all human ills.[181]

Though the epidemic had been a terrible scourge, osteopaths seemed unable to contain their celebratory tone as they outlined what they viewed as their tremendous success during the crisis.

Such celebration, though, was mixed with frustration that so many lives had been lost because the methods of osteopaths had not been employed more broadly, and osteopaths, like homeopaths, spoke openly of the discrimination they faced.[182] Many osteopaths were particularly frustrated that they had not been permitted to serve the men in uniform.[183] "Is it not discrimination" the editors of the *Journal of the American Osteopathic Association* wondered.[184] Or as another particularly frustrated practitioner maintained, "Medical bigotry and medical politics have denied us so far the opportunity of doing in the Army 'the part for which we are best fitted.'"[185] The epidemic had demonstrated just how costly that prejudice had been. As one practitioner proclaimed with passion,

> A great plague has swept, and is still sweeping, our land. A plague whose death-rate is higher than any in the memory of the present generation. Only now we are beginning to compute and reckon the results. Hundreds of thousands have fallen victims of the scourge. Modern medical practice availed but little to check its ravages. Near panics cropped up in many localities. Fear entered into the very heart and soul of man. Serums and vaccines were tried and discarded. . . .

Is there no weapon upon which mankind may rely in this terrible time? *There is.* I repeat, in capital letters, THERE IS. Would that this answer could be indellibly [*sic*] written in letters of fire athwart the heavens, so that *all* might see and know. Would that the hearts and minds of men might be opened to perceive and receive the great truth of osteopathic gospel.[186]

As a result of the epidemic, osteopaths maintained, "osteopathy has gained many friends" and "the peoples' confidence in the efficacy of osteopathy in handling acute diseases" was at new heights.[187] This, then, was the time for the profession to fight for its rights. "Does not our success in handling the recent epidemic cases justify us in demanding the fullest recognition for osteopathy?" an editorial in the *Journal of the American Osteopathic Association* asked.[188] Or, as the same journal queried in a preceding editorial, "Are we going to take advantage of the opportunity the present offers? Are we going to educate the public?"[189] The answer, many declared, was a resounding yes, and they would, in fact, achieve substantial success in gaining the integration of their own practices, and practitioners, into mainstream medicine following the epidemic.[190]

Chiropractors, too, maintained that their treatments could protect Americans from the dangers of influenza more effectively than had orthodox practices. Chiropractic was also a relatively new medical system in 1918. Named "chiropractic," meaning "done by hand," by "the Discoverer," D. D. Palmer first used the appellation in 1896 and opened the Chiropractic School and Cure the following year. Similar to osteopathy in its dedication to manipulation for the treatment of illness, practitioners of chiropractic were sometimes charged with "practicing osteopathy without a license," though it was a distinct and separate profession. Chiropractors based their practice in a belief that disease was caused by "subluxated vertebrae" and directed a more forceful treatment toward single vertebra with the intention of repositioning them to relieve the patient's symptoms.[191] Chiropractors also denounced bacteriology and germ theory.[192] Both MDs and DOs condemned chiropractic with some vehemence and opposed their admission to the medical brotherhood. In 1913 Kansas allowed for the licensing of chiropractors, and by the early 1920s twenty-two states had begun licensing them.[193]

Like other challengers to the dominance of the allopaths, chiropractors sought through the epidemic to establish their own legitimacy as medical practitioners. As one chiropractor, Julius C. Leve, promised in a letter to the Secretary of War, "Chiropractic is making good and will do more than I claim to relieve the sick and safeguard the health of the boys in camps, were it but given the opportunity."[194] Determined to be taken seriously, Leve made clear both his own scientific pedigree and that of his field and did not hesitate to pose it in opposition to allopathy. "Surely when the health boards of several states claim nothing can be done to check the prevailing disease, but to let it run its course, an unbiased investigation of the merits of Chiropractic would not be amiss."[195] Another chiropractor, James F. McGinnis, was more direct in his attack. In an ad entitled "What '2' Do—You want to know when there is no specific for Influenza," which ran in the *Jackson Sentinel* of Maquoketa, Iowa, McGinnis criticized not only the allopaths' failed medical methods but also their hypocrisy in continuing to accept both payment, and cultural authority, for their work. "They tell you to go to bed. They tell you to call a physician," he noted. "But when HE arrives," he jeered, "THERE IS NOTHING HE CAN DO. Yet he asks for pay and insists upon his services being taken. It's a wonderful profession—that of PRACTICING MEDICINE." The solution was obvious for McGinnis: "*The Chiropractic Way to Avoid 'Spanish Influenza'—Be Sure Your Backbone Is Normal. Refuse to Be Panic Stricken. See Your Chiropractor at Once. Get a Spinal Analysis—and Keep Smiling!*"[196] Using the allopaths' own standards for medicine—that it had as its purpose the prevention and cure of disease—chiropractors challenged the allopaths' success in fulfilling that responsibility and offered themselves and their theories of medicine as an alternative.

Though homeopaths, osteopaths, and chiropractors challenged the hegemony of allopaths during the epidemic, these practitioners nevertheless all believed illness was materially real and conducive to treatment by various therapies based in the physical world. Other challengers dismissed altogether this interpretation of illness and of the epidemic, seeing in the emergency a challenge not only to the authority of the allopaths but also to the place of medicine in the culture. Not entirely unlike Billy Sunday, who offered an evangelical narrative of the epidemic and fought it with prayer, Christian Scientists offered an interpretation of the epidemic and a challenge to the allopaths based in religious belief. Because Christian Scientists often understood themselves as medical practitioners offering an alternative approach to healing, they might also be understood as another example of a medical sect.[197] In 1875 Mary Baker Eddy published *Science and Health*, and four years later established the Church of Christ, Scientist, or Christian Science. Struggling with her own illnesses, Eddy had experimented with non-allopathic approaches to health in the middle decades of the nineteenth century.[198] When a serious accident threatened her life in 1866, Eddy found a cure in Bible study. This stunning experience convinced her that Christian teachings offered a remedy to the world's sickness. According to Eddy's teachings, illness did not exist but was only a manifestation of the failure of human insight.[199]

An article in the *Christian Science Monitor* during the early weeks of the epidemic explained that disease occurred because the human mind "accepts material belief and produces the material phenomenon or subjective condition." In other words, "It is this mind which believing in evil, which believing in sickness produces an epidemic, whether of smallpox or influenza."[200] The newspaper routinely referred to the "so-called Spanish Influenza epidemic," or the "alleged epidemic," demonstrating the fundamental belief that disease had no actual physical source.[201] Christian Scientists found in both the epidemic's virulence and traditional medicine's inability to control it clear support for their position. By 1918 the Church of Christ, Scientist was almost forty years old and in the years immediately preceding the epidemic it was the fastest-growing denomination in the United States. Despite Eddy's death in 1910, by 1925 the church claimed at least 200,000 members.[202]

Christian Scientists maintained that "mental contagion" was a pressing risk in American culture. As an article published in the *Christian Science Monitor* in October 1918 entitled "Mad World" suggested, "Let any person who has been brought in contact with the conditions of today ask himself frankly whether it is not fear which is playing such fearful havoc in the world. Everywhere men and women are afraid. . . . A great fear has stricken the world, and it is little wonder if out of this fear there have emerged pestilences and diseases which have mounted on the winds of fear, and scattered their seeds in every direction."[203] Christian Science offered an antidote for this infection: knowledge of the divine Mind, or Truth, as imparted in the Bible through the teachings of Jesus.[204] As another article explained following the epidemic, "No illness of government, of human relations and conditions generally, is too hard or too deeply seated to be healed by the truth. For in its seeming place is divine Mind, which knows all things and knows no evil."[205] Humans needed only to reject the illusions of illness, or evil, and embrace instead the infinite love and goodness of the divine Mind to free themselves from "despotic suggestion" and to enjoy "unassailable health." As one soldier, a practicing Christian Scientist, wrote home to his mother, "If every one could have the same faith in the Father-Mother God everything would be . . . different."[206] In New York, other Christian Scientists made the same argument regarding the power of being in a right mind, noting that Chinese immigrants, unable to read and thereby immune to the terrors of newspaper coverage of the epidemic, remained healthy.[207]

During the epidemic these beliefs led Christian Scientists to vehemently critique the allopathic approach to illness and health and the measures of public health officials. If "the sanest treatment is to do everything possible to destroy fear," then everything from protective masks to church closures, from vaccines to the publication of public health statistics, was wrongheaded. These measures were problematic not only because they were ineffective, but more importantly because they produced fear, cultivating the disease and encouraging the epidemic.[208] What was so surprising, according to some Christian Scientists, was that allopaths were so unwilling to acknowledge the central importance of the mind in fighting disease, or to incorporate such knowledge into their practice.[209]

Physicians, it seemed, could not admit to their own failings.[210] In the end, Christian Scientists' criticism of the allopaths, like those of the other alternative practitioners, reached well beyond their handling of the epidemic to include the allopaths' undemocratic, indeed autocratic, effort to control American medicine.[211]

The number and range of alternative therapies posited by Americans during the epidemic suggests that control of American medical culture remained contested in 1918. Alternative practitioners were ready, when allopathy struggled with epidemic influenza, to assert their own medical influence. Having established their cultural authority on the basis of their success, defined in terms of their efficacy in protecting American health by conquering disease, allopaths had created expectations that their treatments would prove efficacious and they would cure their patients. Failing to meet these standards during the epidemic, allopathic practitioners faced challenges to their cultural dominance.

The Allopathic Counteroffensive

Practicing allopathic physicians soon responded to their alternative medicine opponents with words and actions of their own. The advertisement by the chiropractor, McGinnis, for instance, was lampooned by the editors of *JAMA*, who attempted to make its beliefs seem silly, its practices ridiculous, even unethical. "'Be Sure Your Backbone Is Normal'—'Get a Spinal Analysis—and Keep Smiling!' This is 'The Chiropractic Way to Avoid Spanish Influenza'—Chiropractor McGinnis says so!," the critique began. Honing in on McGinnis's criticism of allopathy, the attack continued, "Not, of course, that there is any such thing as influenza; it is merely 'a new fad, fancy and frill.' 'If it doesn't naturally exist, the doctors artificially make it exist.' And above all—and this is important—'See your Chiropractor at Once'. . . . It's a wonderful 'profession'—Chiropractic."[212] The thick sarcasm evident in this conclusion, designed to mirror McGinnis's own, left no doubt about the position of *JAMA* regarding alternative medical practices.

In other instances the counterattacks were even more direct. In March 1919, the journal critiqued alternative medical practitioners for what it viewed as their manipulation and exploitation of the public during the epidemic in a piece entitled "Figures Never Lie."[213] "Next to the 'patent medicine' exploiters, no class has commercialized the recent epidemic of respiratory disease, or played on the public's fears more skillfully, persistently, and unscrupulously, than the various 'drugless healing' sects and cults," the essay began. Accusing these practitioners of unprincipled behavior, the critique continued, "Following the classic course, 'lies, d—n lies and statistics,' the latest move in this advertising campaign is the publication of statistics. These figures purport to show the vast improvement in the treatment by chiropaths [sic], naprapaths, naturopaths, or some other 'paths,' over that given by scientific medicine, in dealing with the flu and its sequelae." Lashing out with some hostility at a press that too readily accepted these claims, that had "so voraciously swallowed hook, line and sinker" the "bait" cast by these other practitioners, the article engaged in the careful critique it argued the regular press had failed to provide, explaining away the "statistics" that purported to show the success of the "so-called drugless healers" in handling influenza. Returning to sarcasm, the article compared the claims of the irregulars to the claims of a sea captain who promised to "prove by incontrovertible statistics that not one of my passengers was ever run over by a taxicab while in my charge." "Wonderful are the uses to which statistics can be put!" the article concluded. Using terms such as "quacks," "drugless healers" and "sects and cults," the essay's careful enumeration of the fallacies it believed were contained in the claims of these alternative medical systems suggested just how seriously some allopaths took their challenge.

Other mainstream practitioners worried about the practical, and sometimes very real, challenge the medical sects seemed to offer to the public authority of orthodox medicine. When alternative medical theories seemed to lead practitioners to ignore public health regulations, for instance, the response was direct and hostile. A telegram published in the Philadelphia *Public Ledger* that detailed Christian Scientists' beliefs and their holding of "regular services" despite a request for church closures by public health officials prompted one physician to call on the editors of *JAMA* to respond.[214] Noting that "the following of this cult is large," and that "Chicago is a veritable hotbed of Eddyism," the letter writer asked the editors, "Would it not be wise to bend some editorial energies, if any are available, to the scotching or killing of this skunk in lieu of complacently recording dubious impressions?" In noting his own community's response to the Christian Scientists, he hinted at the more active opposition he envisioned.

Beyond the specific problem of the irregulars, allopaths also responded to the challenge posed by patent medicines, folk traditions, and other popular remedies circulating during the epidemic. From the beginning the USPHS warned Americans to be wary of such cures. Its pamphlet, *"Spanish Influenza" "Three-Day Fever" "The Flu,"* for instance, urged Americans to use "only such medicine . . . as is prescribed from the doctor" and argued that "it is foolish to ask the druggist to prescribe and may be dangerous to take the so-called 'safe, sure, and harmless' remedies advertised by patent-medicine manufacturers."[215] The USPHS followed up this message in November with an article in its own *Public Health Reports* detailing the variety of "sure cures" for influenza surfacing around the country. Dismissing the full range of challengers and their cures—from the religious fanatic blaming man's sinfulness to the individual or company offering a cure "for a price," from the food faddist to the amulet wearer—the Health Service urged Americans to "remember that there is as yet no specific cure for influenza, and that many of the alleged 'cures' and remedies now being recommended by neighbors, nostrum vendors, and others do more harm than good." Reasserting the authority of allopathic medicine and its institutional representative, the USPHS, the article concluded, "If any specific like a vaccine or serum is found to have value the Public Health Service will give the matter wide publicity."[216] The editors of *JAMA* joined the USPHS in criticizing the "alleged cures and remedies" gaining attention in the popular press, while local doctors and public health leaders urged Americans to protect their health by avoiding these nostrums.[217] As the Associated Charities of Minneapolis urged, "If you simply must give the much-advertised virtues of patent medicine a trial, try them on the dog. Your children's health and your own is too precious to be tampered with."[218]

Attempting to assert their own authority, establishment physicians traced the appeal of alternative practices and treatments to superstition. Noting that many people could not understand that influenza was spread through personal contact, Simon Flexner of the Rockefeller Institute explained in an issue of *Science* in 1919, "There still resides in the mass of people, even in the more enlightened countries, a large uneradicated residue of superstition regarding disease." Flexner continued, "We have only recently emerged from a past in which knowledge of the origin of disease was scant, and such views as were commonly held and exploited were mostly fallacious. It is indeed very recently, if the transformation can be said to be perfect even now, that the medical profession as a whole has been completely emancipated."[219] Determined to retain their cultural authority, many physicians continued to present themselves as experts and described their abilities in opposition to the superstitions of the past, even though such claims rang hollow for some during the crisis.

For many doctors the epidemic would always remain the low point in their professional lives, a historical moment in which they were forced to abandon the pride in their profession for an unwelcome humility caused by haunting memories of patients lost. That nurses escaped the damage to their personal and professional identities, and found in the epidemic instead a meaningful opportunity for service that only enhanced their personal and professional pride, suggests how complete the gendering of health care roles was by the early twentieth century. As they surveyed the pandemic from the distance of its aftermath, doctors and nurses would share common ground, where they were joined by public health leaders in imagining a positive future for their professions and for the nation's health. The consequences of their triumphant narrative proved both deep and lasting.

5

"The terrible and wonderful experience"

Forgetting and Remembering in the Aftermath

In a lecture before public health professionals in October 1919, Mazyck P. Ravenel, Professor of Preventive Medicine at the University of Missouri and a leader in the field, reviewed the profession's work among American soldiers during the war and admitted to what he viewed as public health's uneven record. Referring specifically to influenza, he conceded, "Any one [*sic*] interested in preventive measures, and wishing to demonstrate the efficiency of modern methods would be glad to pass this disease in silence."[1] Suggesting the epidemic had proven "comparable to the historical plagues of the past, which we are in the habit of connecting with the dark ages of medicine," Ravenel noted that the death rates were sufficient "to demonstrate the ravages of this epidemic, and our lack of control over it."[2] Though recognizing that their protective efforts sometimes seemed to protect the troops from the disease, he nevertheless acknowledged that their successes were limited. "At best," he concluded, "we must admit that no measures adopted controlled the course of the pandemic. It spread with lightning like speed, went where it listed, and ceased its ravages only when available material was exhausted. If any preventive measures prevailed they were local. We must confess that on the whole we made a dismal failure in our attempts to control the spread of influenza."[3] His seemingly chastened narrative was tempered by Ravenel's suggestion that influenza and other "diseases spread by the secretions of the respiratory tract" constituted the toughest foe of public health efforts during the war, that they were, in fact, the "greatest weakness of the Army defense against disease and death by disease."[4] Even so, Ravenel acknowledged in its immediate aftermath the struggle the epidemic had presented to American public health efforts.

Two years later, Ravenel offered a significantly brighter assessment of the field's work. By 1921 Ravenel had reached a pinnacle of professional success, the presidency of the American Public Health Association, and the occasion for his

November lecture was the fiftieth anniversary meeting of the organization. In his lecture, entitled "The American Public Health Association, Past, Present, Future," Ravenel acknowledged the challenges ahead for the public health movement, but ultimately emphasized what he viewed as its extraordinary accomplishments.[5] "We were born at an opportune moment, and have lived in a period which for all time will be remarkable for its scientific achievement," he suggested.[6] Quoting the important leader in medical education, William Osler, on the advancements of the nineteenth century, he continued, "At last science emptied upon him [humanity], from the horn of Amalthea blessings which cannot be enumerated, blessings which have made the century forever memorable; and which have followed each other with a rapidity so bewildering that we know not what next to expect."[7] Ravenel proclaimed, "It is good to have lived in such a period, but it is better to have taken an active part in the events which have made that period notable, and this we can with confidence claim." Looking to the future, he urged continued progress: "We cannot, if we would, stand still and point to our past achievements. *Noblesse oblige.* Our path leads forward, and the difficulties which confront us at this time must serve to stimulate our efforts to even greater accomplishments in the future."[8] Ravenel had recognized the tragedy of the epidemic but did not choose to focus on this past. Rather, he looked confidently to the future, ready to shoulder what he understood as the continuing responsibilities, and opportunities, of the public health profession.

Ravenel was not alone in his perspective. Despite the tragedy that they had witnessed and their own limited ability to control it, in the months and years following the pandemic public health professionals, as well as physicians and nurses, frequently articulated a strikingly optimistic narrative—forward-looking, confident, and full of expressions of the opportunities the future promised. Certainly each group of professionals had concerns as they assessed the pandemic. Doctors worried over the inadequacies of their treatments, while public health experts noted the rapidity and reach of the pandemic's spread. Nurses celebrated their accomplishments during the scourge but feared that their profession might not gain the recognition and status it deserved. Each of these professions, though, soon recast its apparent frustrations into opportunities. Promising that the disaster would lead to continued advancements in American health, physicians, public health leaders, and nurses each articulated a clear link between this brighter future and their own continued, indeed expanded, dominance in the public life of the nation. Looking ever forward, too, they relegated the pandemic to an increasingly irrelevant past, leaving little room for the retention of public memories of its real costs.

If health care professionals voiced an optimistic narrative, the reactions in the aftermath of the pandemic among the broader public proved more complex and varied, and ultimately more troubled. In the public sphere, optimism retained a powerful hold on Americans' imagination. The Red Cross, for instance, indulged in a narrative similar to that of the health care professionals. Though the popular press would at least acknowledge the losses and the long-term consequences of the epidemic, journalists too joined the upbeat chorus of optimism with expressions of faith in modern science and a conviction that progress was sure to follow in the wake of the epidemic. In Congress, too, many elected officials argued in favor of the appropriation of federal funds for influenza research. Here, though, the challenges to the optimistic narrative were more potent, as some members of Congress questioned the past performance of American science and challenged future public appropriations, signaling an undercurrent of unease about activist government. It was in the private sphere, though, that the optimistic narrative was most completely rejected. Particularly among patients who survived and the family and friends of those who did not, the story of the epidemic remained a narrative of loss that ended in lives shattered by dislocation, grief, and despair.

Such a response shadows the memories of Lillian Kancianich, born just a few months before the pandemic on June 6, 1918, in Lidgerwood, North Dakota. A relative recalls seeing Lillian's mother sweeping the family's front porch on Armistice Day. It was the last time she would perform this simple domestic act. The next day she took ill, and on November 17, 1918, she died from influenza. She left behind a husband and two daughters, Lillian and her old sister, Christine. Because local custom discouraged older men from living alone in a household with children, Christine was sent to boarding school, and later to live with her mother's relatives in Minnesota. It took two years for Lillian to be settled. "No one adopted me," she recalls. "I had six different homes. Nobody wanted me. . . . I just went from home to home"[9] Lillian eventually settled in with relatives and was able to see her father every day. Even so, the loss of her mother had an enormous impact on her life. As a child, she often sat on the family's back steps and cried, lamenting, "I wish I had a mother." When asked in school what she wanted to be when she grew up, she staked her future on being "a step-mom." Perhaps most important, she believes, the disruption caused by her mother's death separated her from her sister, who was "very devoted" to her, and complicated their relationship for years afterward. Interviewed in 2003, eighty-five years after her mother's death, Kancianich still maintained that the pandemic had "changed my life completely. . . . It had to." As her story makes clear, while Americans' public culture soon forgot the catastrophe's costs, for some citizens the grief suffered in the darks months of the epidemic were never forgotten. Even some health care providers shared in this narrative, living with a quiet but sustained sense of the costs wielded by the pandemic. But this grief-filled narrative did not suit Americans' sense of themselves and was easily displaced in public life by a collective focus on future triumphs.

Physicians and the Rhetoric of Opportunity

On June 13, 1919, the Section on Industrial Medicine and Surgery of the American Medical Association passed a resolution urging Congress to support influenza research.[10] The resolution began by acknowledging the "approximately 500,000 deaths" the pandemic had caused and the reality that, despite this catastrophe, "medical science is not yet in possession of complete data as to the cause, modes of transmission, prevention, and cure of this disease and its complications." Such ignorance, the resolution made clear, "is of grave social and economic concern to the nation." Quickly turning this problem to their advantage, the American Medical Association (AMA) called on Congress to appropriate $1.5 million to the United States Public Health Service (USPHS) for research into the "causes, modes of transmission, prevention and cure of influenza, pneumonia, and allied diseases." A month later, Otto P. Geier, the Secretary of the AMA's Section on Industrial Medicine and Surgery, shared a supporting informational document and employed a similar strategy for encouraging the funding of medical research.[11] Emphasizing the costs of the epidemic, the supporting statement noted not only the loss of life but also the likelihood of increased mortality over "the next four or five years," as well as the "bad after effects of the disease," the "pathological conditions—bad hearts, bad kidneys and lungs" that followed in the disease's wake. The document even attempted to place an economic value on the epidemic, suggesting that a conservative estimate of the cost of lost lives, lost wages, and lost production would range between $3 billion and $4 billion. These costs were made more frightening as the organization reiterated how little was known about influenza, though "much private research has been carried on," and how certain was the recurrence of influenza. Unless the appropriation were passed, proper research conducted, and its findings distributed to the populace, the informational statement implied, the nation would soon face a repeat of the catastrophe just endured.

This call by the AMA for federally funded research under the auspices of the USPHS illustrates the principle contours of mainstream medicine's response in the aftermath of the epidemic—the acknowledgment of the devastation caused by the crisis, the admission of medicine's inability to control the disease, the linking of this failure with the continued mysteries surrounding influenza, the call for publicly funded research, and the warning that such work could not be postponed because infectious disease remained a pressing danger despite the epidemic's passing. As this public reaction makes clear, many physicians left the epidemic somewhat humbled, willingly acknowledging their failures to avert the crisis. At the same time, those engaged in medical research seemed determined to frame those failures as opportunities, as justifications for future growth of scientific medicine, warning the American public that the nation's health depended on continued support of their work.

Though an occasional physician remembered the epidemic as a time of success, emphasizing medicine's accomplishments during the emergency, in the immediate aftermath of the epidemic such responses were rare.[12] Far more prominent were admissions of the blight influenza had proven in the fall of 1918. Rufus Cole, the first Director of the Hospital of the Rockefeller Institute for Medical Research and an expert on pneumonia, described "an epidemic which in intensity and severity, as measured both by the increased morbidity and mortality, probably exceeded that of any epidemic visitation to civilized people in recent times."[13] Such a result, one physician noted, "had evidently created the most profound respect in the minds of the medical men."[14] As the eminent bacteriologist Milton J. Rosenau admitted, "If we have learned anything, it is that we are not quite sure what we know about the disease."[15] Ignorance of the disease's etiology left doctors, and their patients, in confusion about treatment and at the mercy of the disease.[16] Dr. J. Frank Points admitted a year after the epidemic, "Before its whirlwind onset, cyclonic progress, and hurricane destruction, physicians looked about for a remedy to check the dread monster but without avail, and many times and often did they change their modes of attack in efforts to stop the awful scourge."[17] Given this state of ignorance, some physicians suggested, it was vital that medicine acknowledge the limits of its own understanding of influenza.[18]

As the AMA resolution suggested, it was precisely the inadequacy of their knowledge, made visible in the epidemic, which constituted medicine's opportunity in its wake. Even before the epidemic had run its full course, physicians began to call for research into every aspect of influenza's secrets, from "the cause of the cyanosis of influenza" to its "clinical manifestations," and especially into the cause of influenza itself.[19] Such research, of course, needed to be conducted properly and demanded "the resources of the most expert."[20] Though they had not understood influenza sufficiently in the past, physicians argued, carefully conducted research would allow Americans to protect themselves against future incursions of the disease. Obviously it would be allopaths and their scientific allies who warranted the label of "expert."

As physicians had predicted, influenza did not disappear after the 1918–1919 crisis but continued to prove a scourge, attacking with some severity in a fourth wave in 1920 and again in 1922. As influenza renewed its attack, physicians acknowledged "the pandemic of 1918 is fresh in memory," but maintained optimism about future bouts with the disease, arguing that the attacks in the aftermath of the pandemic would be "less severe than in the primary pandemic."[21] Even so, as late as 1922 physicians continued to express significant interest in the investigation of influenza and to urge further explorations. As an editorial entitled "Interepidemic Influenza" in the *Journal of the American Medical Association* (*JAMA*) explained in late 1922, "If some epidemic diseases have almost vanished, or at least become greatly modified in severity or distribution, there are, nevertheless, others still with us to take their victims, and consequently to demand renewed investigation."[22] As influenza continued to threaten American health, physicians continued to think it would present physicians with "opportunity," with the chance to "test . . . hypotheses" formulated in the wake of the epidemic.[23]

Though a small group of scientists remained dedicated to research on influenza, never losing sight of their purposes, by 1924 the broader interest in influenza was clearly waning. That year the subject index for *JAMA* listed only fifteen entries for influenza, a stunning contrast to the flood of articles published just a few years earlier.[24] "The intense general interest in influenza awakened by the outbreaks of 1918 and 1919 died down rather quickly," an editorial suggested in August 1925.[25]

It is perhaps no coincidence that the declining attention paid to influenza was accompanied by the medical field's growing optimism. *JAMA* offered an encouraging note in January 1925. "The recurring reports of new outbreaks of rapidly spreading disease here and there throughout the world sometimes bring a note of discouragement to those who are interested in the application of scientific research to human welfare," the commentary began.[26] "They are prone to ask themselves whether any real mastery over disease is being acquired." The journal reassured its readers that such dominance was, indeed, under way. "It is still true that there are plague spots and that cholera is on the rampage in India; but influenza is not widely epidemic, and other major 'ills of mankind' are seemingly stationary, if not improved." Noting the encouragement such news should bring, the essay concluded, "Good news gives satisfaction—and courage to meet future emergencies in the world's health."[27] Though physicians often acknowledged their own defeat in the immediate aftermath of the epidemic, their public malaise was short-lived. The epidemic seemed a thing of the past, at least in public.[28] As *Literary Digest* reported in 1927, "Influenza is only serious in the absence of wisdom and prudence."[29]

Public Health and the Rhetoric of Reform

Public health professionals shared with allopaths this positive vision of their future, emerging from the pandemic with a renewed sense of their importance and of their power. Though the lessons of the epidemic were many, these lessons constituted a reform plan for the future, a plan public health advocates viewed with both enthusiasm and a sense of possibility.

In the months following the crisis, some public health leaders argued that their forces had held up well given the difficult conditions of the epidemic. Suggesting that the epidemic's timing had made fighting it especially difficult, for instance, one USPHS surgeon nevertheless concluded "that under the circumstances all possible was done."[30] Others were still more effusive about the success of public health efforts. For some, these accomplishments were measured by their ability to institute public health measures—the provision of public health education to the citizenry, the creation of emergency hospitals, the prevention of crowded conditions, the enactment of quarantines, the closure of public spaces, and the establishment of influenza as a reportable disease.[31] Others went yet further, maintaining that public health efforts had held down death rates and saved lives. Royal S. Copeland, the Health Commissioner for New York City, repeatedly applauded New York's low death rate during the epidemic. "It is gratifying to know," he commented in September 1919, "that our death rate was the lowest of all the Eastern cities, and, indeed among the lowest, if not the very lowest, of any great city in the world."[32] Other public health professionals made similar claims.[33] As a report on the efforts of the USPHS during the epidemic concluded, "Undoubtedly, many lives were saved and much suffering avoided by the combined efforts of the state and local authorities, the Red Cross, and the members of the Volunteer Medical Service Corps acting under the direction of the Public Health Service."[34]

Not all public health professionals expressed such unadulterated confidence in the wake of the epidemic, though, and there were many who openly critiqued their field's performance as they looked back months and years later. In an article published in *The Survey* in December 1919 and subtitled "A General Confession by the Public Health Authorities of a Continent," for instance, George M. Price, a leader in industrial health in New York, criticized the uncertainty he had witnessed at the recent meeting of American Public Health Association (APHA). Noting that "it is but natural that influenza should have been foremost in the thoughts and in the discussion of the more than one thousand health commissioners, administrators, officers and workers" at the meeting, he lamented the limitations the discussion exposed.

> It is unfortunate that more light was not shed upon this most absorbing problem of the hour. In spite of the number of the health authorities present and in spite of the very prolonged and, at times, very heated discussions by those directly dealing with the disease and having the greatest experience with its control—in spite of the numerous committees appointed to sift all data, and, if possible, bring in an authoritative report—one could not but come to the conclusion that the health authorities themselves are not clear where they stand, nor what is to be done.[35]

He continued,

> Again and again it was admitted that the epidemic seemed to care little
> for authorities, showed no respect for its human opponents, that it
> spread in spite of all methods used to prevent it, that it increased in spite
> of the precautions undertaken and the means employed to combat it,
> and declined seemingly without any regard to measures used against
> it.[36]

In the aftermath of the epidemic, public health leaders proved still "at sea as to
the proper methods of treatment, cure and prevention." "It was in the discussion of these questions," Price concluded, "that the total bankruptcy of the present health administrations in the country appeared in full light and was
admitted over and over again."[37] Price's take on the state of the public health
profession surely ranks as one of the most despairing, and yet his sense that
many public health leaders were frustrated was sound.[38] "It is disappointing
that the Epidemiologist was helpless before the great epidemic of influenza,"
William L. Moss, an army epidemiologist, acknowledged. "Such barriers as we
tried to throw on the way of its spread were swept away as chaff before a mighty
tempest. This frightful epidemic seemed to know no bounds, and before its
advance we stood helpless."[39] Or as George Soper, New York City Sanitary
Engineer commented, "Nobody seemed to know what the disease was, where it
came from or how to stop it.... Science, which by patient and painstaking labor
has done so much to drive other plagues to the point of extinction has thus far
stood powerless before it."[40]

Yet such despairing narratives were neither the most dominant nor the most
persistent among public health workers. In a pattern that Price himself adopted,
even those who admitted their own inability to stop or control the disease soon
tied these admissions to a powerful sense of possibility, seeing in the epidemic
both evidence of their own public importance and the opportunity for the
continued growth of their work. For instance, as the president of the APHA,
Lee Frankel, acknowledged in a lecture on "The Future of the American Public
Health Association" in December 1918, "Possibly we too have our shortcomings." And yet, he concluded, "There has been no time in the career of this great
organization when its opportunities have been so brilliant as at present."[41] Similarly, in an article entitled "The Ultimate Benefits to be Derived from the Epidemic," Louis I. Harris of the Department of Health in New York City
acknowledged in the immediate wake of the epidemic both "the tragedy" out
of which his city was "apparently just emerging," and the importance of ensuring that "some measure of good be derived" from it.[42] Noting the importance of preparing for a return of influenza, Harris nevertheless emphasized

the potential value of the epidemic experience. "What counts even more," he argued, "is the ultimate good which this frightful tragedy may be made to yield."[43]

Both the delayed annual meeting of the APHA in 1918, originally scheduled for October but postponed until December, as well as the 1919 meeting, placed significant focus on the epidemic and on influenza.[44] In the pages of their journals, too, public health professionals carried on a lengthy and detailed conversation about the needs of the future and the work yet to be done. The priorities articulated in this discussion ranged widely. Some public health leaders remained dedicated to allaying fear and keeping the public calm.[45] Some looked to broad changes in the field, calling for the development of a greater national presence in epidemic detection, the placement of greater authority in the hands of state departments of health, or greater focus on the respiratory diseases as threats to the nation's health.[46] Others focused more narrowly, advocating for specific projects they felt certain would improve public health. Some commentators argued for the development of community health centers, while others urged recognition of the importance of "steam dishwashing" or regular checkups in combating disease more generally.[47] Four classically Progressive preoccupations, though, dominated the discussions among public health professionals following the epidemic, and gave shape to their proposals in the months that followed: further research, organization, education, and mobilization.

Research remained a priority for many public health leaders, who continued to believe that new and accurate information was crucial to their progress. In an address before the APHA in October 1919, Allen W. Freeman, the State Commissioner of Health for Ohio, told his audience, "Administrative measures for the control of any disease depend for their success upon the possession of specific knowledge regarding that disease."[48] Freeman quickly acknowledged, though, that such knowledge about influenza was still beyond the reach of public health officials. "No one," he continued, "can seriously contend that we have in our possession the specific knowledge necessary to enable us either artificially to raise the mass immunity of the population against influenza, or to break the chain of infection from patient to victim." "What we most need in influenza [*sic*] is research, information, facts from every source and every angle," he urged, adding that federal funds should be made available for this important work.[49] Others agreed. "Much has been learned in the past year about the pandemic," explained Dr. William H. Davis, head of the Bureau of Vital Statistics in New York City and Chairman of the APHA's sub-committee on influenza. "Much more remains to be learned," he continued. "No easy task lies ahead. The battle for knowledge is on in earnest."[50] Only with such facts, public health leaders argued, could officials put in place measures they knew would protect the public.[51] Even before the APHA met in December 1918 it had established a Committee on Statistical

Study of the Influenza Epidemic, a move mirrored by the USPHS in what would become its new Statistical Office.[52]

In addition to deepening their knowledge base, public health advocates argued for more careful, and more complete, organization of their work and their forces. For some the call for greater organization was simply recognition of the need for better enlistment of available resources and better preparedness in anticipation of future problems. The Red Cross Executive Secretary for Kentucky, Lida Hafford, stated in July 1919, "Let us organize our forces so perfectly that a recurrence of this, or any other epidemic, will never find us so unprepared."[53] Recognizing the shortage of doctors and nurses that had plagued efforts to handle the epidemic in Kentucky, she continued, "The only solution to the problem, which is still ours if the influenza is to be with us for the next two years, is to organize our health forces better and to teach the people to care for themselves and their families."[54] For others, such as New York City's Royal S. Copeland, better organization implied a more coordinated and centralized public health system.[55] In Massachusetts, two state health officials criticized the independence of local health agencies and hoped to create better organization for the future—"each wanted to go along in their own accustomed groove"—and suggested the need to "coordinate these forces under one administrative head to work for the common good of all."[56] Far harsher was the criticism of Charles Aiken, a Public Health Service Surgeon. In an essay on the epidemic in South Carolina he scolded the state for its "unpreparedness." "More than 4,000 lives will have been wasted and untold suffering experienced in vain if the people of this State do not make immediate and everlasting use of the terrible lesson so pointedly expressed by the helpless condition into which they were thrown when Influenza struck a population, 90% of which was without adequate health organization."[57] At the national level, too, some commentators called for a more centralized system, with the USPHS serving as the "leader and guide in public health work," while others pleaded for "a permanent organization within the Public Health Service available for emergency work."[58]

Research and organization focused energy and attention on the profession itself, encouraging public health leaders to look at themselves and their work with an eye to reform. While for some in the profession this was a priority, for others attention was turned outward. If there was blame to be distributed in the aftermath of the epidemic, public health leaders willingly shared it with the citizenry. If there was ignorance to be corrected or behaviors to be altered in the epidemic's aftermath, the public was an appropriate target. If public health programs needed some measure of reform, so, too, did the American public.

The simplest criticism targeted the habits of Americans, basic behaviors that defied the most essential rules of hygiene and public health. In January 1920 Mazyck Ravenel offered a "protest against the American habits of promiscuous spitting, and of using saliva as a universal moistener, and also of the general neglect to cover the mouth and nose when coughing or sneezing," concluding, "There is literally no limit to the promiscuous interchange of spit in our daily intercourse with our fellow men."[59] Some health officials hoped such bad habits might be the result of easily corrected ignorance.[60] As Dr. J. W. Duke argued at the annual meeting of the Oklahoma State Medical Association in 1919, "I know you all agree that ignorance is the worst enemy we have to overcome."[61] Education was the obvious solution.[62] The Commissioner of Health in Cleveland, Ohio, suggested in November 1919, "We must learn how to avoid disease by proper methods of living, and, just as unconsciously as we automatically wind the clock before going to bed, we must acquire habits which prevent disease."[63] A physician from Des Moines stated the case even more clearly. "Health education," he declared, "ought to be placed within the reach of millions."[64]

Some public health leaders worried that Americans' misbehaviors were not the result of ignorance but might reflect instead an unwillingness to accept or even acknowledge their responsibilities for community health. As Dr. T. H. Price of Tulsa argued in May 1919, "It seems to me, that we have first of all to combat the decided opinions of the people. We have to educate them that the health authorities must do with them as they see fit."[65] Others shared the concern with Americans' attitudes, emphasizing education rather than coercion as the means to reform. Lee Frankel, the president of the APHA during the epidemic, noted the "indifference and apathy on the part of the public to disease and its results."[66] "While a feeling of dread spread throughout the community," in December 1918, "the epidemic generally was accepted in a spirit of resignation and with a fatalistic philosophy best indicated by the old Italian proverb, 'Che sara sara,' 'what will be will be.'"[67] The solution was clearly education. "We must become a propagandist body, working day in and day out through properly constituted machinery and officials to carry the doctrine of preventive medicine into every city and town," Frankel concluded.[68] Ravenel agreed. Noting the dangers posed by infectious diseases, including influenza, he recognized as well that "the public must experience a change of heart before it will submit to preventive measures which involve much inconvenience, even when death is in full view as a penalty for failure."[69]

Once awakened and educated to the importance of public health expertise, officials hoped, the citizenry might be mobilized in support of public health efforts not only at the personal level but also more broadly. A poem entitled "Some Bugs" published in *Public Health Nurse* in 1922 reflected this desire to awaken the citizenry to the public health movement and its goals. Its early stanzas set context: "Diphtheria, Meningitis, and 'Flu' /We dread their very names, it's true; /But we know these bugs, for they've been caught /Red-handed in the midst of the ruin they've wrought." After listing several other diseases, the poem continued, "Now, we need a real sleuth's patience and skill /To detect these bugs that plunder and kill; /But we also need the co-operation /Of each man and woman and child in the nation." Introducing the notion of the public health movement, the poem proceeded,

> By the way, are you wondering who are "we"?
> Why, your local Board of Health, you see,
> With a doctor chief and a nurse or two
> Who are trying to catch these bugs for you.
> With culture tube and QUARANTINE sign,
> Our purpose is far from being malign;
> On conserving the public health we're bent—
> We are on the deadly disease bug's scent.
> "But," you say, "Our state has no organization
> For Public Health." Then why in creation
> Don't you work for one? Don't be passé;
> Be up with the times, in an up-to-date way.

Reinforcing the importance of the public's commitment to the movement, the poem concluded, "And join with us, the disease bug fighters, /Eschew the example of a few backbiters; /Let us wipe out contagion from the whole U.S. /We can, if we all pull together, I guess."[70] With the American public alerted to the dangers posed by influenza and other infectious diseases, public health forces hoped to create among them advocates and allies for the work.

These new supporters might then play a role in ensuring the financing of public health efforts. "We should take the lessons of the epidemic to heart and go back to our respective communities and demand the apportionment of money for every justified expenditure for the organization of preventive measures, medical care and relief," declared Louis Harris of New York City's Department of Health in early 1919.[71] Making the case even more directly, the State Commissioner of Health for Ohio, Allen Freeman, argued in late 1919, "We must have facts, at whatever cost, and we must secure them now while the public still remembers, funds to carry on field and laboratory research until the truth is found."[72] The USPHS agreed, and called on local municipalities to adjust their future budgets to include emergency funds for use during epidemics and the federal government to set aside research monies.[73]

Despite some criticisms of the citizenry, then, many public health leaders remained optimistic about their ability to move their work of controlling both disease and the public forward. An editorial in the *American Journal of Public Health* suggested, even before the epidemic had concluded, "From the devastation of this epidemic will follow preparations against its repetition which will rival in thoroughness the most efficient planning of a great military offensive."[74]

The editors of the same journal suggested in an editorial in early 1920, "If the intense modern aggregations of humanity are producing new problems of increasing complexity, the means for accomplishing their solution are increasing with them; and the people within the countries represented in the great American Public Health Association can move forward into the new year with ever increasing confidence and hope, knowing that science in the hands of its faithful interpreters will prove yet more and more efficient in providing for their wellbeing."[75] Public health leaders assured the American public that placing their faith, and their resources, in the hands of the medical and public health establishments would reap great benefits.[76]

Despite the dominant optimism, some public health experts continued to express concerns about the profession and to debate its purposes and strategies for the future. The APHA continued to host symposia on topics such as "How to Further Progress in Health Education and Publicity" and publish discussions of "What Is the Matter with Public Health" in the pages of its journal.[77] Concerns about organization and funding persisted as well.[78] While the Sheppard-Towner Act passed Congress in 1921, creating new programs for maternal and infant health, efforts to create a national health insurance program failed, and even the Sheppard-Towner Act faced non-renewal in 1929. Public health activists would have to wait for Franklin D. Roosevelt's New Deal before they would be able to reap the gains they believed their successes in the pandemic had earned them.[79]

And yet in the months and years following the epidemic, public health leaders felt their optimism confirmed as they noted the valuable influence of the epidemic in shaping American perceptions of public health work and in mobilizing support for their efforts. An essay on the American Red Cross Health Center noted in 1921, "The war and the influenza epidemic have created a more general and more earnest interest in physical fitness. National, state and local health officials, private health agencies, doctors, nurses, teachers and social workers, all are endeavoring to make this new interest really count for better health."[80] "There is not the slightest doubt," one nurse exclaimed that same year, "that the average citizen of today is more interested in the subject of public health than he was ten or even five years ago," and further, "America is awake, and with her usual vigor she is bent on seeing to it that public health shall be established and maintained."[81] Algernon Jackson, the director of the School of Public Health at Howard University, reflected this same sense of accomplishment, concluding in 1923,

> Each day gives us a finer and more perfect knowledge of disease, its causes, its cure and its prevention, whose application the modern physician must make in his daily practice in order to render his full duty to those who put their trust in him.... Public Health is lifting the physician

from the position from [*sic*] being merely a watchman over sickness to a place in which he stands as director and guide over life, with the idea of adding to its length, comfort and happiness. What can possibly be more heroic, more scientific and a greater contribution to civilization.[82]

Nurses and the Rhetoric of Professionalization

While physicians sometimes acknowledged their struggles with influenza, and public health officials often noted their struggles with the public, nurses looked both back to their successes in the crisis and forward to the opportunities of the future with a boundless sense of pride, confidence, and optimism. Though the epidemic had been a tragedy, it had proven their effectiveness, their importance, and their promise. Such a performance had opened up opportunities to expand their work and enhance their professional prestige. The only concern troubling these health care workers was the fear that the breadth of their accomplishments might not be fully understood and shared by other health care professionals or the public.

As the director of the Department of Nursing at Columbia University suggested regarding the "rank and file of the nurses of this country" in September 1920, "They have passed in swift succession during the past few years through the awful tests brought by the war and the epidemics. To the courage, endurance and fine spirit of devotion with which they as a body have met these crises no poor words of our's [*sic*] can ever pay a fitting tribute."[83] Others agreed that the achievements were simply beyond words. "To attempt to give an adequate idea of what the nurses accomplished," an account of the work of the Visiting Nurse Society of Philadelphia during the epidemic suggested, "seems an almost hopeless undertaking. It is doubtful if even they themselves dreamed of their capacity."[84] If the nurses had not been aware of their abilities before the epidemic, the crisis seemingly gave them this insight. The report concluded, "Like steel passing through the final test by fire, the Society has come forth infinitely stronger than ever before with a new vigor and redoubled strength."

Nursing's leaders were quick to point out, too, that others shared this sense that the epidemic had highlighted the value and excellence of American nursing. The major nursing journals, for instance, ran stories that illustrated the esteem in which their profession was now held by others, particularly those who knew their work well. Articles from physicians, for instance, frequently appeared in the journals with titles such as "The Future of Nursing Service and Nursing Education" and "Nursing and the Health of the Future."[85] While these pieces often raised significant issues pertaining to the future of nursing, they always remained steadfastly supportive of the profession. Again and again from all corners of the health care landscape came praise for the work of nurses. The Committee on Nursing of the Council of National Defense offered "its highest tribute" to nurses who fell during the epidemic, writing, "To them and to the innumerable volunteers who met every test of fearlessness and self-forgetfulness, for their noble service to the nation and to humanity, this Committee pays its highest tribute."[86] The chairman of the Central Committee of the American Red Cross paid "a tribute to the superb work and service which the nursing profession has given during these past years" in a speech reprinted in the *American Journal of Nursing*, while a patient acknowledged boldly in the same journal a few months later that "to-day it is recognized that a good nurse is as important as a good doctor. . . . The doctor plants the little seed of health, but the nurse is the one who makes it grow. The doctor is a sort of consulting engineer, to change the figure, but the nurse is the official who stays right on the job."[87]

As this last example makes clear, such praise often highlighted the newly discovered importance of nursing in health care. "Society has placed the stamp of approval upon the trained nurse," explained one account of "the position of the nursing profession today," written by a physician and published in late 1920.[88] "She is as necessary a part of the fabric of civilization as are labor, capital, politics and the professions."[89] As an editorial in *Public Health Nurse* suggested, "The accounts of nursing work done in connection with the influenza epidemic which has swept the country with such disastrous effect . . . show the intimate connection which public health nursing organizations sustain to private and municipal activities in time of emergency." And further, "The value of such continuous, well-ordered nursing service is difficult fully to appraise until some such stress . . . throws into relief a structure which has been built upon deep-rooted and well-laid foundations."[90] As another commentator proclaimed more simply, "This epidemic has proved as nothing else the value of our nurse to the community and surrounding towns."[91] Illustrating nurses' new sense of pride in their work and their deep belief that their accomplishments in the epidemic and the war warranted recognition, in the aftermath of the war nurses began calling for military rank for those who served in the armed forces. A protracted debate ensued in which nurses argued that they deserved the respect such rank would bring to them and their work.[92]

Nurses were quite willing to acknowledge that their profession was entering a "period of incredible transition," a "difficult and trying period" in its development.[93] Even before the epidemic, nursing leadership had wrestled with issues related to their field's status as a profession, in particular how to meet the need for nurses while maintaining, indeed improving, nurses' status as educated and highly trained professionals.[94] Leaders in the profession maintained that the demands of the war and then of the epidemic had only exaggerated both the call for nurses and the risk this plea posed to the professionalization of their ranks. As early as 1919 a number of calls for reform emerged. Some advocates called attention to the need for better organization of nursing forces.[95] Specifically, many reformers focused on the complex tension between the need for sufficient nurses and the need to maintain or even raise their standards for entry into the profession. Writing in the midst of a resurgence of influenza in 1920, Lillian D. Wald of the Henry Street Settlement described the problem: "The cry from all was for nurses—more nurses—more nurses!"[96] This kind of demand might invite a lowering of standards. Noting the danger this posed to the nursing ranks, Wald had noted in late 1918,

> Some time when the readjustment period permits, the nurses and their colleagues in public health work must come together and out of the fires of war and epidemic experiences fashion tools to educate better the people in the homes, to use to the greater advantage of society the latent values that lie within the courage and good-will among men and women.[97]

That this need did not reflect failure, but success, was clear in Wald's conclusion. "Those who did so well during the epidemic," she stated simply, "could have done more had they had education for community service."

Wald's optimistic narrative camouflaged deep concerns among the nursing leadership. The need for both "better qualified women" applicants and for ever-higher standards for graduate nurses perplexed professional nursing's leadership and constituted their central struggle in the decades following the influenza emergency.[98] The epidemic had forced professional nurses to accept the assistance of untrained volunteers. In the aftermath, these same professionals looked for a way to raise the standards of nursing education and tighten access to the field. At the same time, nursing's critics complained of shortages and sought to simplify the training of nurses and loosen access, perhaps by creating a two-tiered nursing system.[99] As a response to this range of concerns, in 1919 the Rockefeller Foundation, a philanthropy well known since its founding in 1913 for devotion to health and medicine, established the Committee on Nursing Education.[100] Releasing its findings in 1922 in what became known as the Gold-mark Report in recognition of the group's chair, the Committee confirmed the importance of attracting "young women of high capacity" to the profession, of higher standards in nursing education, and of endowment funding to make possible these new educational opportunities. It also proposed a more controversial development, the creation of a new "subsidiary grade of nursing service," a lower-status attendant who would work under the supervision of physicians or trained nurses.[101] Responding to the report, the editors of the *American Journal of Nursing* concluded, "This is our opportunity for bringing nursing wholly out of the obsolete and wasteful apprenticeship type of training into an ordered, systematic, and dignified educational system comparable to those of the other professions."[102] While the report illustrated both the apparent crisis in nursing and the reform agenda on the minds of many professionals, it had little immediate impact on nursing.[103]

Even such troubling discussions, though, took place in the context of a broader sense of optimism and potential. In 1922 the major nursing organizations—the American Nurses' Association, the National League of Nursing Education, and the National Organization for Public Health Nursing—met together for their annual conventions. Though the president of each group acknowledged the challenges of the future, they also expressed confidence that their professional colleagues were ready to meet those challenges. "It would be folly to think that in a time, such as at present, our system is perfect or what has seemed satisfactory in the past can fit the needs of conditions or of people of today," Anna C. Jamme, the president of the National League of Nursing Education, explained as she began her remarks. "Our civilization is making heavy demands upon us, and we must rise to this challenge and prepare ourselves to meet it effectively by every means which we have at our command. Possibly we have not yet begun to tap the depth of our resources in the richness of what we may contribute to education or service."[104]

Echoing this view, the president of the National Organization for Public Health Nursing, Elizabeth G. Fox, stated simply, "These are indeed interesting times full of thrilling possibilities. We need to have our best wits about us to steer our course straight and safe amidst a multitude of alluring opportunities. Our future is bright before us if we have the wisdom to see it aright and the courage to stay on the track."[105] Clara D. Noyes, the president of the American Nursing Association, detailed just how broadly nursing affected society.

> The work of nursing touches the child, in the home and in the school, it is concerned not only with the care of the sick in the home and institution, but is concerned with the great questions of causation and prevention of disease, and therefore touches the work of other groups, the physician, the nutritional worker, the teacher, the social worker. Its interests are interwoven in the very fabric of civilization. For this reason we cannot go back, neither can we stand still, we must therefore press on.[106]

In stressing the demands that awaited nurses in the future, Noyes concluded by speaking of younger nurses: "In their young hands we must place the torch. To their youthful enthusiasm and devotion we must trust, not only the individual task, but ultimately the affairs of this great organization, knowing full well that they, like those who have preceded them, will find a way."[107]

The Public Narrative of American Health

The optimism of health care professionals found substantial support among the American people. Though the epidemic was recognized as an unfortunate event, such framing was routinely matched in the public sphere by claims that the epidemic's damage was not only reparable, but might prove useful in moving the nation forward in valuable ways. Existing at the crossroads of public health, medicine, and nursing, Red Cross workers had played a substantial role in the coordination and distribution of health care during the epidemic. Even before the end of the crisis, the Gulf Division of the organization suggested, "While the epidemic is deplored by all, the American Red Cross was afforded a tremendous opportunity to demonstrate it is prepared for emergencies at home as well as abroad."[108] In the aftermath, the organization celebrated its successful work and envisioned a great future yet to come. "It is an impossible task to attempt to report the comfort, care and relief rendered the stricken districts by the Red Cross Epidemic Committees through the Southern Division," a typical Red Cross report began, or as another announced, "It would be impossible to do justice to the accomplishments of all the Chapters in the [Atlantic] Division," while in the Northwest, "Red Cross workers . . . made a wonderful record for sane and helpful cooperation."[109] As a report on the work of the Southern Division during the epidemic argued, "It is absolutely certain that without this organization and without the aid rendered by it suffering would have been manifold and the death list terribly augmented."[110]

The Red Cross hoped that the public had become better acquainted with the capabilities of the organization as a result of the epidemic. Echoing the words of health care professionals, one Red Cross report suggested, "Terrible as were the ravages of the disease and the consequent suffering and death it entailed, still the epidemic was an opportunity for the display of a universal and wonderful spirit of helpfulness of the volunteer workers in the Division."[111] "Influenza had made communities stop and take stock of their social problems, and it had shown them the flexibility and power of the Red Cross organization," a report on civilian relief in the Lake Division explained.[112]

Looking ahead, Red Cross officials suggested that this new appreciation would ensure the organization's future vitality and importance in American life. One published report included an entire section entitled "Possible Values of the Epidemic" which highlighted the ways in which both the usefulness of the Red Cross and the health needs of the society had been proven by the epidemic.[113]

A report of the Southeastern Pennsylvania Chapter of the Red Cross suggested that the reports of its work might "serve as a testimonial to the worth of the great organization" and "as a guide and inspiration for future effort in similar emergencies."[114] Some in the Red Cross imagined an expanded role for their organization, recognizing in the needs of families a further opportunity for their Home Service work.[115] Like health care professionals, Red Cross officials expressed their sense of opportunity in a time they believed ripe for their organization's growth.

The popular press coverage seems to have offered some check on such exaggerated optimism in the aftermath as it sometimes emphasized the damage wrought by the disease in its epidemic incarnation.[116] "Flu Jumped Death Rate" the *Los Angeles Times* declared in July 1919, while an article in *Literary Digest* proclaimed, "The Influenza Plague Spread Terror and Death in the South Seas."[117] Even as late as 1928, *Literary Digest* described influenza as "that protean monster," as a "menace" capable of "ravages."[118] Frequent comparisons to the war reminded readers that the epidemic "swept the whole world," and led to more deaths.[119] The press also gave considerable attention to the issue of whether influenza would return.[120]

Even as the press considered the epidemics' costs, though, it also tended to dilute these reports in storylines that recreated the upbeat narrative of health care professionals. Querying "Will the 'Flu' Return?" an article in the *Literary Digest* believed, "The wise physician will prepare for it. We know more about it than we did last year, altho [*sic*] that is not very much." Quickly, though, the magazine went on to express confidence that complemented the voices of health care providers. "We shall be fighting an old foe," it reassured Americans, "with many of whose tricks we are now familiar, and this should give us a certain advantage in the contest." "The next onslaught" would not find Americans so unfamiliar with influenza, or so unprepared to fight it in its epidemic form, the magazine maintained.[121]

The case of the *New York Times* illustrates this shift from concern to complacency particularly well. In the months and years following the pandemic the newspaper reported the number of deaths caused by influenza, both during the epidemic and in subsequent years. From the reports of the Mutual Life Insurance Company to the statistics of the Army's General Staff and the figures released by New York's Department of Health, the paper covered closely the story of the epidemic's costs—both monetary and human.[122] Such articles rarely downplayed the losses but rather declared them boldly. "Ten Million Deaths in 'Flu' Plague a Year Ago" a headline announced in early 1920, and continued, "Half a Million of Them in This Country."[123]

The paper also covered the story of the social and economic problems left in the epidemic's wake. Even as it did so, though, the *New York Times* often diluted the troubling narrative of loss with an upbeat conclusion, portraying Americans responding to the epidemic with strength, succeeding in rebuilding their lives, and ultimately advancing toward an even better future. Pleas for aid for destitute families were balanced by accounts of the reopening of schools, the return of workers to their pre-epidemic routines, and the resumption of public business. Concerns about the long-term health effects of influenza were balanced by accounts of the return of good health to the American public.[124] This tendency to cushion bad news with good, or painful stories with upbeat ones, was especially obvious in the *New York Times*'s accounts of its "Hundred Neediest Cases." Returning to 1918's cases in mid-1919, the paper highlighted the recoveries of influenza's victims. As its account of Case 36 suggested, "Every member of this family had influenza after the father's death." Thanks to extensive medical care and continuing attention to their well-being, though, "a decided improvement has shown itself."[125] Other stories intimated bright futures for influenza's former victims. "Since Christmas three members of this family have had influenza," the report on Case 22 began. "But due to the care we have been able to give the family," it continued, "they recovered quickly." "After two weeks in a convalescent home the children have returned and are doing good work at school."[126] The results for Case 93 were still more promising and illustrated not only the worthiness of those who had received aid but the passing of the epidemic's impact. "This family is now self-supporting," the report began. "The man recovered from his influenza, but could not return to his work until about a month ago, as the doctors feared tuberculosis." Despite this inauspicious start, the family's recovery had soon progressed well. "We supplied an adequate diet, and the man is now in good condition." The broader meaning of this recovery was obvious: "This is a happy and healthy family today."[127]

When the holiday season arrived again in December 1919, the *New York Times* acknowledged that damage from the epidemic continued to trouble some of the most helpless Americans. "Mrs. G. tried to be both breadwinner and mother to her family of seven children after her husband died of influenza last year, but it was too much for her," the story of Case 16 explained. Though her sons were "anxious to grow up and do all the things that the 'charity lady' tells them about when she reads from the gaily covered adventure book," the boys were simply too young to become breadwinners. As a result, the paper explained, "Their mother is faced with the biggest adventure that ever fell to the lot of human being—the care of seven large-eyed sons on no income whatsoever."[128] Again, the paper offered hope. Even in cases such as that of the G. family, the paper suggested, the charity of strangers could prove enough to reverse the epidemic's consequences. "If their cupboard is filled and can be kept filled for them until they grow a little older the story will end with the words, 'and they all lived happily ever after.'"[129] In May 1920, the paper again provided upbeat updates on the progress of the Neediest 100 Cases.[130]

The popular press also retained its interest in developments in the scientific world, and here, too, emphasized the promise of the future contained in modern medicine. The press continued to track the efforts of scientists to discover the causal agent of influenza and to control future epidemics of infectious disease.[131] At times this coverage was tinged with skepticism, emphasizing the reality that influenza remained a "mystery" and "a puzzle."[132] In the spring of 1919 a "Topics of the Times" piece in the *New York Times* was clear about the hard work still ahead for those hunting the causal agent for influenza and several other infectious diseases, declaring in its headline, "Their Task Far From Fully Done."[133] Yet the article also noted that "in the popular mind there exists something like a belief that disease has few secrets or none that still elude the doctors and the biologists" and suggested, "If the curtain that has covered these similar mysteries has at last been raised it is permissible at least to hope that the time has come for another long step toward victory over man's most deadly foes."[134] As this example suggests, the press often shared the optimism of the scientists, repeating, sometimes verbatim, their words of hope. "Discoveries Abounding in Promise," declared another *New York Times* piece.[135] Continuing its upbeat coverage of a report on the purported discovery of the bacilli for influenza, trench fever, nephritis, mumps, measles, and typhus, the story also expressed its confidence in the abilities of the nation's leading scientists, arguing, "The probability that the report is correct is increased by the fact that the Army Medical Corps of the Allies have had at command the very highest professional talent, working with a wealth of material and limitless financial resources, and it is natural enough that they should have solved the problems hitherto unconquered."[136] Other press outlets shared this same hopeful tone about the nation's healthful future.[137]

While the press ended up echoing the optimistic views of American scientists, in another public context, the halls of Congress, those views faced a more critical reception. When scientists turned to Congress for financing both during and after the epidemic, elected representatives discussed, sometimes at length, the merits of those requests. In these debates officials made clear that while many Americans embraced the hope offered by health care professionals, others challenged the dominance of both the professionals and their narrative of optimism and authority.

Having made their earlier appropriation to the USPHS during the pandemic, in early 1919 politicians again expressed interest in the issue. On February 14, a resolution from the Ohio state legislature was offered on the floor of the Senate by the Vice President. In the resolution, the legislature petitioned Congress to "take action for the suppression of influenza," appropriating "an amount not less than $5,000,000 to be devoted to an investigation of the origin and nature of the disease commonly called 'Spanish Influenza' and of the best methods of counteracting it and to the protection of our national life by the total eradication of the germ or germs to which such disease is traceable."[138] Other politicians soon followed Ohio's lead, though few would make such a grand request. Several days later a resolution from the Alabama legislature urged the appropriation of $250,000.[139] In March, Senator Sheppard of Texas urged the appropriation of $500,000 "to discover the virus of influenza."[140] In July Congressman Black as well as Senator Harding, the next president, also urged this appropriation be properly considered.[141] Finally, in 1920 the Senate took up consideration of Joint Resolution 76 with its provision of $1 million to the USPHS for influenza research.[142]

Though their discussions ranged broadly, the rationale provided by petitioners as well as the debates over appropriations in the Senate provide important insight into at least some lay Americans' views regarding both the epidemic and the place of science and medicine in American life. Supportive politicians ultimately reinforced the hopeful narrative of health care professionals. As was the case with many public health experts and physicians, this narrative was often preceded by an acknowledgment of the epidemic's horror, medical science's inability to control it, and its likely return. The state of Alabama, for instance, began their resolution by noting that "our country and the known world are being visited by an awful and death dealing disease commonly called the 'flu,'" an illness about which the "medical world admits its ignorance of the causes and the cure."[143] The petition from the state of Ohio took a similar approach, turning first to the epidemic, and then quickly referencing the country's vulnerability before its powers. "This country has been devastated recently by an epidemic of one of the most deadly diseases known to science," it began, quickly adding, "Medical experts are not agreed either as to its origin nor the proper mode of treatment," and concluding that the "scourge" was bound to return.[144] Like health care professionals, these politicians used medicine's inability to control the epidemic, as well as its pending revival, as justification for appropriations for medical research.[145]

Like many public health officials, senators explained the importance of the involvement of the federal government and the USPHS by pointing out that the problem was "national in scope."[146] "The disease was of such national character and the scourge was so great and appalling," Senator Smith explained, "that I think it justifies the Federal Government in taking cognizance of it and doing all that it can to stamp out or even to ameliorate its ravages."[147] Or as Senator Norris maintained, "We ought not to expect localities to handle it," and further, "The 'flu' does not pay any attention to a State line nor to the line of a municipality."[148] In turn, supporters maintained that, given Americans' helplessness before the disease, reliance on experts offered the best hope of success. As Norris continued,

"It is something new, and we are confronted with the condition and are helpless. If we want to do anything we must go somewhere and trust somebody with the power and authority and equip them with the money to carry out what men who have studied the question think is the proper method to pursue."[149] Similarly, Senator Smith noted the importance of the "Federal medical service" during the epidemic and argued in support of the allocation of funds, "There is hardly a home that is not visited now by this miserable disease, and I do not think it is a time for us to question the experts who come and ask that we do something to help the public at large."[150] Senator Townsend, though uncertain about the specifics involved, nevertheless felt compelled to defer to the experienced. "I am not sure that good will come from the expenditure, but I hope it will," he admitted, and continued, "I must necessarily rely upon men who are familiar with this matter."[151]

Though Townsend was uncertain of the outcomes, other politicians made optimistic claims about the promise of the research their appropriations would fund. Noting that the Surgeon General of the Navy "thinks without a doubt that research would find a remedy," and estimating the financial waste caused by the illness, Congressman Simeon D. Fess of Ohio concluded of the appropriation, "It would be a good investment, indeed."[152] "One could hardly think of a way to expend Federal funds which might be productive of better or more valuable results," Carter Glass, Secretary of the Treasury, confirmed.[153]

But not everyone in Congress shared this enthusiasm for funding medical research. For some who opposed the allocations, the issue was primarily one of opposition to federal encroachment. Critics pointed to the problems of government growth, interference with states' and individuals' rights, and overtaxation.[154] Similarly, others maintained that research was best left to the private sector.[155] These positions mirrored to some extent the rising hostility toward government growth evident during the pandemic among Americans resisting public health encroachment and signaled the rejection of Progressivism that would dominate politics in the 1920s.

Others, though, directed their challenge not at an encroaching federal presence but rather at the USPHS, calling into question the effectiveness of the agency's past research and the wisdom of any further appropriations. As they did so, their narratives of the epidemic reflected not the optimism of health care professionals but a more troubled account. Some believed only that the money could be better spent on nursing, or on direct care, on something "practical" rather than on research.[156] Others were more directly critical of the USPHS itself, arguing that despite sizable appropriations, little of value had resulted. As Senator Gilbert M. Hitchcock argued in January 1920, "It seems to me that when we come to the matter of spending a million dollars, after having expended a million and one-half last year for the purpose, we ought not to vote until we know what was done with the million and a half and what was accomplished."

The reason for Hitchcock's caution was clear: "It is easy enough to waste a million or a million and a half dollars if it is not carefully looked after by Congress."[157]
During the same debate, Senator William H. King of Utah was even more direct
in his expression of concern regarding any further appropriation to the USPHS,
suggesting, "We appropriated a million dollars. What became of the million
dollars? What is there to show for it? What benefit has it derived? Where is the
report? These questions . . . have not been answered, and I doubt whether they
can be satisfactorily answered."[158] Senator Lee S. Overman was more veiled in
his criticism, though his words were hardly less damning. In the midst of the
Senate debate on January 26, 1919, Overman interrupted the discussion to
announce the discovery of a cure. "I want to say, for the benefit of those who are
making this investigation," he reported, "that I was told by a judge of a superior
court that in the mountain country of North Carolina they have discovered a
remedy for this disease."[159] The purported cure implied a critique of modern science and an appreciation for the simple wisdom of simple people. "They say that
common baking soda will cure the disease," he continued, "that they have cured
it with it; that they have no deaths up there at all; and they use common baking
soda, which cures the disease." The dissatisfaction of many with the accomplishments of the USPHS was clear as debates lowered the possible appropriation
from $5 million to $1 million, then $500,000, and eventually to $250,000. In
the end, no specific appropriation was made. For many politicians, the USPHS
had happily spent the public's money without providing any benefits in return,
and had not earned special funding for the investigation of influenza. In this
view the epidemic loomed as a story of failure and waste.

Narratives of Loss

This more critical narrative, though successful in blocking congressional appropriations, never dominated American collective memory, where Americans
imagined instead a history of success and a future of continued triumphs. It was,
though, part of a broader narrative of the pandemic that focused not on the opportunities it opened but on the losses it left in its wake. Though Americans'
public culture embraced an optimistic narrative of recovery and opportunity, as
individuals turned away from issues of professional performance and public
policy and considered their own struggles in the aftermath of the epidemic's horrors, they often articulated narratives that recalled the pain, the losses, and the
dislocation that infused their private memories.

On rare occasions such a perspective found a place in public culture. Perhaps
most appropriately, blues songs about the pandemic emphasized its catastrophic
scale and its powerful impact on American lives. Perhaps best known of these

blues pieces is Essie Jenkins's "1919 Influenza Blues."[160] "People was dying everywhere," she tells us, "death was creeping through the air, and the groans of the rich sure was sad." It was not only the rich who suffered in Jenkins's account, though, as Americans "rich and poor," "North and South, East and West," were stricken. The cause was clear. The epidemic, it seems, was nothing less than an admonition from God. "It was God's almighty plan," she explains, "he is judging this old land," and would surely "kill some more, if you don't turn away from your shame." For Jenkins, the efforts of doctors and nurses were irrelevant in the fight against the pandemic, for influenza was something only God could control: "Down in Memphis, Tennessee, doctors said soon would be / In a few days influenza would be controlled / But God showed that He was head, He sent the doctors on to bed / And the nurses they broke down with the same." In this song the epidemic was remembered as a scourge, a cataclysm for human beings who had no recourse but to God as they faced its trials.

Blind Willie Johnson told a similar story in "Jesus is Coming Soon." "In the year of 19 and 18, God sent a mighty disease / It killed many a-thousand, on land and on the seas," Johnson began. Emphasizing the scale of the disaster, Johnson continued, "Great disease was mighty and the people were sick everywhere / It was an epidemic, it floated through the air." Johnson went on to describe the helplessness not only of the people, but of the medical professionals as well, suggesting, "The doctors they got troubled and they didn't know what to do / They gathered themselves together, they called it the Spanish'in' flu." Having described the terrible blight of the flu and the reactions of the people and their leaders, Johnson concluded, "Well God is warning the nation, He's a-warnin' them every way / To turn away from evil and seek the Lord and pray," and further, "Read the book of Zacharias, Bible plainly says / Said the people in the cities dyin', account of they wicked ways." As the chorus exhorted again and again, "We done told you, our God's done warned you, Jesus comin' soon."[161] As Jenkins and Johnson maintained, the epidemic was a crisis that reflected the nation's failure. Adopting the religious narrative prevalent during the epidemic itself, their lyrics blamed the emergency not on Americans' scientific failures but rather on their spiritual collapse. This accounting did not minimize the epidemic's impact but rather heightened its meaning for the present and the future as a warning for Americans to return to God. In doing so, this narrative offered an interpretation of the pandemic dramatically different from any posed by either the health care professionals or public officials.

Such a narrative resonated with those who suffered most severely as a result of the pandemic—patients who experienced influenza's damage firsthand, and those who lost loved ones to the disease. Here the costs of the epidemic were more readily remembered as individuals and families found their lives remade by the epidemic experience. Former patients' narratives about the epidemic are difficult to locate, and so conclusions about their responses remain tentative. In keeping with the broader cultural dynamic of future-oriented optimism, some patients, especially men, described their certain recovery long before it was assured. "I am all right again," William G. McAdoo, the Secretary of the Treasury, wrote reassuringly to his daughter on November 7, 1918, concluding, "I am up today for the first time and feel sure that I shall have no more trouble now."[162] Others offered upbeat assessments of their progress, but were more willing to admit that their struggles with influenza were nevertheless significant. "I am feeling much better today although I am confined to my home," Joseph P. Tumulty, President Wilson's private secretary, wrote on January 20, 1919. Though he was still housebound, he included a further encouragement in his note, concluding, "I am sure that I am on the road to a complete recovery which I hope will be soon."[163] In a less guarded moment a few days later, though, Tumulty again conceded the difficulty his healing posed. Suggesting that he was "on the way to recovery" in a letter on January 25, he nevertheless acknowledged that "it seems to be rather slow work."[164]

Other patients more readily dispensed with the optimistic narrative and acknowledged that they continued to feel the consequences of the disease even after its passing and found full recovery a slow and even arduous process. "I am still suffering the after effects of that delightful disease," Harold Bowman wrote in a letter in early 1919. "A hard day, such as this has been," he admitted, "tires me out pretty well."[165] In the years that followed, influenza's aftereffects seem to have "left a train of ailing victims with Bright's disease, cardiac irregularities, vascular problems, pulmonary tuberculosis, and a host of nervous and paralytic afflictions."[166] It was immediately following the war and the pandemic, too, that many Americans bought life insurance for the first time, perhaps reflecting their sense of the persistent dangers posed by illness.[167]

While many suffered physical aftereffects of the pandemic, for others its impact was primarily emotional or psychological. Perhaps the best known account of the epidemic by a patient-survivor is that of Katherine Anne Porter (see Figure 5.1), who recounted her experiences in a fictional account, the novella *Pale Horse, Pale Rider*, published in 1936. A journalist writing for the *Rocky Mountain News* in Denver, Porter suffered from a very serious case of influenza during the epidemic and during her illness lost her fiancé to the disease. Porter was sick enough that the newspaper prepared her obituary, and her recovery proved slow and troubled. Even so, six months after her illness she was largely healthy, with the promise of complete recovery assured.[168] Though fictionalized, the autobiographical novella follows Porter's experiences closely and provides unusual insight into the influenza experience from the perspective of both the patient and the survivor, both those who suffered the disease and those who lost loved ones to it. Because she wrote her account years after the pandemic, it also

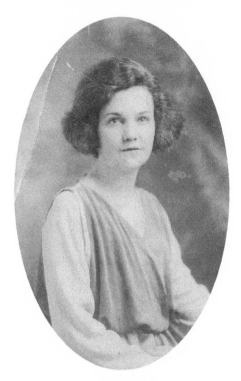

Figure 5.1 Katherine Anne Porter would write the best known account of the epidemic in the United States in a heavily autobiographical novella. This photo of her was taken in the spring of 1918, just a few months prior to the influenza outbreak. (Item #1015), Box 2, Series XII, Katherine Anne Porter Papers, University of Maryland.

opens a window into the post-epidemic lives of those who suffered illness or grief at influenza's hands. Porter's narrative was infused not with rebirth but with death, not with optimism but with despair, not with opportunity but with loss.

The story focuses on Miranda, a 24-year-old woman, and follows first her romance with a young soldier, Adam, and then her struggle with influenza. The novella opens with an unearthly quality, as Miranda dreams she is awakening, strangely certain that something unusual is about to overcome her.[169] The passage is followed by a strange dream in which Miranda races to "outrun Death and the Devil," a race with a pale horse and its rider whose "pale face smiled in an evil trance" beside her. The dreaming Miranda succeeds in escaping the pale rider, declaring "I'm not going with you this time" as she halts and watches the stranger riding on without her.[170] With this opening passage Porter foreshadows Miranda's struggle against influenza, though neither the reader nor Miranda is yet aware of the illness to come.

Porter is masterful in portraying the mood of Americans late in the war—the pressures of the war fever, the exhaustion it produced among the war-weary, and the persistent refusal of the young to allow that weariness to destroy their youthful exuberance. Miranda's struggle against the hysteria of wartime serves as a backdrop for her developing relationship. As Miranda worries that she and Adam "have no time," describes Adam as a "sacrificial lamb," and sees "the face of the man he would not live to be," Porter drives home the danger the war posed to young American men, perhaps distracting the reader from the influenza threat that looms at the edge of the story.[171] At the same time, Porter also hints at both the epidemic coursing through the society and Miranda's own developing illness. In the first account of the young couple walking through the city on Miranda's way to work, for instance, they "waited for a funeral to pass," and then shortly thereafter "hardly glanced at a funeral procession approaching."[172] When Miranda arrives at the newspaper, she finds her colleagues discussing the epidemic, though the characters never name either the disease or its epidemic visitation, and reference only the rumors surrounding its origins among the German enemy.[173] Porter's central characters seem both to acknowledge the epidemic and to steel themselves against the disease with a hopeful, or perhaps naïve, disavowal of its importance.

Avoiding the epidemic, though, soon becomes impossible and Porter slowly submerges Miranda in the symptoms of influenza, allowing the severity of her situation to dawn on the reader only slowly. In the early pages Miranda complains to herself, and thereby the reader, of her heavy sleep and "a burning slow headache," and later admits to Adam that she "can't smell or see or hear today," and that she "must have a fearful cold."[174] Later, on the street with a colleague, Miranda alludes to her mysterious condition in her internal voice. "This is the beginning of the end of something," she thinks to herself, continuing, "Something terrible is going to happen to me. I shan't need bread and butter where I'm going. . . . Oh, Adam, I hope I see you once more before I go under with whatever is the matter with me."[175] Later, Porter again hints at Miranda's growing illness as her internal conversation again considers the words she wishes she might say to Adam: "Come out of your dream and listen to me. I have pains in my chest and my head and my heart and they're real. I am in pain all over, and you are in such danger as I can't bear to think about, and why can we not save each other?"[176]

Though a reader may not yet recognize Miranda's condition, just a few pages later the severity of her situation becomes clear when she acknowledges she is ill with influenza. Gradually Porter provides the reader with an understanding of the broader seriousness of the crisis. Though her neighbor's response is initially only a simple exclamation of "*Horrors*" and a recommendation that she go to bed "at *once!*" her later description of Miranda's influenza as "a plague, a plague, my God" begins to clarify the fear that came to surround this illness.[177] The reader soon learns of the broader emergency as Adam explains it to the ailing

Miranda: "It's as bad as anything can be . . . all the theatres and nearly all the shops and restaurants are closed, and the streets have been full of funerals all day and ambulances all night."[178] Porter's characters struggle, too, with the chaos of the epidemic crisis, reflected in a shortage of doctors, ambulances, and hospital beds.[179]

Even more powerful, though, is Porter's depiction of the experience of those stricken with the disease. Following the conversations of her characters, and later Miranda's internal dialogues, Porter presents the complex and unfamiliar path of one patient through the illness. In Porter's narrative, the sense of fore-boding and of loss looms as the illness develops, suggesting the weight of the war and the epidemic on the consciousness of individuals. As Adam cares for Miranda in the early stages of her illness, their conversation turns to their lives, their plans for what each of them "meant to do," as they consider the hopes that now seem endangered. Miranda celebrates the simple realities seemingly chal-lenged by her sickness. "Don't you love being alive," Miranda asks Adam. "Don't you love weather and the colors at different times of the day, and all the sounds and noises like children screaming in the next lot, and automobile horns and little bands playing in the street and the smell of food cooking?"[180]

When Miranda descends again into fevered dreams, passing back and forth from consciousness to unconsciousness, Porter gives her reader a sense of the peace and the terror, the coherence and the confusion, through which her patient passed. "Her mind, split in two, acknowledged and denied what she saw in the one instant, for across an abyss of complaining darkness her reasoning coherent self watched the strange frenzy of the other coldly, reluctant to admit the truth of its visions, its tenacious remorses and despairs."[181] As death approaches, Miranda is briefly freed from her fears and terrors, and finds comfort, "tranquility," "an amazement of joy," and relaxes, "questioning nothing, desiring nothing, in the quietude of her ecstasy."[182] Perhaps warning the reader of just how painful her life in the aftermath of the pandemic will be, for Miranda death seemed a pleasant prospect in the midst of her illness.

But death is not to be her fate. Porter portrays vividly the malaise, indeed depression, from which influenza victims sometimes suffered in its aftermath.[183] Miranda returns to life, first with the pain of consciousness and then with a sense of loss, struggling to rejoin the living while longing for the heaven of her dream, seeing "with a new anguish the dull world to which she was condemned," and weeping for herself and "her lost rapture."[184] "There was no escape," Miranda realizes.

> Dr. Hildesheim, Miss Tanner, the nurses in the diet kitchen, the chemist, the surgeon, the precise machine of the hospital, the whole humane conviction and custom of society, conspired to pull her inseparable rack

of bones and wasted flesh to its feet, to put in order her disordered mind, and to set her once more safely in the road that would lead her again to death.[185]

Though Miranda would rally for her visitors, smiling and telling them "how gay and what a pleasant surprise it was to find herself alive," she did so only because such was expected of her.[186] As Miranda recovers, she recognizes her gradual adjustment to living, finding herself "not quite dead now . . . one foot in either world now," and knowing that "soon I shall cross back and be at home again."[187] "I shall be glad when I hear that someone I know has escaped from death. I shall visit the escaped ones and help them dress and tell them how lucky they are, and how lucky I am still to have them."[188] The novella ends with an ironic declaration of the promise of the future: "No more war, no more plague, only the dazed silence that follows the ceasing of the heavy guns; noiseless houses with the shades drawn, empty streets, the dead cold light of tomorrow. Now there would be time for everything."[189] Though there would be "time for everything," and life would go on, the epidemic had left at least some survivors stunned by its personal and private tragedies. Miranda's desolation is not the result only of her own illness, of course. Porter's Miranda suffers in the aftermath of the epidemic as a victim of both the illness and the death it left in its wake. Having returned to the living, the loss of Adam seemed a cruel trick. "I wish you had come back," she beseeches him. "What do you think I came back for, Adam, to be deceived like this?"[190]

As Porter's novella suggests, the memory of the pandemic was both vivid and painful for many Americans, recalling the agony of the illness and the grief of its losses that had been central to their own experiences of the crisis. The writer William Maxwell was 10 years old when he lost his mother to influenza, a story he recounts, like Porter, in an autobiographical novel, *They Came Like Swallows*, published in 1937. Focused on the Morison family, the novel exposes the reader to the range of traumas one family suffered as a result of the pandemic. Elizabeth Morison is the heart and soul of her family, and influenza's eventual victim. Maxwell guides his reader through the epidemic experience in three parts, each told from the perspective of a central figure in the story—the sons Bunny and Robert and the husband James. From the beginning the reader is conscious of the peril with which the family lives, as gentle Bunny worries early in the story about what he would do "if his mother were not there to protect him from whatever was unpleasant—from the weather and from Robert and from his father—what would he do? Whatever would become of him in a world where there was neither warmth nor comfort nor love?"[191]

Soon the epidemic arrives at the edges of the story, and one by one family members take sick, first Bunny, and then Robert, James, and Elizabeth. Maxwell lets his reader experience not only the public consequences of the pandemic—closed schools, busy doctors, prohibited church services—but more important the physical, emotional, and psychological costs of the illness and death by which his characters are surrounded. Readers learn something of the experience of influenza itself, as Bunny is "burning up with fever," Robert is "cut loose. . . . adrift utterly in his own sickness," and James listens to his wife's "terrible last hour of . . . breathing."[192] Even more powerful, though, is the accounting of the each character's internal trauma as they suffer through Elizabeth's death. Bunny's grief is matched by Robert's anguish, "his private nightmare," a torment worsened by his belief that he is guilty of causing his mother's illness.[193] James, too, suffers guilt alongside grief, anger, abandonment, and confusion, emotions so deadening that he soon wonders if "he would ever be capable of any emotion again."[194] As Maxwell tells us, "If James Morison had come upon himself on the street, he would have thought *That poor fellow is done for.* . . . But he walked past the mirror in the front hall without seeing it and did not know how grey his face was, and how, all in a few days, sickness and suffering and grief and despair had aged him."[195]

Though the novel prepares the reader for the family's collapse, Elizabeth's influence seems to rescue the family. As Bunny finds light in a new morning and Robert is spared his guilt, even James seems capable of building a new life.[196] In the closing pages of the novel, James looks at his wife in her casket and notices her hands, how "intensely quiet" they were "with the life, with the identifying soul, gone out of them." This is not a tragic observation, though, and the novel ends with the sense that the family would find its way. As James continues, "They would not have been that way . . . if he had not been doing what she wanted him to do. For it was Elizabeth who had determined the shape that his life would take, from the very first moment he saw her. And she had altered that shape daily by the sound of her voice, and by her hair, and by her eyes which were so large and dark. And by her wisdom and by her love."[197] Despite influenza's toll, she had built a family capable of surviving.

As the works of Porter and Maxwell make clear, Americans often remembered the pandemic and its costs, an important counterpoint to the nation's collective memory. Indeed, according to William Maxwell, his memories grew "much more vivid" as he aged. As he suggested in an interview in 1995, "Everything that ever happened to me is there."[198] Memories of the pandemic, of course, were never the province only of writers who intentionally shared their stories with a broader readership. In the 1970s, World War I veterans completed questionnaires as part of a research project on soldiers' experiences conducted by the United States Army Military History Institute, and in their responses to questions about health and health care during the war recalled again and again the epidemic and its consequences. "Flue [*sic*] was extremely bad[.] Hundreds of our men died of Flue," recalled one.[199] "Many never got over it and died," and "the deaths were unbelievable," recalled others.[200] Still others remembered the deaths more vividly. "I can to this day see the 'cords' of bodies stacked in the Base Hospital. They were dying faster than the bodies could be taken care of," remembered Merle Swanter.[201] Or as Private Orville Holman remembered, "When the Influenza hit all men got sick. A man who worked in the morgue said that bodies were stacked as high as your head[,] 700 in there at one time."[202] As one soldier from Fort Custer in Michigan explained simply, "It was awful."[203] More than half a century after the pandemic, these veterans recalled effortlessly the scourge the pandemic had proven.

The memories Americans carried and the narratives that emerged as a result were as varied as the nation's people. As Porter and Maxwell make clear, for some Americans the pandemic brought inconceivable losses and lives changed forever by the deaths of loved ones. In some cases these deaths shattered families, experiences not soon forgotten. In his "Reminiscences: Sawmill City Boyhood," Melvin Frank recalled the agony of the epidemic, and the cost it exacted from his community, his family, and ultimately his childhood. "By whatever name, the disease was a killer and scarcely any household in our north side neighborhood was unaffected," he explained. "It brought eventual tradegy [sic] to our house." It was his father who was "most severely affected."[204] Frank recounted, "While the family feared it was coming, Dad's health crisis did not strike until the spring of 1920 when he became ill with acute cardiac asthma. Heart damage from rheumatic fever attack in his youth had been aggravated by the 1918 flu."[205] The symptoms were horrifying for a young Frank to watch. "That spring he suffered frequent smothering and choking spells that racked him with horrible coughing. It was a terrible thing for a boy to see his father struggle for breath."[206] Eventually his father became a "bed patient," and the entire family suffered over his condition. "Deep anxiety settled over our family. When I came home from school for lunch each day I would ask Mom how Dad was. She just shook her head. It was plain to see that she was troubled. When I went it to see Dad his own deep-set brown eyes expressed his own dismay. Day by day the painful spells took their toll of strength until his strong body was pitifully weak. I was fearful, afraid that my father was dying."[207] Once his father was hospitalized, Frank's family became still more depressed. "Gloom descended," he remembered, "A sob was close to the surface."[208] His father died on June 24, 1920. Though the death came long after his exposure to influenza, Frank's father was nevertheless a victim of the epidemic, and the meaning of his passing no less tragic for its delay. Upon learning of his father's death, Frank found himself "reeling" from the news, "for my world had tumbled in."[209] "I had expected the news," he recognized, "but dreaded it with all my heart." "Those next days," he remembered, "were crowded with events in which I was a spectator witnessing occasions I did not want to be a part of."[210] In his account, Melvin Frank forces us to recognize the pain, grief, and disruption the epidemic wielded.

Other accounts foreground the uncertainty into which the death of one or both parents launched their authors. The writer Mary McCarthy recounted her experiences as an orphan in the wake of the epidemic in her *Memories of a Catholic Girlhood*. If her words name the unfeeling approach of her relatives, the resultant tone illuminates the sense of abandonment and helplessness she suffered as an unwanted child. "Poor Ray's children as commiseration damply styled us, could not afford illusions in the family opinion," she recalled. "Our father had put us beyond the pale by dying suddenly of influenza and taking our young mother with him, a defection that was remarked on with horror and grief commingled, as though as our mother had been a pretty secretary with whom he had wantonly absconded into the irresponsible paradise of the here-after." The reaction of her family and her community did little to ease a young McCarthy's suffering.

> Our reputation was clouded by this misfortune. There was a prevailing sense, not only in the family but among storekeepers, servants, street-car conductors, and other satellites of our circle, that my grandfather, a rich man, had behaved with extraordinary munificence in allotting a sum of money for our support and installing us with some disagreeable middle-aged relations in a dingy house two blocks distant from his own. What alternative he had was not mentioned; presumably he could have sent us to an orphan asylum and no one would have thought the worse of him.[211]

For McCarthy, loneliness and despair were central to the epidemic's impact.

Others, too, noted the expansiveness of the epidemic's costs. The writer Thomas Wolfe recounted the experience of his brother's illness in a fictionalized, but nevertheless closely autobiographical, account in a single chapter of his novel *Look Homeward, Angel*. Like Wolfe, the main character of the book, Eugene, is called home from college when his brother Ben is stricken by influenza.[212] Though the tragedy of young Ben's death rests in the family's dysfunction, it is influenza, nevertheless, that serves as the mechanism for enacting the final stages of the calamity, and Wolfe is unsparing in detailing the misery of an influenza death. The reader learns of each stage of Ben's illness—the initial illness and fever that eventually worsened enough to send Ben to bed, his "apparent convalescent" phase, and then the return to bed "with a high fever" and "pneumonia in both lungs," and the subsequent "brief periods of consciousness, unconsciousness, and delirium."[213] Wolfe provides a grim description of Eugene's first look at his dying brother:

Ben's long thin body lay three-quarters covered by the bedding; its gaunt outline was bitterly twisted below the covers, in an attitude of struggle and torture. It seemed not to belong to him, it was somehow distorted and detached as if it belonged to a beheaded criminal. And the sallow yellow of his face had turned gray; out of this granite tint of death, lit by two red flags of fever, the stiff black furze of a three-day beard was growing. The beard was somehow horrible; it recalled the corrupt vitality of hair, which can grow from a rotting corpse. And Ben's thin lips were lifted, in a constant grimace of torture and strangulation, above his white somehow dead-looking teeth, as inch by inch he gasped a thread of air into his lungs. And the sound of this gasping—loud, hoarse, rapid, unbelievable, filling the room, and orchestrating every moment in it—gave to the scene its final note of horror.[214]

Eugene recognized his brother's "strangulation," and found himself "choked" by "the ugliness and discomfort of the death."[215] Death as Wolfe presents it was not peaceful or easy: "It's messy! Messy! Do you hear?" he demanded of others.[216]

The death seemed no less painful for its witnesses. Eugene's torment seems equal to that of his brother as he witnesses his decline and the broader tragedy of his death. "He [Eugene] felt that he could never again escape from this smothering flood of pain and ugliness, from the eclipsing horror and pity of it all," Wolfe suggested.[217] For Wolfe it was not simply the deaths that were terrible but the broader and more complex meanings those deaths enacted. "The sad prophetic story, a brief and terrible summary of the waste, the tardiness, and the ruin of their lives, silenced them for a moment with its inexorable sense of tragedy," Wolfe wrote.[218] A few pages later, while Ben continues to struggle, his mother collapses into the recognition of that tragedy, "weeping bitterly, helplessly, grievously, for the sad waste of irrevocable years—the immortal hours of love that might never be relived, the great evil of forgetfulness and indifference that could never be righted now."[219] Though Eugene would comfort her, he, too, knew "that it was not, could never be, all right."[220] Wolfe did not offer his readers the promise of a brighter future but rather the anguish of a tragedy, a tragedy that reached beyond innocent loss to the most tormented interpersonal calamities.

For Wolfe influenza was an awful illness, and the death of his brother at its hands was tragic not just for the loss of a young life but also for its thwarting of the possibility of reconciliation or redemption in his dysfunctional family. For some other Americans, too, the epidemic's deaths changed forever their sense of their place in the world. Even for some medical practitioners the meaning of the epidemic could not be easily translated into pronouncements of possibility. Devastated by their ignorance of the disease and the inadequacies of their treatments, some physicians, even long after the pandemic, recounted a narrative not only of frustration or disappointment but also of anguish. Just how deeply some physicians felt the costs of the epidemic is perhaps best illustrated by the experiences of Victor C. Vaughan. Vaughan was a distinguished leader of American medicine by 1918. Dean of the University of Michigan Medical School, he had recently completed a term as the president of the American Medical Association, was the founding editor of the *Journal of Laboratory and Clinical Medicine* and was serving as a colonel in the army, where he led its Division of Communicable Diseases, when the influenza outbreak began.[221] On September 23, 1918, Vaughan had traveled to Ayer, Massachusetts, as part of a team appointed by the Army Surgeon General to look into the apparent outbreak of Spanish Influenza at Camp Devens. Vaughan had extensive experience with epidemic disease, but even so he was stunned by what he discovered on his arrival at the camp. As he suggested a few months later to an audience of public health professionals, "I went to Camp Devens as soon as the epidemic was reported and I might say that I thought my eyes would never see such horror as I saw there. I went through the Spanish-American War; I saw thousands and thousands of cases of typhoid fever, but I never had anything so depress me as the conditions that existed at Camp Devens."[222] Half a year later, in July 1919, Vaughan would recount the epidemic's terrible costs, suggesting the "unparalleled pandemic of influenza" had "been most distressing and disastrous both in military and civilian populations," with its mortality "unparalleled in recent times."[223]

When Vaughan wrote his memoirs in 1926, he largely avoided recounting his experiences in the influenza epidemic. He mentioned it only briefly as he wrote of his service during World War I. Noting the trip to Camp Devens, he continued curtly, "I am not going into the history of the influenza epidemic. It encircled the world, visited the remotest corners, taking toll of the most robust, sparing neither soldier nor civilian, and flaunting its red flag in the face of science."[224] Despite this disclaimer, though, Vaughan recalled the epidemic for his readers as he cast his glance backward to some of the "horrors" of his life. In doing so he exposed the trauma the epidemic had evoked. "In the memory chambers of my brain there hang many pictures. Some are the joy of my life," he began. Others, though, were "ghastly ones which I would tear down and destroy were I able to do so, but this is beyond my power."[225] Among those awful pictures, he explained, hung a canvas of his experience during the influenza epidemic.

> I see hundreds of young, stalwart men in the uniform of their country coming into the wards of the hospital in groups of ten or more. They are placed on the cots until every bed is full and yet others crowd in. The faces soon wear a bluish cast; a distressing cough brings up the blood

stained sputum. In the morning the dead bodies are stacked about the morgue like cord wood. This picture was painted on my memory cells at the division hospital, Camp Devens, in 1918, when the deadly influenza demonstrated the inferiority of human inventions in the destruction of human life.[226]

Despite his efforts to escape the epidemic, Vaughan admitted, he remained haunted by his experiences.

Deeply affected on a personal level by his experiences in 1918, Vaughan also acknowledged the broader impact the epidemic had had on his sense of himself as a medical professional. "The saddest part of my life," he suggested in another context, "was when I witnessed the hundreds of deaths of soldiers in the army camps and did not know what to do. At that moment I decided never again to prate about the great achievements of medical science and to humbly admit our dense ignorance in this case."[227] Having once maintained a heroic image of medicine, Vaughan exchanged this for a cautious humility in the face of the destructiveness of the epidemic and his own helplessness before it. For many Americans, as for Vaughan, the pandemic's meaning lived on, silently haunting its many victims whose injuries remained unspoken and whose losses went publicly unacknowledged in a nation quick to forget the devastation.

Reckoning the Costs of Amnesia

In retrospect, it is tempting to criticize Americans' failure to commemorate the pandemic in their public culture. As they relied on the optimistic narrative that focused only on the promise of the future and erased the dark days of their recent past, Americans' collective memory exhibited a costly amnesia that left too many Americans to suffer in private as they lived out the consequences of the influenza crisis. This dismissal of the memory, indeed of the experiences, of so many seems both cruel and careless. And yet this tendency toward national amnesia and the resulting contradiction between public and private culture, between national forgetting and personal remembering, was not unique to the period following the pandemic but appears instead as a mainstay of American culture. In the wake of the influenza scourge, it seems, Americans were only acting out a process common in the nation's history, drowning out narratives of anguish with the noise of public optimism.

In his book on the aftermath of the 1995 bombing of the federal building in Oklahoma City, Edward Linenthal identified the preferred narratives that emerged as Americans responded to this more recent cataclysm. The narratives he discovered in the wake of the bombing—what he termed the "progressive," "redemptive," and "toxic" narratives—bear a striking similarity to those developed following the pandemic, suggesting that Americans may often resort to an established set of interpretations as they develop understandings of the worst moments in their national story. Linenthal describes a progressive narrative that finds hope in Americans' communal response to catastrophe and imagines a nation made stronger and more cohesive through the shared process of struggle and recovery. "New life," in this view, "springs from death."[1] With its upbeat tenor and its focus on a bright future, this response mirrors almost exactly the optimistic narrative provided by American health care professionals and embraced by the nation's public culture in the aftermath of the epidemic.

Some Americans developed an alternative understanding of the bombing, a redemptive narrative that allowed them to find a place for this experience in their religiously infused world view. Christianity guided the responses of many Oklahomans, leading them to believe the losses of loved ones could be redeemed if those they left behind might love and live more fully, if the scars of loss might serve as a "sacrament—an outward and visible sign of an inward and invisible grace."[2] Such a narrative, too, was evident among Americans in the aftermath of the epidemic as they sought to imbue the catastrophe and its losses with meaning. While for some the redemption was civic, as they believed the emergency had led the nation to embrace its better democratic self, for others the possibility of redemption lay in responding to the pandemic as God's work.

Though in both 1918 and 1995 Americans' public culture found optimism and civic and religious redemption a salve for wounded souls, such a response was meaningless or worse for some of those who suffered most deeply from the tragedies. For Americans like Katherine Anne Porter and Thomas Wolfe, memories of the pandemic experience remained both painful and persistent, offering a narrative strikingly similar to Linenthal's third narrative, the toxic. This narrative emphasizes the terrible event and its lasting costs, the "visible and invisible scars" that produced "enduring pain and loss" for many Americans.[3] In the aftermath of the epidemic, too, some Americans felt only grief, and lived quietly for decades to come with a profound sense of loss. The close parallel in these responses, separated by seventy-seven years, illustrates the recurrence of particular patterns in American reactions to catastrophe.

In fact, the patterns evident as Americans interpreted the epidemic experience resonate not only with the preferred narratives of Oklahoma City in 1995 but with our shared interpretations of other pieces of the American past as well. As a culture, the United States has exhibited a profound tendency to evade, misrepresent, or even mythologize those parts of its past that are difficult, that do not fit somehow with their view of themselves.[4] The history of slavery is a classic case, as Americans have sought to hide its horror behind misrepresentations, to "deny its presence, minimize its seriousness, and ignore its enduring scars."[5] Indeed, the entirety of some groups of Americans' history—one thinks immediately of African Americans, or of the indigenous people of this continent—has gone untold or mistold to make possible a narrative of the nation's unified march from goodness to perfection.[6] In other examples, World War II has been made to stand as our "good war," the contests over its meaning long forgotten and replaced with a simple memory in which the war's personal terrors, family trauma, constitutional failures, and ethical doubts are trumped by individual and national heroism and moral certainty.[7] Even the history of the civil rights movement has too often come to serve the myth of a nation always dedicated to universal freedom, equality, and justice, its complexity and its struggles rewritten to stand as a "shining example of the success of American democracy."[8] More recently, responses to the terrorist attacks of 9/11 suggest that the optimistic and redemptive narratives remain dominant strains in American culture.[9]

Given these parallels, it may seem only fair to excuse the Americans of the early twentieth century for their tendency to find the silver lining in the tragedy of the influenza crisis, for their determination to turn their attention to the future before them. It may be too harsh, or too cynical, for instance, to dismiss the responses of health care professionals as simply self-serving, or the broader culture's response as naïve and uncaring.[10] Though their optimism was coupled with significant opportunism, health care professionals' responses to the influenza catastrophe were nevertheless, at least for some, entirely sincere. Though the epidemic had shown the limitations of modern health care, these professionals, like other Americans facing other disasters, nevertheless believed in a brilliant future—for their professions and for the nation's health. In addition, many other Americans likely welcomed the upbeat narrative, finding in the optimism of public health leaders, physicians, and nurses the requisite strength and encouragement necessary to live full lives in the wake of incomprehensible loss. A classically American response to tragedy, then, the optimistic narrative employed in the aftermath of the pandemic was not unusual, and it may have served some people well.

But it is precisely Americans' repeated tendency to rewrite their past in order to make it tolerable, their continued willingness to embrace a single set of memories, to accept what is inevitably a sanitized and upbeat version of their country's history, that makes this phenomenon both important and troubling. How a people remember their past has real, lived consequences. Perhaps most important is the forgetting such remembering imposes, the silencing of other narratives the preferred storylines demand. In the case of the pandemic, the simplified and singular memory of the complex events of the crisis forestalled deeper analysis of the meaning of those events. In the case of health care professionals, the positive and ultimately triumphant narrative of their experience in the pandemic quieted the more troubled voices among them. Though for some scientists the mystery of the flu became a lifelong challenge that they pursued with dedication and diligence, for medicine and public health as a whole the chastening experience of the pandemic was soon dismissed as an exception or reconceptualized as a step on the way to further scientific, public health, and medical successes. Forgetting or rewriting the history of the pandemic as a medical and public health success had real costs. Official army data on the war, for instance, often cut the death figures in half by eliminating the losses due to influenza, misrepresenting the human costs suffered by the American military in World War I. Such a dismissal did little to prepare the army to control infectious disease during the next war. Though the military would prove far better at keeping their sick alive in World War II, outbreaks of tropical diseases in the

Pacific theatre ran rampant through the American forces and sometimes hampered American military efforts.[11]

Of broader significance, perhaps, is the way the narratives of democratic striving and opportunity hushed the realities of different and disparate circumstances during the pandemic.[12] Invisible in this account are the socioeconomic factors that shaped Americans' experiences of the pandemic. In this version, racism plays no role. Its victims, suffering from the cumulative consequences of centuries of white supremacy and consigned to shoddy facilities and inadequate care on the margins of the American community, are simply erased by a tale of shared suffering and a promising future. Similarly eliminated are the poor, their struggles to survive not only illness but also poverty glazed over in an uplifting tale of brotherhood and opportunity.

Finally, the optimistic and redemptive narratives ignore the importance of more than half a million influenza deaths in the United States. In the aftermath of the epidemic American public culture embraced a positive account of the pandemic—forward-looking, upbeat, and full of possibility. But this interpretation did not match the experiences of many Americans, those who continued to suffer either the physical or the emotional costs of the pandemic for decades afterward. What did the preference for the optimistic and redemptive narratives mean for those who did not embrace them but who experienced instead the dissonance of popular interpretations that shared nothing with their own?[13] How would the sense of opportunity and progress have sounded to someone who had lost a mother, a brother, a wife, a son? Is it possible that the upbeat narrative, embraced by many and clearly comforting to some, might have exacted steep costs for others?

An answer to these questions must prove elusive. Even when the sources are available, it is difficult to really imagine the suffering of others. Writing about the aftermath of his wife's sexual assault in a book first published in 1999, Jamie Kalven acknowledges the difficulty of really understanding the internal world of those who have suffered terrible events. "Day after day, week after week, month after month, year after year, what can it have been like for her?" he wondered of his wife. "I must strain to imagine it, to glimpse the sweep of it, and I have been here beside her every day."[14] How much harder it is for those of us who write about the distant peoples and events of the past. Is it possible for us to bring into focus the actions, experiences, and emotions of those we have never known, of those who lived so long before us, including those who suffered unimaginable tragedies such as the influenza pandemic?

Recent explorations of the aftermath of other catastrophes—from the individual and private trauma of rape to the communal and public tragedy of the Oklahoma City bombing, the 9/11 attacks, and Hurricane Katrina—offer some clues for thinking about those who suffered grievously in the epidemic, and who faced the conflict between public pronouncements of recovery and progress and their own persistent experiences of grief and loss. Perhaps most significantly, the cultural preference for optimistic narratives often seems to include a corollary, the expectation that everyone can and should heal from trauma and tragedy, the sooner the better. Even the diagnosis of post-traumatic stress disorder produces the expectation that people will be "cured," that a "healing process" will produce "closure."[15] The problem, though, is that such a perspective leaves no place for those who do not "heal."[16] For these Americans, the upbeat narrative neglects entirely the reality of their circumstances and can make their persistent pain appear "abnormal," even "pathological." For influenza survivors the dominance of the optimistic narrative left little room for their own narratives of loss. And yet the ability to tell one's story, to share one's narratives of trauma, is a fundamental requirement of recovery, offering the possibility not of returning to "normal" but of creating a new life that accepts the realities of the traumatic experience.[17] As survivors of the epidemic struggled through lives remade by grief and loss, they confronted a culture in which the optimistic narrative trumped their more painful rendition of the pandemic experience. As upbeat optimism suppressed the voices of trauma, many Americans were left to suffer in silence, their suffering likely deepened by that very silence.

Since 1997 a great deal of public attention has been turned to the pandemic of 1918, bringing this once-forgotten event slowly into Americans' public consciousness. A flurry of works on the pandemic has been published, illustrating a growing interest in all of its aspects and in its worldwide reach.[18] Even the genome of the 1918 virus has now been fully constructed. In the 1990s, two groups of scientists set out to find surviving samples of the virus responsible for the 1918 pandemic. One group headed by Kirsty Duncan, a geographer from Canada, planned to exhume bodies of miners who died of the flu while working on an island in the Norwegian Sea with the hope that the permafrost conditions might have preserved the virus in the victims' soft tissue. Though Duncan succeeded in getting permission to do the digging and garnered substantial media attention in the process, her 1998 expedition proved unsuccessful. Meanwhile, in 1995 Jeffery K. Taubenberger, a scientist working at the Armed Forces Institute of Pathology, began searching for the 1918 virus in lung samples taken from military victims of the epidemic, tissue preserved in paraffin and formaldehyde and stored at the institute for almost eighty years. Using a process called PCR, or polymerase chain reaction, Taubenberger and his lab technician, Ann Reid, knew they could build the virus if they could locate even fragmentary genetic remains of the 1918 killer. In 1996 they discovered pieces of the influenza virus in the lung tissue taken from a twenty-one-year-old private, Roscoe Vaughan, who had been stationed at Camp Jackson in South Carolina when he sickened and died from the flu. This breakthrough allowed them to begin constructing the virus bit by bit, work encouraged by the discovery of viable material in a second soldier's preserved lung tissue and in tissue removed from a body contained in permafrost in Brevig, Alaska, and discovered in a quiet and virtually solitary expedition by retired pathologist John Hultin.[19] As a result of this research, which is ongoing, the genomes of several 1918 influenza viruses have now been reconstructed.[20]

Even with this comprehensive knowledge of its genetic make-up, though, the influenza virus of 1918 continues to withhold some of its secrets. Despite the extensive historical, epidemiological, and genetic data now available, experts such as Taubenberger and his colleague David M. Morens of the National Institutes of Health suggest that the geographic genesis of the pandemic remains unknown.[21] And though it now seems reasonably certain that the virus that emerged in pandemic proportions that spring and fall was entirely new to humans, developing from an avian source, its path to human infection and to pandemic capabilities is not yet clear, and the explanation for its stunning pathogenicity and its patterns of fatality "remain[s] obscure."[22]

Even as these mysteries continue to provide scientists with puzzles to solve, influenza remains a continuing danger to an evermore-connected world. An H5N1 avian influenza virus captured worldwide attention in 1996. Originating in China and producing a shocking death rate among humans, the outbreak led to the slaughter of millions of waterfowl in Asia. Though the virus has now traveled to Eurasia and Africa, a human catastrophe has so far been avoided because of the virus's failure to adapt for human-to-human infection.[23] This H5N1 virus has had to share the public's attention since 2009, when a novel H1N1 influenza virus emerged and proved itself frighteningly infectious. By the end of 2009 it had reached 208 countries and cost over 12,000 lives. Fortunately, this virus, which moves easily from human to human, did not produce high mortality rates in its first wave, and its second wave, too, has proven much milder than expected.[24] Influenza is not alone in endangering human health today. A series of new and emerging infectious diseases such as Ebola, SARS (severe acute respiratory virus), and the West Nile Virus has created substantial problems for public health efforts even as older diseases such as tuberculosis have developed new and troubling antibiotic resistant strains.[25] We cannot pretend that another epidemic will not someday emerge to race around the globe and stun humankind as Spanish influenza did in 1918.

The question that confronts us is whether it, too, will be forgotten. The AIDS (acquired immune deficiency syndrome) epidemic suggests that it need not be. In late June 1987, Cleve Jones and several others in the San Francisco gay community established the NAMES Project Foundation and began work on the AIDS Memorial Quilt, a project that grew out of a need for public remembering, out of what Jones described as "a deep yearning not only to find a way to grieve individually and together but also to find a voice that could be heard beyond our community, beyond our town."[26] Announcing itself with just forty squares and the promise of a display on the National Mall later in the year, the project took off in the summer of 1987 with a pace suggesting the need it filled. By the time the Quilt arrived in Washington, D.C., for its first public display on October 11, 1987, it had grown to 2,000 squares, a number that continued to grow exponentially, reaching 32,000 in the Quilt's first eight years.[27] For many Americans, it seems, the Quilt served its creators' purposes. As the historian John D'Emilio, who saw the Quilt during that first showing on the National Mall, wrote in a letter to a friend months later, "Instead of individual, silent, pent-up grief, the quilt had made it possible for grief to be shared, released, and finished with in a collective fashion—and for the lives of those who had died to be remembered with dignity and respect." And further, "The NAMES Project was a way to grieve publicly and collectively, to affirm the value of the lives of those who died, and to call attention to the severity of the epidemic."[28]

The AIDS Quilt is not an uncontested memorial. Even in its origins, the gay community of San Francisco out of which it first emerged offered a diversity of responses to it. How much more complex were the reactions it engendered across a country fighting the culture wars of the 1980s.[29] Today, too, the Quilt remains a focus for debate as scholars and activists alike explore its meanings and its consequences, its functions and its limits.[30] Even with this promising attention, the history of the AIDS epidemic is not yet remembered or written with the fullness that the complexity of that tragedy requires. And of course that tragedy continues, made worse by the way inequities have ensured disparate experiences of the disease. As Richard Kim suggested in 2002, "The current demographic of AIDS, marked as they are by severe economic and racial inequality, were not preordained. AIDS is a preventable and treatable disease, and it exists as it does because it was allowed to unfold this way."[31] Today AIDS ravages some communities but not others, some continents suffer deaths in the millions while others benefit from retroviral drugs, its sufferers too frequently suffer the marginalization of stigmatizing, and educational efforts around the world remain stalled by moral and political authorities unwilling to care enough to save lives. And yet the Quilt does offer one example of an epidemic kept alive in public life and memory through intentional memorializing efforts. Even the debates it has engendered have served to keep our eyes and our minds on the pandemic.

There is no simple way to prepare for the pandemics of the future. As a recent volume on influenza and public health reminded its readers, "Each pandemic unfolds in a different way."[32] While we will turn to scientists to determine the best way to contain disease, and public health leaders to determine the best way to protect and educate the public, it will be left to others of us to remember and act on the human lessons of the 1918 pandemic. Should we face such an eventuality, let us prove better prepared to admit to a tale of sorrow and loss, to acknowledge the trauma such a tragedy leaves in its wake, and to provide the support and understanding sufferers would need in its wake.

ABBREVIATIONS

AA	*Afro-American* (Baltimore)
AJN	*American Journal of Nursing*
AJPH	*American Journal of Public Health*
AC	*Atlanta Constitution*
APHA	American Public Health Association
ARC	American Red Cross
CSJM	*California State Journal of Medicine*
CT	Chicago Tribune
CSM	*Christian Science Monitor*
HM	*Hahnemannian Monthly*
IMJ	*Illinois Medical Journal*
JAMA	*Journal of the American Medical Association*
JAOA	*Journal of the American Osteopathic Association*
JLCM	*Journal of Laboratory and Clinical Medicine*
JNMA	*Journal of the National Medical Association*
KMJ	*Kentucky Medical Journal*
LAT	*Los Angeles Times*
LD	*Literary Digest*
MH	*Modern Hospital*
MO	*Morning Oregonian* (Portland)
MRR	*Medical Review of Reviews*
MS	*Military Surgeon*
NA	National Archives
NA (PAR)	National Archives, Pacific-Alaska Region (Seattle, Washington)
NAJH	*North American Journal of Homeopathy*

NLM   National Library of Medicine
NYMJ   *New York Medical Journal*
NYT   *New York Times*
PHN   *Public Health Nurse*
PHR   *Public Health Reports*
PI   *Post-Intelligencer* (Seattle, Washington)
USAMHI   U. S. Army Military History Institute, Carlisle Barracks
           (WWORP: World War One Research Project)
           (AEQC: Army Experiences Questionnaire Collection)
USPHS   United States Public Health Service
WN   *World News* (Roanoke, Virginia)

NOTES

Introduction

1. Niall P. A. S. Johnson and Juergen Mueller, "Updating the Accounts: Global Mortality of the 1918–1920 'Spanish' Influenza Pandemic," *Bulletin of the History of Medicine* 76 (Spring 2002): 114–115; Jeffery K. Taubenberger and David M. Morens, "1918 Influenza: the Mother of All Pandemics," *Emerging Infectious Diseases* 12 (January 2006): 15. The term "epidemic" refers to an outbreak of a disease that affects large numbers simultaneously throughout a particular community or region. The term "pandemic" refers to still larger events.

2. Ibid., 107; Jeffery K. Taubenberger and David M. Morens, "Influenza: The Once and Future Pandemic," *Public Health Reports* (hereafter *PHR*) 125 (2010, Supplement 3): 19–20; Dorothy A. Pettit and Janice Bailie, *A Cruel Wind: Pandemic Flu in America, 1918–1920* (Murfreesboro, TN: Timberlane Books, 2008), chap. 7. I would like to thank Howard Markel for illuminating the idea of a fourth wave.

3. Taubenberger and Morens, "Influenza: The Once and Future Pandemic," 20; Taubenberger and Morens, "1918 Influenza: the Mother of All Pandemics," 15.

4. Andrew Noymer and Michel Garenne, "Long-term effects of the 1918 'Spanish' influenza epidemic on sex differentials of mortality in the USA: Exploratory findings from historical data," in *The Spanish Influenza Pandemic of 1918–19: New Perspectives*, ed. Howard Phillips and David Killingray (London: Routledge, 2003), 202.

5. Taubenberger and Morens, "Influenza: The Once and Future Pandemic," 20–21.

6. James D. Bristow, interview by the author, August 6, 2004.

7. Alfred W. Crosby, *Epidemic and Peace, 1918* (Westport, CT: Greenwood Press, 1976), 311.

8. Alfred W. Crosby, *America's Forgotten Pandemic: The Influenza of 1918* (New York: Cambridge University Press, 1989), 314–315.

9. See for instance Philip C. Ensley, "Indiana and the Influenza Pandemic of 1918," *Indiana Medical History Quarterly* 9 (1983): 3; Kim Allen Scott, "Plague on the Homefront: Arkansas and the Great Influenza Epidemic of 1918," *Arkansas Historical Quarterly* 47 (1988): 319; Jack Fincher, "America's Deadly Rendezvous with the 'Spanish Lady,'" *Smithsonian* 19 (1989): 139; Russell R. Elliott, "The Influenza Epidemic of 1918–1919," *Halcyon* 14 (1992): 256; Gina Kolata, *Flu: The Story of the Great Influenza Pandemic of 1918 and the Search for the Virus That Caused It* (New York: Farrar, Straus and Giroux, 1999), x; John Barry, *The Great Influenza: The Epic Story of the Deadliest Plague in History* (New York: Viking, 2004), 393–394; Carol R. Byerly, *Fever of War: The Influenza Epidemic in the U.S. Army During World War I* (New York: New York University Press, 2005), 187–190; Ilana Lowy, "Comment: Influenza and Historians: A Difficult Past" in *Influenza and Public Health: Learning from Past Pandemics*, ed. Tamara Giles-Vernick and Susan Craddock (London: Earthscan, 2010), 91, 95–96.

10. See for instance Gabriel W. Kirkpatrick, "Influenza 1918: A Maine Perspective," *Maine Historical Society Quarterly* 25 (1986): 173–175; Ann McLaurin, "The Influenza Epidemic of

1918 in Shreveport," *North Louisiana Historical Association* 13 (1982): 11; Pettit and Bailie, *A Cruel Wind*, 228; Barry, *The Great Influenza*, 393.

11. Crosby, *America's Forgotten Pandemic*, 322–323.

12. Michael R. Bristow, interview with author, August 6, 2004.

13. James D. Bristow, interview with author, August 6, 2004.

14. Kathleen S. Bristow, interview with author, August 6, 2004.

15. Edward T. Linenthal, *The Unfinished Bombing: Oklahoma City in American Memory* (New York: Oxford University Press, 2001), 41, 253; Lawrence Langer, *Admitting the Holocaust; Collected Essays* (New Haven: Yale University Press, 1995); Lawrence Langer, *Preempting the Holocaust* (New Haven: Yale University Press, 1998).

16. For a broad introduction to collective memory studies see Jeffrey K. Olick, Vered Vinitzky-Seroussi, and Daniel Levy, *The Collective Memory Reader* (New York: Oxford University Press, 2011); Susanna Radstone and Bill Schwarz, *Memory: Histories, Theories, Debates* (New York: Fordham University Press, 2010). For excellent examples of the study of American memory by historians, see for instance John Bodnar, *The "Good War" in American Memory* (Baltimore: Johns Hopkins University Press, 2010); Karl Jacoby, *Shadows at Dawn: A Borderlands Massacre and the Violence of History* (New York: Penguin, 2008); Renee C. Romano and Leigh Raiford, eds., *The Civil Rights Movement in American Memory* (Athens: University of Georgia Press, 2006); James Oliver Horton and Lois E. Horton, *Slavery and Public History: The Tough Stuff of American Memory* (Chapel Hill: University of North Carolina Press, 2006); David W. Blight, *Race and Reunion: The Civil War in American Memory* (Cambridge, MA: Harvard University Press, 2001); W. Fitzhugh Brundage, ed., *Where These Memories Grow: History, Memory, and Southern Identity* (Chapel Hill: University of North Carolina Press, 2000); John E. Bodnar, *Remaking America: Public Memory, Commemoration and Patriotism in the Twentieth Century* (Princeton, NJ: Princeton University Press, 1992).

17. Crosby, *Forgotten Pandemic*, 321–322; Scott, "Plague on the Homefront," 319–320.

18. Kirkpatrick, "Influenza 1918," 175.

19. David M. Kennedy, *Over Here: The First World War and American Society* (New York: Oxford University Press, 1980); Christopher Capozzola, *Uncle Sam Wants You: World War I and the Making of the Modern Citizen* (New York: Oxford University Press, 2010).

20. Crosby, *America's Forgotten Pandemic*, 320.

21. Ensley, "Indiana and the Influenza Pandemic of 1918," 12; Joann P. Krieg, *Epidemics in the Modern World* (New York: Twayne Publishing, 1992), 19.

22. H. L. Mencken, quoted in Richard Collier, *The Plague of the Spanish Lady: The Spanish Influenza Pandemic of 1918–1919* (New York: Atheneum, 1974), 304. See also Krieg, *Epidemics in the Modern World*, 2–12.

23. Barry, *The Great Influenza*, 394.

24. James Longrigg, "Epidemic, Ideas and Classical Athenian Society," in *Epidemics and Ideas: Essays on the Historical Perception of Pestilence*, ed. Terrence Ranger and Paul Slack (New York: Cambridge University Press, 1992), 27.

25. Susan J. Brison, *Aftermath: Violence and the Remaking of a Self* (Princeton, NJ: Princeton University Press, 2002), 9.

26. Linenthal, *The Unfinished Bombing*, 253. Linenthal was discussing the work of Lawrence Langer.

27. Crosby, *America's Forgotten Pandemic*, 319.

28. Kolata, *Flu*, 6.

29. Carol Byerly illustrates the military medical staff's effort to rewrite the history of the epidemic as a success in Byerly, *Fever of War*, chap. 6 and conclusion.

30. W. A. Brooks, "Out-Door Treatment of Spanish Influenza," *The Modern Hospital* 11 (December 1918): 427.

Chapter 1

1. "Europe's Latest Scourge," *New York Times* (hereafter *NYT*) December 11, 1889, 5; "The Epidemic of Influenza," *Chicago Tribune* (hereafter *CT*), December 12, 1889, 6; "The Influenza Epidemic," *NYT*, December 12, 1889, 2; "The Influenza Epidemic," *Los Angeles Times* (hereafter

LAT), December 13, 1889, 1; "Spread of Influenza," *CT*, December 13, 1889, 6; "Europe's Epidemic," *NYT*, December 14, 1889, 2; "The Influenza," *LAT*, December 26, 1889, 1.

2. "Everybody Is Sneezing," *CT*, December 15, 1889, 4.

3. "The Influenza Epidemic in Europe," *CT*, December 15, 1889, 12.

4. Editorial, *NYT*, December 11, 1889, 4.

5. "The Influenza Here," *NYT*, December 19, 1889, 1.

6. "Influenza's Fatal Phase," *NYT*, December 27, 1889, 2; "Virulence in Europe," *NYT*, December 28, 1889, 1.

7. "Gaining a Foothold Everywhere," *CT*, December 29, 1889, 2.

8. "First Fatal Case in Chicago," *CT*, December 29, 1889, 2.

9. "West Virginia Has It," *CT*, January 4, 1890, 2.

10. "All Baltimore Seized," *CT*, January 5, 1890, 3.

11. "It Has a Firm Grip on Milwaukee," *CT*, January 5, 1890, 3.

12. "Sickness in Oregon," *Morning Oregonian* (hereafter *MO*), January 2, 1890, 2.

13. "Dying by Hundreds . . . Raging in Dakota," *Newark Daily Advocate* (Ohio), January 9, 1890, 1.

14. "La Grippe—The Disease Has a Firm Hold on San Francisco," *LAT*, January 17, 1890, 5.

15. "It Is Spreading—The Influenza Is the Biggest Thing in Atlanta Just Now," *Atlanta Constitution* (hereafter *AC*), January 30, 1890, 5.

16. "Rough on the Indians," *Oregon Statesman*, January 31, 1890, 4.

17. "The Fatal Influenza," *San Antonio Daily Express*, January 16, 1890, 1.

18. "An Official Warning," *NYT*, January 1, 1890, 1.

19. Editorial, *NYT*, January 2, 1890, 4.

20. "They Have the Grip—New York and Philadelphia Policemen Down with the Russian Disease," *AC*, December 31, 1889, 1; "March of La Grippe—Bad in Detroit," *AC*, December 29, 1889, 11.

21. "March of La Grippe—Bad in Detroit," 11.

22. "March of La Grippe—Post Office Employees Prostrated," *AC*, December 29, 1889, 11; "Der Blitzen Krankheit," *San Antonio Daily Express*, January 24, 1890, 5.

23. "It Ends in Death," *AC*, January 3, 1890, 1; "La Grippe Among the Convicts," *Marshall Daily Chronicle* (Michigan), January 11, 1890, 1.

24. "It Hits the Cops—Bad in Milwaukee," *AC*, January 7, 1890, 1.

25. "Effects of Influenza," *Newark Daily Advocate* (Ohio), January 4, 1890, 1.

26. "La Grippe Holds the Town," *San Antonio Daily Light*, January 28, 1890, 1.

27. "It was supposed that Astoria . . .," two sentence article without title, *Daily Astorian* (Oregon), January 24, 1890, 3; "Railroadings," *LAT*, January 20, 1890, 2; "Down with the 'Grippe,'" *AC*, January 15, 1890, 1.

28. "Monmouth Notes," *Oregon Statesman*, January 31, 1890, 1; Brief article, no author, no title, *Daily Astorian*, January 26, 1890, 3.

29. Michael B. A. Oldstone, *Viruses, Plagues, and History* (New York: Oxford University Press, 1998), 178.

30. Jeffery K. Taubenberger and David M. Morens, "Influenza: The Once and Future Pandemic," *PHR* 125 (2010, Supplement 3): 17; August Hirsch, *Handbook of Geographical and Historical Pathology*, I, cited in William H. McNeill, *Plagues and Peoples* (New York: Anchor Books, 1998), n. 90, 353; Madeline Drexler, *Secret Agents: The Menace of Emerging Infections* (New York: Penguin Books, 2003), 161; John Barry, *The Great Influenza: The Epic Story of the Deadliest Plague in History* (New York: Penguin/Viking, 2004), 113–114.

31. Roy Porter, *The Greatest Benefit to Mankind* (New York: W.W. Norton and Co., 1998), 164.

32. McNeill, *Plagues and Peoples*, 218.

33. Oldstone, *Viruses, Plagues and History*, 178–179; Dorothy A. Pettit and Janice Bailie, *A Cruel Wind: Pandemic Flu in America, 1918–1920* (Murfreesboro, TN: Timberlane Books, 2008), 22–24.

34. Arno Karlen, *Man and Microbes: Disease and Plagues in History and Modern Times* (New York: Touchstone, 1995), 144.

35. The term "allopath" had its origins with the homeopaths, who used it to portray practitioners of regular medicine as "merely one type of physician." Though the term as defined

by Hahnemann, the founder of homeopathy, had a specific meaning, describing "one who would offer treatments that produce completely opposite effects of the disease when administered in health," over the decades the term lost this specific meaning, and came to serve as a generic term for "regular" physicians. Norman Gevitz, *The D.O.'s: Osteopathic Medicine in America* (Baltimore: Johns Hopkins University Press, 1982), 8.

36. Nancy Tomes, *The Gospel of Germs: Men, Women, and the Microbe in American Life* (Cambridge, MA: Harvard University Press, 1998), 33, 38–43.

37. Lester S. King, *Transformations in American Medicine: From Benjamin Rush to William Osler* (Baltimore: Johns Hopkins University Press, 1991), 142; Porter, *The Greatest Benefit to Mankind*, 10; Tomes, *The Gospel of Germs*, 29. A brief word on terminology is appropriate here. The terms "infectious," "contagious," and "communicable" have very distinct meanings. As Nancy Tomes explains, "'Infectious' denotes a disease that may spread from person to person without actual contact between them; in contrast, a contagious disease is directly transmitted from person to person. 'Communicable' is a more general term that covers both infectious and contagious diseases." Complicating these understandings, though, is the reality is that these terms were often used interchangeably in the late nineteenth and early twentieth centuries, in part because it was so difficult for physicians to determine the proper category for many of the diseases with which they wrestled in that period. For that reason, I agree with Nancy Tomes that the terms should not be read too literally or precisely in materials from this time. Tomes, *The Gospel of Germs*, 20.

38. Barry, *The Great Influenza*, 49.

39. Tomes, *The Gospel of Germs*, 27, 29.

40. John Duffy, *The Sanitarians: A History of American Public Health* (Chicago: University of Illinois Press, 1990), 99.

41. David Rosner, "Introduction," *Hives of Sickness: Public Health and Epidemics in New York City*, ed. David Rosner (New Brunswick, NJ: Rutgers University Press, 1995), 9.

42. Sheila Rothman, *Living in the Shadow of Death: Tuberculosis and the Social Experience of Illness in American History* (New York: Basic Books, 1994), 17; Tomes, *Gospel of Germs*, 4.

43. Duffy, *The Sanitarians*, chap. 6 and 93; David Rosner, "'Spanish Flu, or Whatever It Is. . . .': The Paradox of Public Health in a Time of Crisis," *PHR* 125 (2010, Supplement 3): 39–40.

44. Rosner, "'Spanish Flu, or Whatever It Is. . . .,'" 39–40. On garbage see Martin V. Melosi, *Garbage in the Cities: Refuse, Reform, and the Environment*, 3rd ed. (Pittsburgh: University of Pittsburgh Press, 2005).

45. Elizabeth Fee, "Public Health and the State: The United States," *The History of Public Health and the Modern State*, ed. Dorothy Porter (New York: Clio Medica, 1994), 225–227, 229; Duffy, *The Sanitarians*, 96, 99.

46. Duffy, *The Sanitarians*, 66–67.

47. Rosner, "'Spanish Flu, or Whatever It Is,'" 41.

48. Dorothy Porter, *Health, Civilization and the State: A history of public health from ancient to modern times* (New York: Routledge, 1999), 146–162; Rosner, "'Spanish Flu, or Whatever It Is,'" 42.

49. Duffy, *The Sanitarians*, chaps. 7 and 8.

50. Ibid., 120–123, 138–147, 149–154; Porter, *Health, Civilization and the State*, 154–155. The southern region lagged behind the rest of the country as it struggled through recovery from the Civil War, and continued to neglect its African American citizens even as urban public health efforts began to gain traction.

51. Duffy, *The Sanitarians*, chap. 11 and 240–242.

52. James H. Cassedy, *Medicine in America: A Short History* (Baltimore: Johns Hopkins University Press, 1991), 117–119.

53. Duffy, *The Sanitarians*, 130, 162; Porter, *Health, Civilization and the State*, 156.

54. King, *Transformations in American Medicine*, chaps. 7–9; Duffy, *The Sanitarians*, chap. 13; Tomes, *The Gospel of Germs*, 6.

55. Charles Chapin, quoted in Barry, *The Great Influenza*, 53. Chapin would go on to serve as the Superintendent of Health of the City of Providence, Rhode Island, and to a distinguished career as a leader in the developing science of public health administration. He would play a substantial public role during the pandemic of 1918. See James H. Cassedy,

Charles V. Chapin and the Public Health Movement (Cambridge, MA: Harvard University Press, 1962).

56. Rosner, "Introduction," *Hives of Sickness,* 9–11.
57. C. Edson, "Defenses Against Epidemic Diseases," *Forum* 9 (June 1890): 475.
58. Tomes, *Gospel of Germs,* 6.
59. Edson, "Defenses Against Epidemic Diseases," 481.
60. Gina Kolata, *Flu: The Story of the Great Influenza Pandemic of 1918 and the Search for the Virus That Caused It* (New York: Farrar, Straus and Giroux, 1999), 47; Tomes, *The Gospel of Germs,* 45.
61. Unfortunately, there was little public health response to the pandemic in the United States in 1889–1890. See Nancy Tomes, "'Destroyer and Teacher': Managing the Masses During the 1918–1919 Influenza Pandemic," *PHR* (2010, Supplement 3): 50.
62. "The Epidemic," in "Miscellany," *Journal of the American Medical Association* (hereafter *JAMA*) 14 (January 25, 1890): 143.
63. *Index Medicus: A Monthly Classified Record of the Current Medical Literature of the World* (Boston: George S. Davis, 1891). See for instance pages 105, 544. The heading "Influenza and Dengue" appeared under the category "General Diseases—A. (Diseases Dependent on Morbid Poisons)."
64. "Domestic Correspondence—Letter from Philadelphia (From our own correspondent)," *JAMA* 16 (June 13, 1890): 862. See also Alex. L. Hodgdon, "A Few Observations on the Treatment of Epidemic Influenza," *Maryland Medical Journal* 26 (February 13, 1892): 881.
65. C. F. Ulrich, "Some of the Vagaries of the Grippe," *JAMA* 15 (October 4, 1890): 495.
66. William Porter, "Epidemic Influenza," read before the St. Louis Academy of Medicine, *JAMA* 14 (January 25, 1890): 114–115.
67. L. F. Bryson, "The Present Epidemic of Influenza," and responses at the New York Academy of Medicine, recounted in "Society Proceedings—New York Academy of Medicine—Section on Theory and Practice of Medicine," *JAMA* 14 (March 22, 1890): 427–428; "Topics of the Week—Ocular Complications in Influenza," *JAMA* 14 (June 7, 1890): 834; E. Fletcher Ingals, "The Epidemics of Influenza of 1890 and 1891 in Chicago," *Climatologist* 2 (1892): 225–226; "Editorial—Influenza," *JAMA* 13 (March 26, 1892): 397; N. S. Davis, "Report on the Meteorological Conditions and Their Relations to the Epidemic Influenza, and Some Other Diseases in Chicago During the Six Months Ending March 31, 1890," *JAMA* 14 (June 7, 1890): 818.
68. See for instance "On Psychoses After Influenza," *JAMA* 15 (September 13, 1890): 398; C.H. Hughes, "The Epidemic Inflammatory Neurosis; or, Neurotic Influenza" (read before the St. Louis Medical Society, January 30, 1892), *JAMA* 13 (February 27, 1892): 245–249; F.D. Thompson, "La Grippe, as It Prevailed in North Texas," *Virginia Medical Monthly* 18 (1891–1892): 366, 367; George Allen, "Cases of Insanity Following 'La Grippe,'" *North American Journal of Homeopathy* (hereafter *NAJH*) 6 (1891): 718–721; Charles K. Mills, "The Nervous and Mental Phenomena and Sequelae of Influenza," *JAMA* 18 (January 30, 1892): 121–127.
69. Morell Mackenzie, "Influenza," *Living Age* (August 1, 1891): 299. Mackenzie founded the field of laryngology in England and was also co-founder of the *Journal of Laryngology.* For a complete biography, see R. Scott Stevenson, *Morell Mackenzie: The Story of a Victorian Tragedy* (London: Heinemann Medical, 1946).
70. "Editorial—Influenza," *JAMA* 18 (March 26, 1892): 397. See also Ulrich, "Some Vagaries of the Grippe," 496; F. D. Thompson, "La Grippe, as It Prevailed in North Texas," 367; S. J. Radcliffe, "Epidemic Influenza with Cases Illustrating Some of Its Peculiar Complications," *Virginia Medical Monthly* 18 (1892): 1048, 1050–1051.
71. Mackenzie, "Influenza," 300; "Society Proceedings—New York Academy of Medicine," *JAMA* 14 (March 22, 1890): 426–427; John Eyler, "The State of Science, Microbiology, and Vaccines Circa 1918," *PHR* 125 (2010, Supplement 3): 28.
72. A. C. Davidson, "La Grippe: Its Etiology, Clinical History, and Treatment," *Southern Medical Record* 21 (October 1891): 473.
73. Taubenberger and Morens, "Influenza: The Once and Future Pandemic," 18. For a fuller discussion of the research leading to the discovery of the influenza virus, see John Barry,

The Great Influenza: The Epic Story of the Deadliest Plague in History (New York: Viking, 2004), Part X.

74. The author thanks Dr. James D. Bristow for his essential contributions to this discussion. See also "Flu Pandemics," http://www.flu.gov/individualfamily/about/pandemic/index. html [accessed March 7, 2011]; Taubenberger and Morens, "Influenza: The Once and Future Pandemic," 18–19.

75. "Editorial—The Epidemic," *JAMA* 14 (January 11, 1890): 60.

76. "Influenza in England," in "Editorial Notes and Items," *JAMA* 16 (June 20, 1891): 894"; "Editorial—Influenza," *JAMA* 18 (March 26, 1892): 397.

77. Tomes, *The Gospel of Germs*, 7, 34.

78. "Editorial—The Epidemic," *JAMA* 14 (January 11, 1890): 61.

79. Davidson, "La Grippe," 474. *Ignis fatuus* is the gaseous haze that builds above marshes and swamps. It can also refer to a "will-o-the-wisp," hence suggesting Davidson's dismissal of germ theory as a mysterious and fleeting theory.

80. One clear indication of this tendency to connect the atmosphere and the epidemic was the appearance in the journal *Climatologist* of articles related to the epidemic. The *Climatologist* described itself as "A Monthly Journal of Medicine Devoted to the Relation of Climate, Mineral Springs, Diet, Preventive Medicine, Race, Occupation, Life Insurance, and Sanitary Science to Disease." See for instance Ingals, "The Epidemics of Influenza of 1890 and 1891 in Chicago," 223–230; John C. Munro, "The Epidemiology of Influenza," *Climatologist* 2 (1892): 231–235; Roland G. Curtin and Edward W. Watson, "Epidemic of Influenza in Philadelphia in 1889, '90, '91," *Climatologist* 2 (1892): 77–94.

81. "Topics of the Week—Epidemic Visitation," *JAMA* 15 (September 27, 1890): 476.

82. "Editorial Notes—The Influenza Epidemic of 1889," *JAMA* 14 (January 4, 1890): 25.

83. "Miscellany—Mortality by Influenza Influenced by Humidity," *JAMA* 24 (March 9, 1895): 379; "The Present Epidemic of Influenza," in "Miscellany," *JAMA* 21 (December 16, 1893): 951; "Cold Comes Through the Feet," *Marshall Daily Chronicle* (Michigan), April 25, 1890, 1; "Dr. Richardson on Chloroform and Influenza," *Review of Reviews* 5 (June 1892): 598.

84. "La Grippe," *JAMA* 17 (December 26, 1891): 993.

85. "Society Proceedings—New York Academy of Medicine," *JAMA* 14 (March 22, 1890): 427, 428.

86. "Letter from Philadelphia (From our own correspondent)," in "Domestic Correspondence," *JAMA* 16 (June 13, 1891): 862; "Practical Notes—The Treatment of Influenza," *JAMA* 14 (January 25, 1890): 137; "Practical Notes—The Treatment of Influenza," *JAMA* 14 (February 8, 1890): 209; Davidson, "La Grippe," 478.

87. James M. Anders, "Clinical Features of the Present Epidemic of Influenza," *Medical and Surgical Reporter* 66 (1892): 448; "Practical Notes—The Treatment of Influenza," *JAMA* 14 (February 8, 1890): 209.

88. For a fuller discussion of the competition among medical practitioners in the nineteenth century, see William Rothstein, *American Physicians in the Nineteenth Century: From Sects to Science* (Baltimore: Johns Hopkins University Press, 1972).

89. Cassedy, *Medicine in America*, 37; Martin Kaufman, "Homeopathy in America," in *Other Healers: Unorthodox Medicine in America*, ed. Norman Gevitz (Baltimore: Johns Hopkins University Press, 1988), 99–101; James C. Whorton, *Nature Cures: The History of Alternative Medicine in America* (New York: Oxford University Press, 2002), 61.

90. Whorton, *Nature Cures*, 51–52; Kaufman, "Homeopathy in America," 99.

91. Kaufman, "Homeopathy in America," 99–100; Whorton, *Nature Cures*, 49, 64.

92. Whorton, *Nature Cures*, 64–68.

93. "Homeopaths Tackle La Grippe—They Blame the Brethren of the Old School for This Among Other Things," *CT*, January 26, 1890, 4.

94. Allen, "Cases of Insanity Following 'La Grippe,'" 720, 721.

95. "The Psychology of Epidemics," excerpted from *The Lancet*, published under "Topics of the Week," *JAMA* 14 (March 15, 1890): 387, 388.

96. Tomes, *Gospel of Germs*, 50.

97. Tomes, *Gospel of Germs*, 26–29, 34–38, 49–58.

98. "La Grippe," *CT*, December 28, 1889, 4.

99. "The Source of La Grippe—Russian Influenza Caused by an Infusorial Parasite," *CT*, January 3, 1890, 9 (Supplemental section).

100. "Chicago Is Stricken," *CT*, January 7, 1890, 1.

101. "The Microbe and Its Mission," *CT*, January 12, 1890, 12.

102. J. H. Kedzie, "The Grip and Sun Spots," *CT*, January 13, 1890, 6.

103. "La Grippe and Microbes," *CT*, January 14, 1890, 9 (supplemental sheet).

104. See for instance "Sneezing's the Fad," *CT*, December 18, 1889, 1; "Chicago in for It," *CT*, December 28, 1889, 1; "Dr. Rauch Discusses 'La Grippe,'" *CT*, January 4, 1890, 2; "Chicago Is Stricken—All the Doctors Agree That the Influenza Is Here," *CT*, January 7, 1890, 1; "Doctors Disagree," *CT*, January 11, 1890, 1.

105. "Paris in a Real Panic," *CT*, December 29, 1889, 2; "Got 'Em in the Grip," *AC*, January 26, 1890, 22; "A Doctor on the Grippe," *AC*, January 27, 1890, 4.

106. "Philadelphia Has Not Escaped," *CT*, December 28, 1889, 1.

107. "A Remedy for La Grippe," *Eastern Oregon Republican*, January 30, 1890, 3. See also "Influenza's Victim," *CT*, January 20, 1890, 1.

108. "Is Grippe Contagious?" ad for Paine's Celery Compound, *CT*, January 30, 1890, 5.

109. "Here It Is!" ad for Hunnicutt's Throat and Lung Cure, *AC*, January 1, 1890, 3.

110. "Ubiquitous La Grippe," *LAT*, December 31, 1889, 4; "The Great Leveler," *San Antonio Daily Light*, January 8, 1890, 1; "All Europe A-Sneeze—Russian Influenza Has Its Grip on the People—High, Low, Rich and Poor Alike Affected," *San Antonio Daily Express*, December 25, 1889, 1; "The Progress of the World," *Review of Reviews* 1 (February 1890): 87.

111. Editorial, no title, *CT*, December 19, 1989, 4.

112. "First Fatal Case in Chicago," *CT*, December 29, 1889, 2.

113. "New Cases Without Number—Five Thousand Cases in Cleveland, O.—In Other Cities," *CT*, January 4, 1890, 2; "La Grippe's Doings—The List of Its Victims Is Increasing," *LAT*, December 30, 1889, 1; "Dying by the Hundred—The Deadly La Gripe Decimating the City of New York," *Daily Astorian*, January 10, 1890, 3.

114. "State Board of Health—Facts Contained in Its Annual Report Just Issued," *NYT*, February 7, 1890, 2.

115. "La Grippe," *LAT*, January 4, 1890, 4. See also "Editorials," *LAT*, January 6, 1890, 7; "Editorials," *LAT*, January 25, 1890, 7; "Now Here or Coming?" *LAT*, January 15, 1890, 7; "Editorials," *LAT*, February 7, 1890, 7.

116. "They Have the Grip," *AC*, December 31, 1889, 1.

117. "It Is One of Fashion's Fads," *CT*, January 3, 1890, 2.

118. "Have They La Grippe?" *Des Moines Homestead* (Iowa), January 24, 1890, 14.

119. "The Rear Guard of the Grippe," *San Antonio Daily Express*, January 21, 1890, 2.

120. "March of the Malady," *NYT*, January 7, 1890, 1. See for instance "La Grippe," *LAT*, January 4, 1890, 4; "The Grippe," *NYT*, January 26, 1890, 4; "La Grippe a Century Ago," *NYT*, January 12, 1890, 5; "Obesity and La Grippe," *NYT*, January 22, 1890, 3; "Sneezing's the Fad—A Century of the Epidemic," *CT*, December 18, 1889, 1; "First Fatal Case in Chicago," *CT*, December 29, 1889, 2; "Views of North Side Physicians," *CT*, January 7, 1890, 2; no title, *Lafayette Advertiser* (Louisiana), April 5, 1890, 2; "Jacob the Patriarch—Had La Grippe—Consumption as Old as the Hills," *LAT*, February 26, 1891, 7.

121. Both during and after the pandemic, medical observers sometimes criticized Americans for their lackadaisical response to its dangers. See for instance "Topics of the Week—The Influenza Epidemic in Germany," *JAMA* 14 (January 18, 1890): 100; Mackenzie, "Influenza," 296; Ingals, "The Epidemics of Influenza of 1890 and 1891 in Chicago," 557; "La Grippe," *JAMA* 17 (December 26, 1891): 993.

122. "The Little Grip—It Has Been Coming—It Is Now Here," *AC*, January 25, 1890, 5.

123. "Brevities," *Marshall Daily Chronicle* (Michigan), April 21, 1891, 3.

124. "What's the Matter with Him, Doctor?" *Harper's Weekly* 34 (January 11, 1890): 23.

125. "Between Sneezes," *CT*, December 29, 1889, 12; "La Grippe," *CT*, December 30, 1889, 4.

126. See for instance "Grip and Gondoliers—Both Disease and Opera Have Captured New York," *AC*, January 12, 1890, 9; "Preparing for Battle," *Des Moines Homestead* (Iowa), May 30, 1890, 14; "Why Not Get at the Facts," *NYT*, October 5, 1891, 4; No title, *San Antonio Daily Light*, January 17, 1890, 8.

127. See for instance ad for Wilbor's Cod Liver Oil and Phosphates, *CT*, January 13, 1890, 8; ad for Jacoby Brothers, Retail Department, *LAT*, January 18, 1890, 8; "Let Me Influenzu," ad for Herman Wise, The Old Reliable Clothier and Hatter, *Daily Astorian*, January 10, 1890, 3; ad for Sunset Wood Company, *San Antonio Daily Light*, January 25, 1890, 9.

128. "The Doctor's Prescription," ad for Golden Eagle Clothing Company, *LAT*, January 30, 1890, 3.

129. Ad for Andrew J. Miller and Son, *AC*, February 2, 1890, 1.

130. Barry, *The Great Influenza*, 70–71.

131. Tomes, *The Gospel of Germs*, 92, 94; McNeill, *Plagues and Peoples*, 278–279, 284–286, 289; Karlen, *Man and Microbes*, 139.

132. "La Grippe," *JAMA* 17 (December 26, 1891): 993; "Editorial Notes—Treatment of Influenza," *JAMA* 16 (May 9, 1891): 675; Porter, "Epidemic Influenza," 115.

133. E.J. Blair, brief excerpt published in "Selections," *JAMA* 18 (May 14, 1892): 628.

134. "Editorial Notes—The Epidemic," 60, 61; "Note on the Bronchitis of Influenza," from *The Practitioner*, in "Selections," *JAMA* 18 (February 27, 1892): 277.

135. Eyler, "The State of Science, Microbiology, and Vaccines Circa 1918," 28–29.

136. Ibid., 28–29.

137. For stories confirming his discovery see Arthur MacDonald, "Latest Details Concerning the Germs of Influenza," *Science* 19 (February 12, 1892): 90; Arthur MacDonald, "Confirmation of the Discovery of the Influenza Bacillus," *Science* 19 (February 19, 1892): 100; George H. F. Nuthall, Letter to the Editor, "The Bacillus of Influenza," *Science* 19 (April 1, 1892): 193–194.

138. Eyler, "The State of Science, Microbiology and Vaccines, Circa 1918," 29–30. See for example John B. Huber, "A Doctor's Point of View—Influenza," *Collier's* 56 (March 11, 1916): 40; Review of P.C.C. Hubschmann, "Influenza," from *Munchener Medizinische* in "Current Medical Literature," *JAMA* 65 (September 25, 1915): 1147–1148; Charles H. Duncan, "A Remedy of Precision in Influenza," *The Medical Standard* 39 (January 1916): 97; H. E. Robertson, "Influenzal Sinus Disease and Its Relation to Epidemic Influenza," *JAMA* 70 (May 25, 1918): 1533.

139. William Osler and Thomas McCrae, *The Principles and Practice of Medicine: Designed for the Use of Practitioners and Students of Medicine*, 8th ed. (New York: D. Appleton and Company, 1912), ix, xi.

140. Eyler, "The State of Microbiology and Vaccines, Circa 1918," 30.

141. George Mathers, "Etiology of the Epidemic Acute Respiratory Infections Commonly Called Influenza," *JAMA* 68 (March 3, 1917): 678; F. X. Mahoney, quoted in "Influenza and Pneumonia—A Symposium presented before the Massachusetts Association of Boards of Health, Boston, Mass., January 27, 1916," *AJPH* 6 (April 1916): 307, 314.

142. Isaac A. Abt, quoted in "Abstract of Discussion," following Lawrence A. Royster, "Grip in Children," *JAMA* 67 (October 28, 1916): 1267.

143. Joseph A. Capps, and A. M. Moody, "The Recent Epidemic of Grip," *JAMA* 67 (November 4, 1916): 1350.

144. Eyler, "The State of Science, Microbiology and Vaccines, Circa 1918," 30; "Therapeutics—The Cause and Treatment of the Present Epidemic of 'Grip,'" *JAMA* 66 (January 15, 1916): 189; A. M. Moody and J. A. Capps, "Notes on Grip Epidemic in Chicago," *JAMA* 66 (May 27, 1916): 1696; A. M. Moody and J. A. Capps, "The Recent Epidemic of Grip," 1350; Louis M. Warfield, "Acute Ascending Paralysis Following Grippe," *Wisconsin Medical Journal* 14 (1916): 508.

  Some scientists had begun, by 1918, to acknowledge the possibility that a "filterable virus" might be responsible for influenza, but the argument remained muted. See for instance Mathers, "Etiology of the Epidemic Acute Respiratory Infections Commonly Called Influenza," 679; Capps and Moody, "The Recent Epidemic of Grip," 1350.

145. "Therapeutics—The Cause and Treatment of the Present Epidemic of 'Grip,'" 190. See also "Abstract of Discussion" following Royster, "Grip in Children," 1268.

146. "Deaths from Grip Increase Fivefold," *NYT*, December 29, 1915, 6.

147. Robert P. Hudson, *Disease and Its Control: The Shaping of Modern Thought* (Westport, CT: Greenwood Press, 1983), 188–190.

148. Tomes, *The Gospel of Germs*, 6.

149. Fee, "Public Health and the State," 233–234; Howard Markel, *When Germs Travel: Six Major Epidemics That Have Invaded America Since 1900 and the Fears They Have Unleashed* (New York: Pantheon, 2004), 67–68.

150. This is not to suggest that the social concerns of public health reformers disappeared. Rather, bacteriology offered new mechanisms for the practice of a socially inflected field. See Judith Walzer Leavitt, "'Typhoid Mary' Strikes Back: Bacteriological Theory and Practice in Early 20th-Century Public Health," in *Sickness and Health in America: Readings in the History of Medicine and Public Health*, 3rd ed., rev., ed. Judith Walzer Leavitt and Ronald L. Numbers (Madison: University of Wisconsin Press, 1997), 555–572.

151. Fee, "Public Health and the State," 236; Duffy, *The Sanitarians*, 193–196, 199–200, 216. As Fee notes, throughout the Progressive era "alternative" approaches to public health persisted. Alice Hamilton's research into industrial illness, for instance, reflected a continued appreciation for the important role environment played in health.

152. Fee, "Public Health and the State," 241; Duffy, *The Sanitarians*, 159–161, 239–242.

153. Cassedy, *Medicine in America*, 116–117.

154. M. J. Rosenau as quoted in "Influenza and Pneumonia—A Symposium presented before the Massachusetts Association of Boards of Health, Boston, Mass., January 27, 1916," 307.

155. "Col. Gorgas Called to Africa to Fight Grippe Plague," *NYT*, October 26, 1913, SM9. Gorgas made his reputation in the battle against yellow fever, first in Havana beginning in 1898 and then in his work as Chief Sanitary Engineer on the Panama Canal. He was appointed Surgeon General of the Army in April 1914, serving until his mandatory age-related retirement in early October 1918, in the midst of the influenza pandemic. John M. Gibson, *Physician to the World: The Life of General William C. Gorgas* (Durham, NC: Duke University Press, 1950).

156. See for instance Paul M. Allen and Paul L. Hudson, Students, College of Physicians and Surgeons, Columbia University, New York City, "The Present Influenza Epidemic in New York," *Journal of the South Carolina Medical Association* 12 (February 1916): 51.

157. M. J. Rosenau, quoted in "Influenza and Pneumonia—A Symposium," 309–310; "Fight Against Grip to Get Police Aid," *NYT*, January 8, 1916, 18; "456 Grip Spreaders Arraigned in Court," *NYT*, January 13, 1916, 8; Royster, "Grip in Children," 1267; "Therapeutics—The Cause and Treatment of the Present Epidemic of 'Grip,'" 189.

158. "Deaths from Grip Increase Fivefold," *NYT*, December 29, 1915, 6.

159. "A Revival of Shot-Gun Methods in Epidemic Control," *American Journal of Public Health* (hereafter *AJPH*) 6 (September 1916): 932.

160. David M. Kennedy, *Over Here: The First World War and American Society* (New York: Oxford University Press, 1980), 13–14.

161. John Dewey, "The Social Possibilities of War," in *Characters and Events: Popular Essays in Social and Political Philosophy*, vol. 2, ed. Joseph Ratner (New York: H.H. Holt, 1929), 551–560.

162. Carol R. Byerly, *Fever of War: The Influenza Epidemic in the US Army During World War I* (New York: New York University Press, 2005), 22–25.

163. William Gorgas, "Report of the Surgeon General," *War Department Annual Report, 1917*, quoted in Byerly, *Fever of War*, 21.

164. William Colby Rucker, "The Influence of the European War on the Transmission of the Infections of Disease with Special Reference to Its Effect upon Disease Conditions in the United States," quoted in Byerly, *Fever of War*, 4.

165. According to Paul Starr, "Of 3,760,000 men examined, about 550,000 were rejected as unfit; and of the 2.7 million called into service, about 47 percent were said to have physical impairments." Paul Starr, *The Social Transformation of American Medicine: The Rise of a Sovereign Profession and the Making of a Vast Industry* (New York: Basic Books, 1982), 193.

166. Irving Fisher, "Health and War," *AJPH* 8 (August 1918): 560.

167. Byerly, *Fever of War*, chap. 2, "Building a Health Army: Government Control and Accountability."

168. Ibid., 51–56.

169. Nancy K. Bristow, *Making Men Moral: Social Engineering and the Great War* (New York: New York University Press, 1996).

170. Neil A. Wynn, *From Progressivism to Prosperity: World War I and American Society* (New York: Holmes and Meier, 1986), 120.

171. Fee, "Public Health and the State," 242.

172. Frank Parker Stockbridge, "Health at Home to Help the Army: Improving the Sanitary Conditions in the United States in Order that the Flow of Munitions and Other Supplies will be Sufficient to Help the Army Win the War," *World's Work* 35 (April 1918): 608. See also George M. Price, "The Nationalization of Public Health," *Survey* 41 (October 19, 1918): 62.

173. Isaac W. Brewer, "The Control of Communicable Diseases in Camps," *AJPH* 8 (February 1918): 121. See also S.B.G., "Editorial—Health Protection After the War," *AJPH* 7 (October 1917): 825–826.

174. Gertrude Seymour, "The Health of Soldier and Civilian—Some Aspects of the American Health Movement in War-Time," *Survey* 40 (April 27, 1918): 89.

175. Peter H. Bryce, "History of the American Public Health Association," *AJPH* 8 (May 1918): 335.

176. "Guarding Against Infection from War Epidemics," *Review of Reviews* 51 (February 1915): 231. See also "The Progress of Science: The Control of Epidemic Diseases and the Causes of Death," *Scientific Monthly* 3 (October 1916): 410; D. Greenberg, "Two Historic World-Pestilences Robbed of Their Terrors by Modern Sanitation," *Scientific Monthly* 4 (June 1917): 554.

177. Frank Hunter Potter, "Prevention First: What the Health Department Is Doing for New York City," *Outlook* 117 (September 5, 1917): 17.

178. See for instance "Hunting the Bacteria," *NYT*, February 3, 1895, 24.

179. "Dooley Has 'The Lah Grippe,'" *LAT*, September 30, 1899, 7.

180. Grace Eckley, *Finley Peter Dunne* (Boston: Twayne Publishers, 1981), 9–10, 15, 72.

181. Elizabeth Peck, "The Grip," *NYT*, January 12, 1916, 12.

182. "How to Cure a Cold," *LAT*, May 15, 1898, B2; "The Public Health," *NYT*, March 4, 1904, 8; "The Paramount Issue," *Independent* 85 (January 1916): 144; "Chicago Prays for Cold Snap," *LAT*, January 15, 1907, 11; "Not Losing Its Grip," *LAT*, February 20, 1898, A10; Richard Cole Newton, "How We Can All Avoid the 'Grippe,'" *Ladies' Home Journal* 25 (October 1908): 34.

183. "Warns Public How to Avoid the Pneumonia," *San Antonio Light*, March 3, 1918, 5. See also "A Doctor's Point of View," *Collier's* 56 (March 11, 1916): 40.

184. "Drink Hot Lemonade and go to bed," ad for Sunkist lemons, *Marshall Evening Chronicle*, February 9, 1917, 5.

185. "An Influenza Preventive," *NYT*, April 9, 1905, 14; "Cinnamon for Influenza," *LAT*, June 19, 1907, II: 7; "Onions for a Cold," *LAT*, October 23, 1913, II: 6.

186. See for instance "Grip Bacillus Coming Westward," ad for Peruna, *LAT*, March 14, 1902, 4; "Grippe Germs," ad for Johnson's Tonic, *AC*, February 7, 1904, 13; "Grim Grip's Grasp," ad for Dr. Miles' Nervine, *AC*, February 7, 1900, 6. For some these ads may have been their first exposure to germ theory. See James Harvey Young, *The Toadstool Millionaires A Social History of Patent Medicines in America Before Federal Regulation* (Princeton, NJ: Princeton University Press, 1961), 144.

187. See for instance "Mortality of the State," *NYT*, July 1, 1891, 9; "The Thousand Deaths, *NYT*, May 6, 1892, 1; "Health Board Statistics," *NYT*, December 31, 1893, 3; "Many Deaths from Pneumonia," *NYT*, December 17, 1893, 16; "Vital Statistics of the Week," *NYT*, May 6, 1894, 13; "A Week's Vital Statistics," *NYT*, January 10, 1897, 13; "Fight Against Grip to Get Police Aid," *NYT*, January 8, 1916, 18; "Fewer Die from Grip," *NYT*, January 23, 1916, 18; "February Births 4142," *San Antonio Light*, March 21, 1916, 4; Louis I. Dublin, "The 'Grip' Epidemic of the Winter of 1915–1916," *AJPH* 6 (May 1916): 485–487; "Many Die of Pneumonia," *NYT*, January 28, 1917, E3.

188. "Influenza Is Not Harmless Disease," *AC*, June 16, 1913, 2.

189. "Not Losing Its Grip," *LAT*, February 20, 1898, A10.

190. "Hon. Josiah B. Allen," ad for Pe-ru-na, *LAT*, January 1, 1899, E14.

191. "Influenza Bugs Are Leaving Town," *LAT*, January 23, 1901, A1.

192. "Thirty-three Diseases Chiefly to Blame for New York's Death Roll," *NYT*, December 14, 1913, SM12.

193. Huber, "A Doctor's Point of View—Influenza," 40; "State Board of Health," *NYT*, March 31, 1892, 3; "Death Rate of the State," *NYT*, January 29, 1897, 4; "Influenza in Chicago," *NYT*,

February 20, 1898, 1; Filson Young, "Influenza," *The Living Age*, 277 (May 3, 1913): 306; Dublin, "The 'Grip' Epidemic of 1915–1916," 485.

194. See for instance "Grip Is Spreading over United States," *AC*, January 4, 1916, 1; "The Influenza Epidemic," *LAT*, January 4, 1916, sec. I, 1; "Epidemic of Grippe Sweeping the Country," *San Antonio Light*, January 4, 1916, 1; "The Paramount Issue," *The Independent* 85 (January 31, 1916): 144.

195. Holworthy Hall, "Grippe!" *McClure's* 46 (January 1916): 24–26, 58–59.

196. Ibid., 24.

197. Ibid., 25.

198. Ibid. See also "Chicago Sneezes and Weeps," *NYT*, September 9, 1897, 1; "The Contagiousness of the 'Grip,'" *NYT*, December 20, 1898, 6; "White Sox Pitcher Taken to Hospital," *Nevada State Journal*, May 5, 1915, 5; "To Avoid Grippe," *NYT*, April 12, 1909, 6.

199. See for instance "A Godsend to All Humanity," ad for the Quaker Bath Cabinet, *LAT*, January 29, 1899, B5; "How Catarrh Can Be Cured," ad for Dr. Geo. Leininger's For-Mal-De-Hyde Inhaler, *AC*, February 25, 1900, 21; "Are There Cold Spots In Your House?" ad for Atlanta Steam Heating Co., *AC*, October 23, 1909, 3; "The Ruthless Rule of Boreas!" ad for Eiseman Bros. Overcoats, *AC*, January 8, 1910, 7; "Look Out for the Blizzard," ad for R.M. Rose Co., "The Old Reliable Distillers," *AC*, January 24, 1906, 9.

200. "Grippe—You May Recoil With Horror, But You Cannot Escape!" ad for Johnson's Tonic, *AC*, February 10, 1904, 3.

201. "Danger Follows Attack of Grip," ad for Dr. Williams' Pink Pills for Pale People, *LAT*, March 5, 1918, sec. I, 4. See also "Grip Deals Hard Blows," ad for Duffy's Pure Malt, *NYT*, March 10, 1896, 2; "Appalling! The Sudden and Overwhelming Increase of Grippe and Pneumonia," ad for Duffy's Pure Malt, *NYT*, December 16, 1898, 3.

202. "The Grippe," *LAT*, April 3, 1894, 4.

203. Margaret Murphy, "Grip Don'ts," *JAMA* 66 (February 5, 1916): 449. The article was first published in the *University Missourian*.

204. "Mortality from Influenza—Chicago Health Department Wants the Disease More Actively Fought," *NYT*, April 28, 1901, 3.

Chapter 2

1. Edith Potter, Application for Enrollment in a Nonreservation School, Edith Potter File (5017), Student Files, Chemawa Indian School, Box 66, RG 75, NA (PAR).

2. David Wallace Adams, *Education for Extinction: American Indians and the Boarding School Experience, 1875–1928* (Lawrence: University of Kansas, 1995), chap. 1; Sonicray Bonnell, *Chemawa Indian Boarding School: The First One Hundred Years, 1880–1980*, MA Thesis, Dartmouth College, 1997, chaps. 2 and 3, available as an e-book.

3. Letter from Harwood Hall, Superintendent, to W. W. McConihe, Superintendent, Round Valley Agency, October 18, 1918, Edith Potter File (5017), Student Files, Chemawa Indian School, Box 66, RG 75, NA (PAR).

4. Chemawa Indian School Annual Report, 1919, Box 86, Annual and Special Reports 1916–1940, Chemawa Indian School, RG 75, NA (PAR).

5. Telegram from Hall, Superintendent to McConihe, Superintendent, October 19, 1918, Edith Potter File (5017), Student Files, Chemawa Indian School, Box 66, RG 75, NA (PAR).

6. Telegram from Hall, Superintendent to McConihe, Superintendent, October 20, 1918, Edith Potter File (5017), Student Files, Chemawa Indian School, Box 66, RG 75, NA (PAR).

7. Letter from Hall, Superintendent, to Mrs. Jessie Barker, October 28, 1918, Edith Potter File (5017), Student Files, Chemawa Indian School, Box 66, RG 75, NA (PAR).

8. Ibid.

9. Letter from McConihe, Superintendent, to Hall, Superintendent, Chemawa Indian School, November 19, 1919, Edith Potter File (5017), Student Files, Chemawa Indian School, Box 66, RG 75, NA (PAR).

10. Letter from Hall, Superintendent to McConihe, Superintendent, November 24, 1919, Edith Potter File (5017), Student Files, Chemawa Indian School, Box 66, RG 75, NA (PAR).

11. I use the terms "Native American" and "Indian" interchangeably for people indigenous to the territory that makes up the United States, recognizing these are both contested terms. Today, many Native people refer to themselves as Indians, giving dignity to a term that acknowledges centuries of genocide and oppression.

12. Bonnell, *Chemawa Indian Boarding School*, chaps. 2 and 3. For a fuller history of the experience of children at Indian Schools, see Adams, *Education for Extinction*; K. Tsianina Lomawaima, *They Called It Prairie Light: The Story of Chilocco Indian School* (Lincoln: University of Nebraska Press, 1994); Brenda J. Child, *Boarding School Seasons: American Indian Families, 1900–1940* (Lincoln: University of Nebraska, 1998).

13. Child, *Boarding School Seasons*, 55, 60–68; Adams, *Education for Extinction*, 124–125, 130–133.

14. Adams, *Education for Extinction*, 134–135; Hospital Record, 1917–1924, Box 134, Chemawa Indian School, RG 75, NA (PAR).

15. Child, *Boarding School Seasons*, 55.

16. Alfred W. Crosby, *America's Forgotten Pandemic: The Influenza of 1918* (New York: Cambridge University Press, 1989), 18–19; Gina Kolata, *Flu: The Story of the Great Influenza Pandemic of 1918 and the Search for the Virus That Caused It* (New York: Farrar, Straus and Giroux, 1999), 10–11. For a useful account of the first spring wave of the epidemic, see John Barry, *The Great Influenza: The Epic Story of the Deadliest Plague in History* (New York: Viking, 2004), chap. 14.

17. Crosby, *America's Forgotten Pandemic*, 18; Carol R. Byerly, *Fever of War: The Influenza Epidemic in the U.S. Army During World War I* (New York: New York University Press, 2005), 70–71.

18. Crosby, *America's Forgotten Pandemic*, 18, 21–25.

19. Ibid., 25–32; Barry, *The Great Influenza*, 170–174.

20. Kolata, *Flu*, 12–13; Crosby, *Forgotten Pandemic*, 39–40.

21. "Chronological map of the influenza epidemic of 1918," illustration in Edgar Sydenstricker, "Preliminary Statistics of the Influenza Epidemic," *PHR* 33 (December 27, 1918): 2310.

22. J.J. Keegan, "The Prevailing Pandemic of Influenza," *JAMA* 71 (September 28, 1918): 1051.

23. "Therapeutics—Epidemic Influenza," *JAMA* 71 (October 5, 1918): 1136; George A. Soper, "Military Medicine and Surgery—The Pandemic in the Army Camps," *JAMA* 71 (December 7, 1918): 1901.

24. "Therapeutics—Epidemic Influenza," 1136.

25. E. R. LeCount, "The Pathologic Anatomy of Influenza Bronchopneumonia," *JAMA* 72 (March 1, 1919): 650; M. W. Lyon, Jr., "Gross Pathology of Epidemic Influenza at Walter Reed General Hospital," *JAMA* 72 (March 29, 1919): 925. As LeCount's example makes clear, many physicians at the time did not distinguish between the influenza and pneumonia deaths, making only more mysterious the combination of symptoms and outcomes.

26. Kolata, *Flu*, 4, 12; Lynette Iezzoni, *Influenza 1918: The Worst Epidemic in American History* (New York: TV Books, 1999), 16, 49–51; Crosby, *America's Forgotten Pandemic*, 5–9.

27. Letter from Roy (Surgical Ward No. 16, Camp Devens) to Burt, September 29, 1918, available on PBS Website, http://www.pbs.org/wgbh/americanexperience/features/primary-resources/influenza-letter/ [accessed February 28, 2011].

28. LeCount, "The Pathologic Anatomy of Influenza Bronchopneumonia," 650.

29. Keegan, "The Prevailing Pandemic of Influenza," 1052; "Therapeutics—Epidemic Influenza," 1136.

30. Entry for January 12, 1919, Diary of Martin Franklin, 1914–1919, History of Medicine Division Collection, National Library of Medicine.

31. Ibid., entry for January 13, 1919.

32. Ibid., entry for January 13, 1919.

33. Letter from Harold S. Barr to "Darling Mother," November 17, 1918, Folder 7: November–December 1918, Box 2, Harold Standish Barr Manuscript Collection, Manuscripts Section, Indiana State Library.

34. Clifford Adams, quoted in Barry, *The Great Influenza*, 232.

35. Robert Frost, quoted in Dorothy A. Pettit and Janice Bailie, *A Cruel Wind: Pandemic Flu in America, 1918–1920* (Murfreesboro, TN: Timberlane Books, 2008), 151.

36. Questionnaire of William Otto Reimann, HQ Det., 16th Division, Army Experiences Questionnaire Collection [hereafter AEQC], World War One Research Project [hereafter WWORP], US Army Military History Institute, Carlisle Barracks, Carlisle, Pennsylvania [hereafter USAMHI].

37. Harvey Cushing, M.D., *From a Surgeon's Journal, 1915–1918* (Boston: Little, Brown and Co., 1936), 469.

38. Harvey Cushing, quoted in Barry, *The Great Influenza*, 233.

39. William Maxwell, quoted in Barry, *The Great Influenza*, 233.

40. Bill Sardo, quoted in Barry, *The Great Influenza*, 233.

41. George Hoyt Whipple in *A Dozen Doctors: Autobiographical Sketches*, Dwight J. Ingle, ed. (Chicago: Chicago University Press, 1963), 224; Questionnaire of Oliver L. Bell, 60th FA, 20th Division, AEQC, WWORP, USAMHI.

42. Crosby, *America's Forgotten Pandemic*, 50–51, 71, 96–97.

43. Morgan Brawner, "REPORT OF MR. MORGAN BRAWNER," "Epidemics, Influenza—Reports and Statistics—Lake Division," File 803.8, Box 688, RG 200, NA. See also "War-Reports from the Influenza Front," *Literary Digest* (hereafter *LD*) 60 (February 22, 1919): 62; Eugene H. Fellows, Executive Secretary, "Lackawanna County Report," November 30, 1918, in "Emergency Service of the Pennsylvania Council of National Defense in the Influenza Crisis—Report of the Vice-Director, Department of Medicine, Sanitation and Hospitals," 25, PAM 173, College of Physicians (Philadelphia); Mrs. S. J. Kinkead, "Report of Mrs. S. J. Kinkead . . . November 7th, 1918," "Epidemics, Influenza—Reports and Statistics—Lake Division," File 803.08, Box 688, RG 200, NA.

44. Charles E. Rosenberg, "Introduction: Community and Communities: The Evolution of the American Hospital," in *The American General Hospital: Communities and Social Contexts*, ed. Diana Elizabeth Long and Janet Golden (Ithaca, NY: Cornell University Press, 1989), 4–11; Morris J. Vogel, *The Invention of the Modern Hospital, Boston 1870–1930* (Chicago: University of Chicago Press, 1980), Introduction and chaps. 1–6; Charles E. Rosenberg, *The Care of Strangers: The Rise of America's Hospital System* (New York: Basic Books, 1987); Sandra Opdycke, *No One Was Turned Away: The Role of Public Hospitals in New York City since 1900* (New York: Oxford University Press, 1999), chap. 1. See also Harry F. Dowling, *City Hospitals: The Undercare of the Underprivileged* (Cambridge, MA: Harvard University Press, 1982); David Rosner, *A Once and Charitable Enterprise: Hospitals and Health Care in Brooklyn and New York 1885–1915* (New York: Cambridge University Press, 1982).

45. J. Prentice Murphy, "Meeting the Scourge—How Massachusetts Organized to Fight Influenza Told for the Benefit of Other States," *Survey* 41 (October 26, 1918): 98.

46. Charles V. Aiken, "Influenza in South Carolina 1918," *Journal of the South Carolina Medical Association* 15 (January 1919): 347.

47. Rupert Blue, "Epidemic Influenza and the U.S. Public Health Service," *Modern Hospital* (hereafter *MH*) 11 (December 1918): 426.

48. Questionnaire of H. Louis Brooks, 12th Division, 42nd Infantry, AEQC, WWORP, USAMHI.

49. Interview with Josie Mabel Brown, "A Winding Sheet and a Wooden Box," *Navy Medicine* 77 (May–June 1986): 18–19. At http://www.history.navy.mil/library/online/influenza%20wind.htm [accessed May 6, 2011].

50. Gust B. Westby, Btty. C. 42nd Field Artillery, 14th Field Artillery Brigade, 14th Division, AEQC, WWORP, USAMHI.

51. Miss Hall, "Personal experiences during the epidemic," Student nurse epidemic accounts, Folder 1, Box 8, RG 22.1, Department of Nursing, Academic Departments, College Archives, Simmons College. With thanks to the Influenza Digital Archive, Center for the History of Medicine, University of Michigan.

52. "War-Reports from the Influenza Front," 62.

53. Oral history, Dr. William B. Bean (#RG-26/4), Special Collections Department, University of Virginia.

54. Elizabeth Gregg, "Emergency Nursing Service During the Epidemic: Care Given to Patients During the Epidemic of Influenza by the Nurses of the Bureau of Preventable Diseases," *Monthly Bulletin of the Department of Health, City of New York* 8 (December 1918): 289.

55. Millicent Edwards, Supervisor of Nursing, "American Red Cross—Baltimore Chapter— Report of the Red Cross Nursing Center during Epidemic of Spanish Influenza October 1918," "Epidemic, Influenza, Maryland," File 803.11, Box 689, RG 200, NA.

56. Mrs. W. R. Mercer, Chairman, "Coatesville," in *Southeastern Pennsylvania Chapter of the American Red Cross in the Influenza Epidemic, September–October 1918*, 21, "Epidemics, Influenza, Pennsylvania," File 803.11, Box 689, RG 200, NA.

57. Letter from Will to Squeechy, October 26, 1918, Folder October 26, 1918 WOF to EKF w/ env. (Charlottesville), Box 1, Ella Katherine Fife Letters, Special Collections Department, University of Virginia Library; "Private Johnson Leaves Two Sisters," *Baltimore Afro-American* (hereafter *AA*), October 18, 1918, 2.

58. Pettit and Bailie, *A Cruel Wind*, 115.

59. J. R. Steward, Field Director, American Red Cross, Camp Dodge, Iowa, "Field Director's Report—Camp Dodge, Iowa—Period Covering Influenza Epidemic," October 17, 1918, "Epidemics, Influenza, Iowa," File 803.11, Box 689, RG 200, NA.

60. Ibid.

61. Mrs. Annie Murphy to Mr. Harwood Hally [*sic*], October 16, 1918, Mary Murphy File, Student Files, Chemawa Indian School, Box 66, RG 75, NA (PAR).

62. Pettit and Bailie, *A Cruel Wind*, 146.

63. Letter from Arthur T. Hadley to Colonel Craig, October 7, 1918, Series II—Box 130, Arthur T. Hadley Papers, Record Group YRG 2-A-13, Sterling Memorial Library, Yale University; Royal Brougham, "And Now the Flu Cancels Big Contest," *PI*, October 9, 1918, 11.

64. "News from the Artillery Regiments," *Pass in Review* (Camp Bowie, Texas), October 5, 1918, 19; Kathleen Edtl Hampton, "The 1918 Spanish Influenza: A Pandemic Strikes Cowlitz County," *Cowlitz Historical Quarterly* 38 (1996): 11.

65. Letter from L. F. Knowles to Leopold Bruenner, October 21, 1918; letter from R. C. Jones to Leopold Bruenner, October 14, 1918; letter from F. H. Burgert to Leopold Bruenner, October 16, 1918; all in Folder: Director of Liberty Choruses and Community Singing (Leopold Bruenner), Correspondence-September–October, 1918, "Correspondence of the Director of Liberty Choruses and Community Singing, 1917–1918," Minnesota Commission of Public Safety, Minnesota Historical Society; letter from Frederic A. Hall, Chancellor, Washington University to Opie, November 6, 1918, US Army—Correspondence #2, Eugene Lindsay Opie Papers (B/OP3), American Philosophical Society; "Hampton Postpones Anniversary Celebration," *Baltimore Afro-American* (hereafter *AA*), November 1, 1918, 1; Laura Stephenson Carter, "Cold Comfort," *Dartmouth Medicine* (Winter 2006): 38–39, available at: http://dartmed. dartmouth.edu/winter06/html/cold_comfort.php [accessed March 28, 2011].

66. "Influenza Fast Passing Away," *WN*, November 2, 1918, 1.

67. "'There Wasn't a Mine Runnin' a Lump O' Coal': A Kentucky Coal Miner Remembers the Influenza Pandemic of 1918–1919," available on the History Matters website, http://historymatters.gmu.edu/d/107 [accessed January 27, 2011]; Pete Davies, *The Devil's Flu: The World's Deadliest Influenza Epidemic and the Scientific Hunt for the Virus That Caused It* (New York: Henry Holt, 2000), 86.

68. J. Frank Dreher, "Monroe County Report," in "Emergency Service of the Pennsylvania Council of National Defense in the Influenza Crisis—Report of the Vice-Director, Department of Medicine, Sanitation and Hospitals," PAM 173, Philadelphia College of Physicians.

69. Teamus Bartley, in "'There Wasn't a Mine Runnin' a Lump O' Coal."

70. Letter from Roy (Surgical Ward No. 16, Camp Devens, MA) to Burt, September 29, 1918. Primary Resources: A Letter from Camp Devins [*sic*], MA., Influenza, 1918, WGBH American Experience, available online at http://pbs.org.wgbh/americanexerience/features/primary-resources/influenza-letter/.

71. The Reminiscences of Gardner Jackson, (1959), 92, in the Oral History Collection of Columbia University.

72. Questionnaire of Merle E. Swanger, 68th Infantry, 18th Infantry Brigade, 9th Division, AEQC, WWORP, USAMHI.

73. The Reminiscences of A. R. Dochez (1957), 73, in the Oral History Collection of Columbia University.

74. Questionnaire of George C. Dobbs, 50th M.G. Bn., 33rd Infantry Brigade, 17th Division, AEQC, WWORP, USAMHI; "Death Grip of Epidemic Broken, Following Toll of 483 Dead and 1438 Serious," *Camp Sherman News*, October 9, 1918, 1.

75. "The Burial Situation During the Epidemic," in "What the Health Department Has Done to Curb the Epidemic of Influenza," *Monthly Bulletin of the Department of Public Health and Charities of the City of Philadelphia* 3 (October–November 1918): 18.

76. George H. Meeker, "Descriptive," in "Southeastern Pennsylvania Chapter of the American Red Cross in the Influenza Epidemic, September–October 1918," 11, File 803.11, Epidemic, Influenza, Pennsylvania, Box 689, RG 200, NA.

77. Robert D. Dripps, "Philadelphia County Report," in "Emergency Service of the Pennsylvania Council of National Defense in the Influenza Crisis," Report of the Vice-Director, Department of Medicine, Sanitation and Hospitals, 35, PAM 173, Philadelphia College of Physicians.

78. Ibid., 36; "The Burial Situation During the Epidemic," 18.

79. "The Burial Situation During the Epidemic," 19; Dripps, "Philadelphia County Report," 36.

80. Louise Apuchase in "'Please Let Me Put Him in a Macaroni Box': The Spanish Influenza of 1918 in Philadelphia," History Matters website, available at http://historymatters.gmu.edu/d/13 [accessed January 27, 2011].

81. "The Burial Situation During the Epidemic," 18; Dripps, "Philadelphia County Report," 36–37.

82. James Higgins, "Keystone of an Epidemic," unpublished manuscript, September 16, 2011, 103–107.

83. "The Closing Order—October 3, 1918," in "Resolutions of the Board of Health," in "What the Health Department Has Done to Curb the Epidemic of Influenza," *Monthly Bulletin of The Department of Public Health and Charities of the City of Philadelphia* 3 (October–November 1918): 7.

84. On Lawrence, Massachusetts, for instance, see Jane Brox, "Influenza, 1918," *Five Thousand Days Like This One: An American Family History* (Boston: Beacon Press, 1999), 101.

85. Elizabeth Gregg, "Emergency Nursing Service During the Epidemic," *Monthly Bulletin of the Department of Health, City of New York* 8 (December 1918): 289.

86. "Foreword," "Southeastern Pennsylvania Chapter of the American Red Cross in the Influenza Epidemic September–October 1918," Folder Epidemic, Influenza, Pennsylvania, File 803.11, Box 689, RG200, NA.

87. "Report of Superintendent of Schools," *Annual Report of the Commissioners of the District of Columbia, Year Ended June 30, 1919, vol. IV: Report of the Board of Education* (Washington, D.C.: n.p., 1919), 17.

88. Emphasis in the original. Letter from Blanche to Lloyd, October 16, 1918, Folder 1: 1918–1950: Family Correspondence—Letters, Genealogy, Box 1, Lloyd Campbell Bird Papers, Special Collections Department, University of Virginia Library.

89. Marian Moser Jones, "The American Red Cross and Local Response to the 1918 Influenza Pandemic: A Four-City Case Study," *PHR* 125 (2010, Supplement 3): 93–94.

90. Ibid., 93, 95–96; "Foreword," "Southeastern Pennsylvania Chapter of the American Red Cross in the Influenza Epidemic September–October 1918."

91. "Red Cross News—Influenza Relief," *World News (hereafter WN)*, November 4, 1918, 4; "Influenza Shows Let-Up in Roanoke," *WN*, October 28, 1918, 2.

92. "Report of Superintendent of Schools," *Annual Report of the Commissioners of the District of Columbia, Year Ended June 30, 1919, vol. IV: Report of the Board of Education*, 17.

93. J. R. Steward, "Field Director's Report—Camp Dodge, Iowa—Period Covering Influenza Epidemic," October 17, 1918, "Epidemic, Influenza, Iowa," File 803.11, Box 689, RG 200, NA.

94. "In The Present Emergency," ad for The Owl Drug Co., *LAT*, October 21, 1918, sec. I, 3.

95. "Honesty and Fairness to the Bitter End: A Depression Victim's Story," oral history of William Iverson Wilson, WPA Federal Writers' Project Collection, Manuscript Division, Library of Congress, available online at http://memory.loc.gov/ammem/ammemhome.html [accessed March 25, 2004].

96. "Always Flowers," Life History of Charles L. Sligh, WPA Federal Writers' Project Collection, Manuscript Division, Library of Congress, available online at http://memory.loc. gov/ammem/ammemhome.html [accessed March 25, 2004].

97. "The Burial Situation During the Epidemic," 19.

98. Health Officer Fowler of Washington, D.C., quoted in A. A. Hoehling, *The Great Epidemic* (Boston: Little, Brown and Co., 1961), 118.

99. Elizabeth, oral history included in "'Please, Let Me Put Him in a Macaroni Box': The Spanish Influenza of 1918 in Philadelphia."

100. Pettit and Bailie, *A Cruel Wind*, 109–110.

101. "Big Firms Take up Fight on Influenza," *NYT*, October 23, 1918, 8.

102. Hampton, "The 1918 Spanish Flu: A Pandemic Strikes Cowlitz County," 12.

103. Account quoted in American Red Cross, *The Mobilisation of the American Red Cross During the Influenza Pandemic 1918–1919* (Geneva: Printing Office of the Tribune de Geneve, 1920), 24.

104. "Personal Experiences During the Epidemic," Accounts of Miss Franklin, Miss Delano, and Miss Purbrick, Folder 1, Box 8, Student Nurse Epidemic Accounts, Academic Departments, College Archives, Simmons College.

105. Telegram from R. C. Ballard, Asst. Mgr. Lake Division, American Red Cross to Mr. Jas. L. Fieser, American Red Cross, Cleveland, October 31, 1918, Folder: Epidemics, Influenza— Reports and Statistics—Lake Division, File 803.03, Box 688, RG200, NA.

106. Letter from Sue G. Whitmore to Harry and Bettie, October 20, 1918, Folder: 1918 August— December Susan Gregory Whitmore to Harry Gregory Whitmore, Box 4, Papers of the Gregory—Whitmore Family (#10754-d), Special Collections Department, University of Virginia Library; Letter from Ella to Dearest Papa, no date, Folder: [1919] EKF to RHF w/ env. (St. Denis), Box 2, Ella Katherine Fife Letters (#5943-e), Special Collections Department, University of Virginia Library.

107. Letter from Katherine to Jamie, October 13, 1918, Folder: October 13, 1918 Katherine Mae Reynolds Fife to JDF, Box 1, Ella Katherine Fife Letters (#5943-e), Special Collections Department, University of Virginia Library.

108. Letter from Ella to Madge, January 15, 1919, Folder: January 15, 1919, EKF to MWF w/env. (St. Denis), Box 2, Ella Katherine Fife Letters (#5943-e), Special Collections Department, University of Virginia Library.

109. Letter from Nell to Mrs. Fife, December 5, 1918, Folder: December 5, 1918 Nellie Nash to SAGSF w/env. (Leith, Scotland), Box 1, Ella Katherine Fife Letters (#5943-e), Special Collections Department, University of Virginia Library; letter from Blanche to Lloyd, October 16, 1918, Folder 1: 1918–1950: Family Correspondence—Letters, Genealogy, Box 1, Lloyd Campbell Bird papers (#MSS-9854), Special Collections, University of Virginia Library; letter from Katherine to Jamie, October 13, 1918, Folder: October 13, 1918 Katherine Mae Reynolds Fife to JDF, Box 1, Ella Katherine Fife Letters (#5943-e), Special Collections Department, University of Virginia Library.

110. Letter from Elizabeth to Mother dear, October 29, 1918, Folder: Correspondence 1918— October 17–31, Series I: Box 28, William Kent Family Papers, MSS Group #309, Sterling Memorial Library, Yale University.

111. Letter from Amelia Earhart to Kenneth Griggs Merrill, March 13, 1919, Kenneth Griggs Merrill Papers, 1918–1919 (A/M571), Schlesinger Library, Radcliffe Institute for Advanced Study, Harvard University.

112. Letter from Amelia Earhart to Kenneth Griggs Merrill, December 26, 1918, Kenneth Griggs Merrill Papers, 1918–1919 (A/M571), Schlesinger Library, Radcliffe Institute for Advanced Study, Harvard University. While Earhart was certain she suffered from influenza, historians have disagreed. Mary S. Lovell accepts Earhart's diagnosis in *The Sound of Wings: The Life of Amelia Earhart* (New York: St. Martin's Press, 1989), 27. Other accounts disagree, for instance Jean L. Backus, *Letters from Amelia 1901–1937: An Intimate Portrait of Amelia Earhart* (Boston: Beacon Press, 1982), 49–50; Susan Butler, *East to the Dawn: The Life of Amelia Earhart* (Reading, MA: Addison-Wesley, 1997), 86.

113. Letter from James M. Howard to wife, November 20, 1918, Folder 1—Correspondence, Howard, G.H., Box 1, Series 1, James M. Howard Papers, Sterling Memorial Library, Yale University; letter from Rob to Dearest Mother, October 9, 1918, Folder "October 9, 1918

Robert Herndon Fife II to SAGSF (Middletown, CT)" Box 1, Ella Katherine Fife Letters, Special Collections Department, University of Virginia Library; Virginia Wilson Wallace, ed., "An Ohioan in the Great War—Letters from the Front: The Correspondence of Lieutenant Willard W. Wilson of Hillsboro, Ohio," included in Willard W. Wilson, 323rd Field Artillery Hq. Co., 83rd Division, AEQC, WWORP, USAMHI; Diary entry, October 17, 1918, Evan J. Miller, Medical Corps, Base Hospital #8, AEQC, WWORP, USAMHI. See also examples in Byerly, *Fever of War*, 119.

114. Michael Kimmel, *Manhood in America: A Cultural History* (New York: Free Press, 1996), 100 and chaps. 4 and 5; E. Anthony Rotundo, *American Manhood: Transformations in Masculinity from the Revolution to the Modern Era* (New York: Basic Books, 1993), chaps. 10 and 11.

115. Questionnaire of Merle E. Swanger, Battalion Sergeant Major, 9th Division, 68th Infantry Brigade, AEQC, WWORP, USAMHI; letter from Harney to Papa, September 25, 1918, Folder: Stover, Urban C.—Letters, August–September 1918, Urban C. Stover Manuscript Collection (#L151), Manuscript Section, Indiana State Library.

116. "In Memoriam," *The Dooins—of U.S. Reserve Base Hospital No. 2*, December 7, 1918, in file of J. E. Croman, Medical Corps, Base Hospital #2 (WWI—403), AEQC, WWORP, USAMHI.

117. Letter from Pvt. Victor W. Jones to Mother, September 25, 1918, 8th (45th) Co., Camp Lewis, 166th Depot Brigade (WWI—2999), AEQC, WWORP, USAMHI.

118. Letter from Greg to "Yare" (Mrs. Greg M. Auger), November 17, 1918, Folder: "Correspondence of Greg N. Auger (Private) 1918 October–December, Box 2, World War I American Soldiers' Correspondence and Diaries, 1917–1945," Joseph M. Bruccoli Great War Collection, Special Collections, University of Virginia.

119. Letter from Joe (St. Paul, MN) to Max Winkel, November 10, 1918, Folder: Winkel (Max and Family) Papers—Correspondence, 1916–1919, Max Winkel and Family Papers, 1850–1963, Minnesota Historical Society.

120. Letter from Charles H. Stenger to Mother, October 24, 1918, included in Charles H. Stenger, Battery B, 81st Field Artillery, 8th Field Artillery Brigade, 8th Division, (WWI—2125), AEQC, WWORP, USAMHI.

121. Letters from Harney to Mother, September 15 and 16, 1918, Folder: Stover, Urban C.—Letters, August—September 1918, Urban C. Stover Manuscript Collection, Manuscript Section, Indiana State Library.

122. See for instance Bill McAdoo Jr. to sister Sally, October 8, 1918, Container 57, William G. McAdoo Papers, Manuscript Division, Library of Congress. Some men employed humor to disarm anxiety. See discussion of exchange between Robert Frost and Louis Untermeyer in Pettit and Bailie, *A Cruel Wind*, 135.

123. Letter from Joseph M. Turbyfill to My Dear old Sweetheart and Wife, October 22, 1918, Letter #XX, Joseph M. Turbyfill, 1st Lieutenant, 306th Ammunition Train, 81st Division, (WWIS—6965), Folder 2, AEQC, WWORP, USAMHI.

124. Letter from Joseph M. Turbyfill, 1st Lieutenant to My Dear Old Wonder Girl, Letter #XXI, October 25, 1918, included Joseph M. Turbyfill, 1st Lieutenant, 306th Ammunition Train, 81st Division (WWIS—6965), Folder 2, AEQC, WWORP, USAMHI.

125. Letter from Joseph M. Turbyfill to My Dear Old Sweetheart, October 28, 1918, Letter #XXII, Joseph M. Turbyfill, 1st Lieutenant, 306th Ammunition Train, 81st Division (WWIS—6965), Folder 2, AEQC, WWORP, USAMHI.

126. Letter from Joseph M. Turbyfill to My Dear Old Wonder Girl, October 25, 1918, Letter #XXI, and letter from Joseph M. Turbyfill to My Dear Old Sweetheart & Wife, October 22, 1918, Letter #XX, both in Joseph M. Turbyfill, 1st Lieutenant, 306th Ammunition Train, 81st Division (WWIS—6965), Folder 2, AEQC, WWORP, USAMHI.

127. Letter from Thomas L. Sidlo to Newton D. Baker, November 7, 1918, Record #50, Reel #5, Papers of Newton D. Baker, Manuscript Division, Library of Congress.

128. Letter from Charles H. Stengler to My dear Mother, September 30, 1918, Charles H. Stengler, PFC, Battery B, 81st Field Artillery, 8th Field Artillery Brigade, 8th Division, AEQC, WWORP, USAMHI.

129. For a brief overview of the development of domestic ideology see Sara M. Evans, *Born for Liberty: A History of Women in America* (New York: Free Press, 1997), chaps. 4 and 5. On

the use of domestic ideology to justify women's participation in the public sphere, see Paula Baker, "The Domestication of Politics: Women and American Political Society, 1780–1920," *American Quarterly* 89 (June 1984): 620–647.

130. "Editorial—The Spanish Influenza," *NYT*, October 7, 1918, 12.

131. "Editorial—Here Is a Chance for Service," *NYT*, October 28, 1918, 10.

132. Ad detailed in Lillian D. Wald, "The Work of the Nurses' Emergency Council," *Public Health Nurse* (hereafter *PHN*) 10 (December 1918): 306.

133. "Foreword," "Southeastern Pennsylvania Chapter of the American Red Cross in the Influenza Epidemic September–October 1918," File 803.11, "Epidemic, Influenza, Pennsylvania," Box 689, RG200, NA.

134. Ibid.; "How the Red Cross Met the Influenza Epidemic," *Potomac Division Bulletin* I (Illustrated Supplement, November 22, 1918), bound volume: *Potomac Division 1918*, File 494.2—Division Bulletins, Box 521, RG200, NA; "How the Influenza Epidemic was Fought by the Red Cross Nurse," *American Red Cross Central Division Bulletin*, I (November 16, 1918): 7, Hazel A. Braugh Records Center of the American Red Cross.

135. "Foreword," "Southeastern Pennsylvania Chapter of the American Red Cross in the Influenza Epidemic September–October 1918."

136. "War-Reports from the Influenza Front," 62; "Excerpt from the September Monthly Report of the New England Bureau of Civilian Relief on Influenza," October 28, 1918, "Epidemics, Influenza—Reports and Statistics—New England Division," Box 688, File 803.08, RG 200, NA; memorandum from Mr. Shelly D. Watts to Mr. James L. Fieser, "Subject: Aftermath of the Influenza Epidemic in Kentucky Mountains," February 12, 1919, "Epidemics, Influenza, Kentucky," File 803.11, Box 689, RG 200, NA.

137. "The Year of the Plague," *The Bulletin* (published weekly by the Associated Charities of Minneapolis) 4 (April 21, 1919): 1–2, Folder: [3:6—Associated Charities/Family Welfare Association—Corporate and General Historical—"The Bulletin," Vol. 4, 1919–1920], Box 3, Minneapolis Family and Children's Services, Social Welfare History Archives, University of Minnesota Libraries.

138. Memorandum from Mr. Shelly D. Watts to Mr. James L. Fieser, "Subject: Aftermath of the Influenza Epidemic in Kentucky Mountains," February 12, 1919, "Epidemics, Influenza, Kentucky," File 803.11, Box 689, RG 200, NA.

139. "City Provides Free Medical Service for Poor During the Epidemic," "What the Health Department Has Done to Curb the Epidemic of Influenza," *Monthly Bulletin of The Department of Public Health and Charities of the City of Philadelphia* 3 (October–November 1918): 19–20.

140. Opdycke, *No One Was Turned Away*, chap. 2; Rosenberg, *The Care of Strangers*, 6, 293–297.

141. Pettit and Bailie, *A Cruel Wind*, 111; Higgins, "Keystone of an Epidemic," 103–107.

142. "Nurses Report," in *Fifth Annual Report of the Social Service Society of West Chester, Pennsylvania, 1918–1919*, Folder 3: "Neighborhood VNA Social Service Society of West Chester, Annual Reports—1916–1924," Series 1, Subgroup IV, Box 9, Neighborhood Visiting Nurse Association Records (MC100), Center for the Study of the History of Nursing, School of Nursing, University of Pennsylvania.

143. Letter from Mrs. J. M. Russell to Mrs. Bruce, November 8, 1918, "Epidemic, Influenza, Kentucky," File 803.11, Box 689, RG 200, NA.

144. Letter from Reldia Holt to Miss Bruce, December 2, 1918, "Epidemic, Influenza, Kentucky," File 803.11, Box 689, RG 200, NA.

145. Case #13906, Reel #197, Family Welfare, Minneapolis Family and Children's Service Case Records, 1895–1945, Social Welfare History Archives, University of Minnesota Libraries; Oscar Jewell Harvey, *The Spanish Influenza Pandemic of 1918: An Account of Its Ravages in Luzerne County, Pennsylvania, and the Efforts Made to Combat and Subdue It* (Wilkes-Barre, PA: n.p., 1920), 45–49.

146. Case #13906, Reel #197—Family Welfare, Minneapolis Family and Children's Service Case Records 1895–1945, Social Welfare History Archives, University of Minnesota Libraries.

147. See also "50,000 Children Examined," *NYT*, February 24, 1919, 5.

148. "Spanish Stonecutter's Widow," in "Four Women," American Life Histories, Manuscripts from the Federal Writers' Project, 1936–1940, American Memory Project, Library of

Congress, available at http://lcweb2.loc.gov/cgi-bin/query/D?wpa:2:./temp/~ammem_ kwLX [accessed July 8, 2011].

149. Melvin Lynn Frank, "Reminiscences: 'Sawmill City Boyhood,'" 83, undated, Minnesota Historical Society.

150. Starr Cadwallader, Division Director, Civilian Relief, Lake Division to James L. Fieser, Association Director General National Headquarters, August 12, 1919, "Report of the Department of Civilian Relief," "Lake Division—Civilian Relief Reports-July–December 1918," File 149.18, Box 216, Entry 27130D, RG 200, NA; "Report of the Influenza Epidemic—Lake Division," "Epidemics, Influenza—Reports and Statistics, Lake Division," File 803.08, Box 688, RG 200, NA; "Report of Bureau of Civilian Relief Lake Division—American Red Cross for the Month of October 1918," "American Red Cross Report of Division Directors of Civilian Relief for the Month of October 1918," "Civilian Relief Reports-All Divisions-September–October 1918," File 149.18, Box 201, Entry 27130D, RG 200, NA.

151. "Report of Mrs. Ella May Huber and Mrs. C. A. Dolan, who went to Pineville, Bell Co., Ky. To nurse influenza," "Epidemics, Influenza—Reports and Statistics—Lake Division," File 803.08, Box 688, RG 200, NA.

152. "An Account of the Influenza Epidemic in Perry County, Kentucky," in "Report of the Influenza Epidemic—Lake Division," "Epidemics, Influenza—Reports and Statistics—Lake Division."

153. Ibid. See also "Report of Mrs. S. J. Kinkead, who volunteered to nurse Influenza in the mountains. Report made in the office of R. C. Ballard Thurston, November 7, 1918," "Epidemics, Influenza—Reports and Statistics—Lake Division."

154. Starr Cadwallader, Division Director, Civilian Relief, Lake Division to James L. Fieser, Association Director General National Headquarters, August 12, 1919.

155. Starr Cadwallader, Division Director, Civilian Relief, Lake Division, American Red Cross, "Report of the Department of Civilian Relief, July 1—December 31, 1918," "Lake Division—Civilian Relief Reports July—December 1918," File 149.18, Box 216, Entry 27130D, RG 200, NA.

156. Letter from Shelly D. Watts, Field Supervisor, to James L. Fieser, Department of Civilian Relief, November 13, 1918, "Epidemics, Influenza—Reports and Statistics—Lake Division."

157. Memorandum, Shelly D. Watts, Field Supervisor, to James L. Fieser, "Subject: Report to date on the Influenza situation in Perry Co. Kentucky," November 11, 1918, "Epidemics, Influenza—Reports and Statistics—Lake Division."

158. Letter from MacKenzie R. Todd, Executive Secretary, Lake Division for Kentucky to James L. Fieser, Director, Civilian Relief Committee, November 13, 1918, "Epidemics, Influenza—Reports and Statistics—Lake Division."

159. "New York's 100 Neediest Cases," *NYT*, December 15, 1918, 73.

160. Ibid., 76.

161. Ibid.

162. Ibid.

163. Ibid., 75.

164. Ibid., 74.

165. Ibid.

166. Ibid., 76.

167. Ibid.

168. Ibid.

169. Case #13369, Reel #194—Family Welfare, Minneapolis Family and Children's Service Case Records 1895–1945 (SWF19), Social Welfare History Archives, University of Minnesota Libraries.

170. "What the Visiting Nurse Does," front-page story in *The House on Henry Street* (publication of the Visiting Nurse Service), vol. 1, no. 1 (December 1921), Folder 4: "Publicity, Flyers 1918, 1920–1927," Box 1, Henry Street Visiting Nurse Service (SW63), Social Welfare History Archives, University of Minnesota Libraries.

171. Miss Condell, "Personal experiences during the epidemic," Student nurse epidemic accounts, Folder 1, Box 8, RG 22.1, Department of Nursing, Academic Departments, College Archives, Simmons College.

172. Miss Delano, "Personal experiences during the epidemic," student nurse epidemic accounts, Folder 1, Box 8, RG 22.1, Department of Nursing, Academic Departments, College Archives, Simmons College.

173. Miss Underwood, "Personal experiences during the epidemic," student nurse epidemic accounts, Folder 1, Box 8, RG 22.1, Department of Nursing, Academic Departments, College Archives, Simmons College.

174. Miss Donahue, student nurse epidemic accounts, Folder 1, Box 8, RG 22.1, Department of Nursing, Academic Departments, College Archives, Simmons College.

175. Miss Coolidge, "Personal experiences during the epidemic."

176. Miss Condell, "Personal experiences during the epidemic."

177. See for instance Case #3041, Reel #16 and Case #13025, Reel #192, Family Welfare, Minneapolis Family and Children's Service Case Records 1895–1945, Social Welfare History Archives, University of Minnesota Libraries; Miss Coolidge, "Personal experiences during the epidemic"; Miss Dailey, "Personal experiences during the epidemic," student nurse epidemic accounts, Folder 1, Box 8, RG 22.1, Department of Nursing, Academic Departments, College Archives, Simmons College.

178. Miss Franklin, "Personal experiences during the epidemic," student nurse epidemic accounts, Folder 1, Box 8, RG 22.1, Department of Nursing, Academic Departments, College Archives, Simmons College.

179. See for instance Howard Markel, *When Germs Travel* (New York: Pantheon Books, 2004); Nayan Shah, *Contagious Divides: Epidemics and Race in San Francisco's Chinatown* (Berkeley: University of California Press, 2001); Susan Craddock, *City of Plagues: Disease, Poverty and Deviance in San Francisco* (Minneapolis: University of Minnesota Press, 2000); Howard Markel, *Quarantine! East European Jewish Immigrants and the New York City Epidemics of 1892* (Baltimore: The Johns Hopkins University Press, 1997); Alan M. Kraut, *Silent Traveler: Germs, Genes, and the "Immigrant Menace"* (Baltimore: Johns Hopkins University Press, 1995); Alan M. Kraut, *Huddled Masses: The Immigrant in American Society, 1880–1921* (Arlington Heights, IL: Harlan Davidson, 1982).

180. Alan M. Kraut, "Immigration, Ethnicity, and the Pandemic," *PHR* 125 (2010, Supplement 3): 124–127. Kraut notes that Denver was the lone exception, where Italians were targeted for abuse and seen as "primitive and willfully noncompliant." On immigrants and World War I, see also Nancy Gentile Ford, *Americans All! Foreign-Born Soldiers in World War I* (College Station, TX: Texas A & M University Press, 2001); Christopher M. Sterba, *Good Americans: Italian and Jewish Immigrants during the First World War* (New York: Oxford University Press, 2003).

181. J. Frank Dreher, "Monroe County Report," "Emergency Service of the Pennsylvania Council of National Defense in the Influenza Crisis—Report of the Vice-Director, Department of Medicine, Sanitation and Hospitals," Charlton Yarnall, 30, PAM173, College of Physicians of Philadelphia.

182. Miss Coolidge, "Personal experiences during the epidemic," 1.

183. Kraut, "Immigration, Ethnicity and the Pandemic," 127–132.

184. Case #3126, entry for November 26, 1918, Reel #16, Children's Protective Society, Minneapolis Family and Children's Service Case Records 1895–1945, Social Welfare History Archives, University of Minnesota Libraries.

185. Case #3126, entries for December 17, 1918 and December 18, 1918.

186. Case #3126, entry for January 20, 1919.

187. Case #3126, entry for January 23, 1919.

188. Case #3126, entry for January 27, 1919.

189. Case #3126, entry for February 3, 1919.

190. Case #3126, entry for February 28, 1919.

191. Case #3126, entry for May 17, 1919.

192. Case #3126, entries for June 2, 1919 and June 18, 1919.

193. Case #3126, entry for June 27, 1919.

194. Case #3126, entries for June 30, 1919, July 22, 1922, August 19, 1922, February 16, 1924, June 18, 1925.

195. Case #3126, entry for January 23, 1919, December 18, 1918, January 20, 1919.

196. Case #3126, entry for February 11, 1919. For another example, see Case #13786, Reel #196—Family Welfare, Minneapolis Family and Children's Service Case Records 1895–1945, Social Welfare History Archive, University of Minnesota Libraries.

197. Edna Hoffer, Register of Death, Bureau of Vital Statistics, Washington State Board of Health, Death Certificates 1917–1930, Box 276. Yakima Indian Agency, RG 75, NA (PAR).

198. Letter from D. A. Richardson, M.D., to P. T. Lonergan, Superintendent, December 20, 1918, Subject: Influenza Epidemic at Pueblos of Albuquerque Day School Section, in "The Deadly Virus—The Influenza Epidemic of 1918," National Archives and Records Administration Online Exhibit, available at http://www.archives.gov/exhibits/influenza-epidemic/records-list.html [accessed February 15, 2011].

199. Ibid.

200. "Another type of dwelling in Virginia City," photo of Indian dwelling and description of conditions, File—Influenza Epidemic, Box 33, Reno Agency Records Related to Agency Health and Social Services, 1910–1923, Bureau of Indian Affairs, RG 75, NARA (SF).

201. "The best house in camp" and "Group of Paiutes and Ed Clous, Chief of Police, Virginia City," photos and descriptions, File—Influenza Epidemic, Box 33, Reno Agency Records Related to Agency Health and Social Services, 1910–1923, Bureau of Indian Affairs, RG 75, NARA (SF).

202. Vanessa Northington Gamble, "'There Wasn't a Lot of Comforts in Those Days:' African Americans, Public Health, and the 1918 Influenza Epidemic," *PHR* 125 (2010, Supplement 3): 115–116; Vanessa Northington Gamble, *Making a Place for Ourselves: The Black Hospital Movement, 1920–1945* (New York: Oxford University Press, 1995), chap. 1; Keith Wailoo, *Dying in the City of the Blues: Sickle Cell Anemia and the Politics of Race and Health* (Chapel Hill: University of North Carolina Press, 2001), 32–35. See also James Summerville, *Educating Black Doctors: A History of Meharry Medical College* (Tuscaloosa: University of Alabama Press, 1983).

203. Samuel Kelton Roberts, Jr., *Infectious Fear: Politics, Disease, and the Health Effects of Segregation* (Chapel Hill: University of North Carolina Press, 2009), 4, 34–35, 68–70.

204. Gamble, "'There Wasn't a Lot of Comforts in Those Days,'" 117; Wailoo, *Dying in the City of the Blues*, 30. See also Tera W. Hunter, *To 'Joy My Freedom: Southern Black Women's Lives and Labors after the Civil War* (Cambridge, MA: Harvard University Press, 1997), chap. 9.

205. Gamble, "'There Wasn't a Lot of Comforts in Those Days,'" 117–120; "'"Flu" Shuns Us,' Says Health Doctor," *Cleveland Advocate*, November 2, 1918, 6, available on the African American Experience in Ohio, 1850–1920 website, http://dbs.ohiohistory.org/africanam/page.cfm?ID=7741 [accessed January 27, 2011]; "Influenza and Pneumonia in Philadelphia during the Recent Epidemic," *JNMA* 11 (January–March 1919): 20.

206. Gamble, "'There Wasn't a Lot of Comforts in Those Days,'" 119; Darlene Clark Hine, "The Call That Never Came: Black Women Nurses and World War I—An Historical Note," *Indiana Military History Journal* 8 (January 1983): 23–25.

207. Marian Moser Jones, "The American Red Cross and Local Response to the 1918 Influenza Pandemic: A Four-City Case Study," *PHR* 125 (2010, Supplement 3): 101; Gamble, "'There Wasn't a Lot of Comforts in Those Days,'" 119.

208. Gamble, "'There Wasn't a Lot of Comforts in Those Days,'" 119.

209. "Influenza and Pneumonia Claims Many Victims," *AA*, October 18, 1918, 1; William G. Jordan, *Black Newspapers and America's War for Democracy, 1914–1920* (Chapel Hill: University of North Carolina Press, 2001), 8, 32, 35.

210. "Influenza and Pneumonia Claims Many Victims," 1.

211. Reverend Francis J. Grimke, "Some Reflections, Growing Out of the Recent Epidemic of Influenza That Afflicted Our City," November 3, 1918, Manuscript Department, Moorland-Spingarn Research Center, Howard University.

212. Ibid.

213. William Pickens, "God's a Nigger," *AA*, December 20, 1918, 4.

214. "Fighting on Two Fronts—At Home and 'Over There,'" Supplement to the *Gulf Division Bulletin* November 1, 1918), File 803.7—"Epidemics, Influenza, Publicity and Publications," Box 688, RG 200, NA; Mary E. Lent, Directing Nurse, USPHS, "The Extent and Control of Influenza in Washington D.C.," *PHN* 10 (December 1918): 296.

215. Frances Hayward, "A Brotherhood of Misericordia," *Survey* 41 (November 9, 1918): 148, 149. See also Lillian D. Wald, "The Work of the Nurses' Emergency Council," *PHN* 10 (December 1918): 307.

216. Rev. Francis J. Grimke, "Some Reflections, Growing Out of the Recent Epidemic of Influenza."

217. Sister Georgiana Ennison, President, "Report of St. Ann's Infant Asylum," in *Annual Report of the Commissioners of the District of Columbia, Year Ended June 30, 1919, Vol. I: Miscellaneous Reports* (Washington, D.C.: n.p., 1919), 516.

218. Richard Collier, *The Plague of the Spanish Lady: The Spanish Influenza Pandemic of 1918–1919* (New York: Atheneum, 1974), 199; letter from Urban C. Stover from [indecipherable] in Los Angeles, September 29, 1918, Folder: Urban C. Stover—Letters, August–September, 1918, Urban C. Stover Manuscript Collections, Manuscript Section, Indiana State Library.

219. Eugene H. Fellows, Executive Secretary, "Lackawanna County Report," November 30, 1918, in "Emergency Service of the Pennsylvania Council of National Defense in the Influenza Crisis—Report of the Vice-Director, Department of Medicine, Sanitation and Hospitals," 25, PAM 173, Philadelphia College of Physicians.

220. Letter from Katherine to Jamie, October 13, 1918, Folder: October 13, 1918 Katherine Mae Reynolds Fife to JDF, Box 1, Ella Katherine Fife Letters, Special Collections Department, University of Virginia Library; letter from Will to "Squeechy," October 26, 1918, Folder October 26, 1918 WOF to EKF w/env. (Charlottesville), Box 1, Ella Katherine Fife Letters, Special Collections Department, University of Virginia Library.

221. J. R. Steward, "Field Director's Report—Camp Dodge, Iowa—Period Covering Influenza Epidemic," October 17, 1918, 3, "Epidemic, Influenza, Iowa," File 803.11, Box 689, RG 200, NA.

222. Letter from Sam and Clara, October 20, 1918, Herbert Greenfelder collection, HQ Company, 325th Field Artillery, 84th Division, WEQC, WWORP, USAMHI.

223. "War-Reports from the Influenza Front," 62; J. R. Steward, "Field Director's Report—Camp Dodge Iowa—Period Covering Influenza Epidemic" (October 17, 1918), 76.

224. "Editorial—Don't Help the Plague," *Tacoma News Tribune*, October 11, 1918, 14; G. A. Stirling, "The Superintendent," in "Report of the Board of Trustees of the National Training School for Boys," in *Annual Report of the Commissioners of the District of Columbia, Year Ended June 30, 1919—Vol. I: Miscellaneous Reports* (Washington, D.C.: n.p., 1919), 426; letter from Madge to Ella, November 7, 1918, Folder: "November 7, 1918 —MWF to EKF w/env. (Charlottesville)," Box 1, Ella Katherine Fife Letters (5943-e), Special Collections Department, University of Virginia Library; Mazyck P. Ravenel, "Preventive Medicine and War," *AJPH* 10 (January 1920): 28.

225. Guy W. Latimer, M.D., President, Board of Trustees, "The School Physician," in "Report of the Board of Trustees of the National Training School for Boys," in *Annual Report of the Commissioners of the District of Columbia, Year Ended June 30, 1919—Vol. I: Miscellaneous Reports* (Washington, D.C.: n.p., 1919), 426; Letter from Mother to "My precious daughter," October 29, 1918, Folder "1918 October 29 SAGSF to EKF (Charlottesville)," Box 1, Ella Katherine Fife Letters, Special Collections Department, University of Virginia Library.

226. Royal S. Copeland, Commissioner of Health of the City of New York, "General Survey of the Influenza Epidemic" (reprinted from the *New York Medical Journal* for October 26, 1918), NYC Vertical Files, City of New York Municipal Reference and Research Center; letter from "Your Sailor Boy, Herb" to "Dearest Mother," October 31, 1918, Folder: August 1918–March 1919, Carl R. and Edwin J. Jones and Family Papers, Minnesota Historical Society; Anne L. Colon, "Influenza at Cedar Branch Camp," in "Experiences During the Epidemic," *American Journal of Nursing* (hereafter *AJN*) 19 (May 1919): 605; letter from Alfred F. Hess to Biggs, November 8, 1918, Governor's Commission on Epidemic Influenza (New York): Correspondence 1918–1919, Series III—Box 79, Charles-Edward Amory Papers, Sterling Library, Yale University; Georgette Moses, "Report of the Activities of the Chapters and Branches of the Atlantic Division of the American Red Cross during The Epidemic of Spanish Influenza, December 20, 1918," File 803.08—Epidemics, Influenza, Reports and Statistics, Atlantic Division, Box 688, File 803, RG 200, NA.

227. See Susan Sontag, *Illness as Metaphor* (1978 reprint), combined edition, *Illness as Metaphor and AIDS and Its Metaphors* (New York: Anchor Books, 1990), 3–4, 66–67; Deborah

Oates Erwin, "The Militarization of Cancer Treatment in American Society," in *Encounters with Biomedicine: Case Studies in Medical Anthropology*, ed. Harold O. Baer (New York: Gordon and Breach Science Publishers, 1987), 201–227; Arthur Kleinman, *Patients and Healers in the Context of Culture: An Exploration of the Borderland between Anthropology, Medicine and Psychiatry* (Berkeley: University of California Press, 1980), 108–109; Deborah Lupton, *Medicine as Culture: Illness, Disease and the Body in Western Societies*, 2nd ed. (Thousand Oaks, CA: Sage, 2003), 61–64; Howard F. Stein, *American Medicine as Culture* (Boulder, CO: Westview Press, 1990), 67–68; Barron Lerner, *Breast Cancer Wars: Hope, Fear, and the Pursuit of a Cure in Twentieth-Century America* (New York: Oxford University Press, 2001).

228. "The Grip's Deadly March," *NYT*, January 17, 1890, 1; Morell MacKenzie, "Influenza," *Living Age* 190 (August 1, 1890): 301; C. F. Ulrich, "Some of the Vagaries of the Grippe," *JAMA* 15 (October 4, 1890): 497. See also T. H. Buckler, Sr., "Influenza, From a Sanitary Point of View," *Maryland Medical Journal* 27 (1892): 580; "The Grip," *NYT*, February 22, 1903, 6.

229. Filson Young, "Influenza," *The Living Age* (May 3, 1913): 306–308.

230. Crosby, *America's Forgotten Pandemic*, 73, 77–78; Kim Allen Scott, "Plague on the Home-front: Arkansas and the Great Influenza Epidemic of 1918," *Arkansas Historical Quarterly* 47 (1988): 320; Russell R. Elliott, "The Influenza Epidemic of 1918–1919," *Halcyon* 14 (1992): 249; Ann McLaurin, "The Influenza Epidemic of 1918 in Shreveport," *North Louisiana Historical Association Journal* 13 (Winter 1982): 1; Philip C. Ensley, "Indiana and the Influenza Pandemic of 1918," *Indiana Medical History Quarterly* 9 (1983): 12; Leonard J. Arrington, "The Influenza Epidemic of 1918–1919 in Southern Idaho," *Idaho Yesterdays* 32 (1988): 22. Barron H. Lerner notes the distinct impact of World War II and the Cold War on the use of military metaphor, suggesting another context in which the existence of actual wars made more complicated the meaning of military metaphors. Barron H. Lerner, *The Breast Cancer Wars: Hope, Fear, and the Pursuit of a Cure in Twentieth-Century America* (New York: Oxford University Press, 2001), 41.

231. The tendency to blame epidemics on outside enemies is a common theme across cultures and centuries. See Paul Slack, "Introduction," *Epidemics and Ideas: Essays on the Historical Perception of Pestilence*, ed. Terrence Ranger and Paul Stack (New York: Cambridge University Press, 1992), 3–4.

232. Letter from B. R. Hart, Chief, Eastern District to Chief, Bureau of Chemistry, October 28, 1918 and Letter, Assistant Surgeon General to B. R. Hart, November 15, 1918, both in File 1622, Box 144, RG 90, NA.

233. Letter from Mrs. N. A. Field, Socorro, New Mexico, to War Department, September 1918, File 710 Influenza—September 1918, Box 394, Decimal 710, Subseries 1917–1927, Entry 29, Record Group 112, NA.

234. Letter from George F. Murphy to Surgeon General's Department, September 17, 1918, File 710 Influenza September 1918, Box 394, Decimal 710, Subseries 1917–1927, Entry 29, Record Group 112, National Archives.

235. Alfred M. Brooks, Bloomington, Indiana, "The GERMAN PLAGUE—Give a New Name to the Prevalent Epidemic," Letter to the Editor, signed October 13, 1918, *NYT*, October 20, 1918.

236. Sunday quoted in William G. McLoughlin, Jr., *Billy Sunday Was His Real Name* (Chicago: University of Chicago Press, 1955), 259–260.

237. Other historians have acknowledged the valuable role placing blame has played historically as cultures struggle against diseases beyond their understanding. See for instance Dorothy Nelkin and Sander L. Gilman, "Placing Blame for Devastating Disease," *Social Research* 55 (1988): 362.

238. Letter from Victor W. Jones to "Mother, Squickie and Dad," November 3, 1918, Victor W. Jones, Camp Lewis, 8th (45th) Co., 166th Depot Brigade, WWORP, AEQC, USAMHI; Editorial, *WN*, December 3, 1918, 6.

239. "The Epidemic Over," *Red Cross Clippings* (Penn-Del Div.), December 5, 1918, p. 7, Bound Volume—Penn vol. 1–2, Box 521, File 494.2—Div. Bulletins, Entry 27130D, Record Group 200, National Archives.

240. Hermann M. Biggs, "The Recent Epidemic of Influenza," *American Review of Reviews* 59 (January 1919): 69.

241. "WALLACE YOUTH DIES SUDDENLY—Harry R. Kinkead Victim of Pneumonia Which Follows Influenza Attack," *Wallace Press-Times*, October 29, 1918, 1; "Will the 'Flu' Return?" *LD* 63 (October 11, 1919): 26; "Uncle Sam's Advice on Flu," *Shenandoah Valley* (New Market, Virginia), October 17, 1918, 1.

242. Wesley T. Lee, *The Battle of Pougues-Lels-Eaux: A History of U.S. Army Base Hospital No. 44* (New York: Globe Press, 1923), 41; News Release #2569 "RELEASED FOR MORNING PAPERS OF SUNDAY SEPTEMBER 29TH," contained in bound volume: News Releases nos. 1861–2821, 1918, vol. III, File 020.1801 News Releases, Box 4, Entry 27130D, Record Group 200, National Archives; "How to Fight Spanish Influenza," *LD* 59 (October 12, 1918): 13–14; letter from Hugh to "Folks," no date, Folder 9—Correspondence September–October 1918, Box 1, Hugh Arthur Barnhart Manuscript Collection, Manuscript Section, Indiana State Library.

243. George M. Price, M.D., "Influenza—Destroyer and Teacher," *Survey* 41 (December 21, 1919): 367; "Editorial—Influenza Masks," *Daily Californian*, October 22, 1918, 2.

244. Sherman C. Kingsley, "Cleveland and the 'Flu,'" *PHN* 10 (December 1918): 314.

245. "How to Fight Spanish Influenza," ad for Dr. Pierce's Pleasant Pellets, *LAT*, October 12, 1918, II, 6.

246. "FACIAL ARMOR FOR THE INFLUENZA," caption for photographs depicting masks in use, included on same page as "How Influenza Got In," *LD* 59 (November 30, 1918): 23.

247. Lillian D. Wald, "Influenza: When the City Is a Great Field Hospital," *Survey* 43 (February 14, 1920): 581; Cheney C. Jones, Director, Bureau of Civilian Relief, "Report of the Bureau of Civilian Relief, Pennsylvania-Delaware Division, American Red Cross, for the Month of October 1918," in "American Red Cross Report of the Division Directors of Civilian Relief for the Month of October 1918," File 149.18—Civilian Relief Reports—All Divisions—September–October 1918, Box 201, Entry 27130D, RG 200, NA; Raymond Pearl, "Influenza Studies—On Certain General Statistical Aspects of the 1918 Epidemic in American Cities," *PHR* 34 (August 8, 1919): 1744.

248. "Spanish Influenza—A Circular to the Medical Profession," *Weekly Bulletin of the Department of Health, City of New York* 7 (October 26, 1918): 335.

249. "Home Folks Need Not Worry About the Boys in Camp Cody," *Trench and Camp—Camp Cody*, October 31, 1918, 8.

250. Dr. Lee H. Smith, "Health Talk: Spanish Influenza or Grip," *Shenandoah Valley*, November 7, 1918, 4.

251. Sgt. A. H. Brayton, "WITH GERMS IN ROUT, VICTORIOUS HOSPITAL WORKERS REST A BIT," *Camp Dodger*, October 18, 1918, 1; "Base Hospital Flurries," *Camp Jackson Click*, October 19, 1918, 1.

252. "Editorial—Showing the Courage of Soldiers," *NYT*, November 5, 1918, 12.

253. Alfred Crosby argues a similar point. Crosby, *America's Forgotten Pandemic*, 320–321. Carol Byerly complicates this idea, suggesting that while it was often the case that soldiers who died of influenza were viewed as heroes by loved ones, the broader culture tended to view them as somehow less than those who died in battle. Byerly, *Fever of War*, 133–134.

254. "War-Reports from the Influenza Front," 62.

255. See also Hospital Annual Report for Gardiner General Hospital, quoted in Gabriel W. Kirkpatrick, "Influenza 1918: A Maine Perspective," *Maine Historical Society Quarterly* 25 (1986): 170; W.G. Rauch, letter to Spencer C. Gilbert, November 11, 1918, reprinted in "Emergency Service of the Pennsylvania Council of National Defense in the Influenza Crisis—Report of the Vice-Director, Department of Medicine, Sanitation and Hospitals, College of Physicians, Philadelphia, PAM173.

256. Dora Christianson, "Your Chance," *AJN* 19 (January 1919): 275.

257. "The Epidemic Over," *Red Cross Clippings* (Penn-Del Div.), December 5, 1918, p. 7, Bound Volume—Penn vol. 1–2, Box 521, File 494.2—Div. Bulletins, Entry 27130D, RG 200, NA.

258. Portia B. Kernodle, *The Red Cross Nurse in Action* (New York: Harper Bros., 1949), 147.

259. "Our Workers Who Lost Their Lives Fighting the Influenza Epidemic—A Civilian Role of Honor," *Staff News* 6 (December 1, 1918): 1.

260. "The Supreme Sacrifice—Text of Gov. W. L. Harding's Speech at Services Honoring Memory of Camp Dodge Epidemic Victims," *Camp Dodger* (Camp Dodge, Iowa), November 8, 1918, 2.
261. *Corks and Curls* (UVA Yearbook) 32 (1919).
262. "EPIDEMIC CLAIMS 926 HERE," *Camp Sherman News*, October 15, 1918, 1.
263. Such an interpretation was especially appropriate in the early twentieth century, a period during which Americans' cultural responses to death were undergoing profound changes. See Robert V. Wells, *Facing the "King of Terrors": Death and Society in an American Community, 1750–1990* (New York: Cambridge University Press, 2000), 194, 200, 227, 236.

Chapter 3

1. "Man Dies After Attack of Grippe," *World News* (Roanoke, Virginia) (hereafter *WN*), September 30, 1918, 2.
2. "Cases of Influenza," *WN*, September 28, 1918, 2.
3. "Man Dies After Attack of Grippe," 2.
4. "Influenza Spread by Careless Folk," *WN*, September 30, 1918, 4.
5. Editorial, no title, *WN*, October 29, 1918, 6.
6. Editorial, no title, *WN*, November 1, 1918, 6.
7. "Schools of City Reopen Monday," *WN*, November 9, 1918, 1.
8. "Influenza Shows Let-Up in Roanoke," *WN*, October 28, 1918, 2; "Flu 'Flare-Back' Reported Today," *WN*, October 29, 1918, 1.
9. "Dr. Foster Warns Influenza Patients," *WN*, October 23, 1918, 2.
10. "Gradual Decline in Influenza Cases," *WN*, October 30, 1918, 1.
11. Editorial, no title, *WN*, October 29, 1918, 6.
12. Editorial, no title, *WN*, November 1, 1918, 6; editorial, no title, *WN*, November 2, 1918, 6.
13. "'Flu' Shows Signs of a 'Comeback,'" *WN*, November 4, 1918, 2.
14. "'Flu' Epidemic Shows Some Life," *WN*, November 23, 1918, 1.
15. "Influenza Again on Increase Here," *WN*, November 25, 1918, 1.
16. Editorial, no title, *WN*, December 3, 1918, 6; "Most 'Flu' Cases Are in Mild Form," *WN*, December 4, 1918, 1.
17. "Influenza Shows Stubborn Fight," 1.
18. "Most 'Flu' Cases Are in Mild Form," 1.
19. Ibid.; "Eighty-Eight New Influenza Cases Reported to Board," *WN*, December 9, 1918, 1.
20. "Influenza Keeps Up Heavy Record," *WN*, December 10, 1918, 1; "Editorial—Keep Out of Crowds," *WN*, December 10, 1918, 4.
21. "Influenza Shows Stubborn Fight," *WN*, December 7, 1918, 1.
22. "Eighty-Eight New Influenza Cases Reported to Board," 1.
23. "City Council Issues Notice to Public on Influenza Situation," *WN*, December 10, 1918, 10.
24. "Influenza Keeps Up Heavy Record," 1; "'Flu' Lid Will Be Applied in City Thursday," *WN*, December 11, 1918, 1; "Editorial—The Lid Goes on Again Tomorrow," *WN*, December 11, 1918, 6.
25. "'Flu' Lid Will Be Applied in City Thursday," 1; "Editorial—The Lid Goes on Again Tomorrow," 6.
26. "New Warrants Issued for Flu Ban Violators," *WN*, December 14, 1918, 1, 2.
27. Ibid., 2.
28. "Closing Order Debated Before Judge Berkeley," *WN*, December 16, 1918, 1.
29. Ibid.
30. Ibid.
31. "May Repeal the Closing Order," *WN*, December 16, 1918, 8; "Editorial—Dr. Foster's Return," *WN*, December 17, 1918, 6.
32. "Editorial—Dr. Foster's Return," 6.
33. "Weddings and Parties Are Under Influenza Ban," *WN*, December 21, 1918, 1.
34. Ibid.
35. "Someone Will Die Unless Nurses Are Found for the Sick," *WN*, December 23, 1918, 1.
36. Ibid.

37. "Influenza Shows Slight Increase in Recent Days," *WN*, December 24, 1918, 1.
38. "Holiday Delays Influenza Count," *WN*, December 26, 1918, 1; "Flu Decrease Brings Cases to Lowest Level," *WN*, December 27, 1918, 1.
39. "Thirty-One Cases of Flu Reported," *WN*, December 28, 1918, 1; "City Schools Opened Today," *WN*, December 30, 1918, 1.
40. "Influenza Still Holds Its Level," *WN*, January 7, 1919, 1. In the end, sixty people died of influenza in Roanoke in December alone. "Sixty Influenza Deaths in Month," *WN*, January 4, 1919, 1. Infection rates for the epidemic were as follows: September, 28; October, 4,042; November, 1,033; December, 1,474 (up through December 26). "Flu Decrease Brings Cases to Lowest Level," *WN*, December 27, 1918, 1.
41. David Rosner, "'Spanish Flu, or Whatever It Is. . . .': The Paradox of Public Health in a Time of Crisis," *PHR* 125 (2010, Supplement 3): 43–44.
42. Bulletin No. 37, Division of Sanitation, Bureau of Medicine and Surgery, Department of the Navy, "Influenza," reprinted in "Measures for the Prevention of the Introduction of Epidemic Influenza," *PHR* 33 (September 13, 1918): 1542.
43. Letter from C. R. Fellers, Scientific Assistant, Officer in Temporary Charge (Extra-Cantonment Sanitation, Charlotte, North Carolina), to the Surgeon General, October 11, 1918, Box 144, #1622, Record Group 90, NA.
44. V. C. Vaughan to Dr. Royal S. Copeland, October 11, 1918, in response to telegram the preceding day, Box 348, F(States and Cities)—New York, New York City, Subseries 1917–1927, Entry 29, RG 112, NA. There were exceptions to this optimism. Charles V. Chapin, a leading light in public health from Providence, Rhode Island, early on recognized that this was a disease that would be difficult to control. James H. Cassedy, *Charles V. Chapin and the Public Health Movement* (Cambridge, MA: Harvard University Press, 1962), 187–188.
45. Letter unsigned, to Dr. John T. Black, Commissioner of Health, State of Connecticut, October 17, 1918, File 68–0921—Connecticut Department of Health: Correspondence, 1916–1918, Box 68, Series III, Charles-Edward Amory Winslow Papers, Sterling Memorial Library, Yale University.
46. W. A. Evans et al. (Editorial Committee of the American Public Health Association), "A Working Program Against Influenza," *AJPH* 9 (January 1919): 1.
47. Capt. J. G. Townsend, "United States Public Health Service—Spanish Influenza," in *Pass in Review* (Camp Bowie), October 5, 1918, 6; "Influenza Warning from the Academy of Medicine," *New York Medical Journal* (hereafter *NYMJ*) (October 19, 1918): 682; Bulletin No. 37, Division of Sanitation, Bureau of Medicine and Surgery, Department of the Navy, "Influenza," reprinted in "Measures for the Prevention of the Introduction of Epidemic Influenza," 1541–1544; Evans et al., "A Working Program Against Influenza," 1–2; "Editorial—Weapons Against Influenza," *AJPH* 8 (1918): 788.
48. Evans et al., "A Working Program Against Influenza," 1; letter from Rupert Blue, Surgeon General, to Medical Officers in Charge of United States Quarantine Stations, reprinted in "Measures for the Prevention of the Introduction of Epidemic Influenza," 1540; Bulletin No. 37, Division of Sanitation, Bureau of Medicine and Surgery, Department of the Navy, "Influenza," reprinted in "Measures for the Prevention of the Introduction of Epidemic Influenza," 1543.
49. Evans et al., "A Working Program Against Influenza," 1.
50. Commission on Epidemic Influenza, appointed by the Governor of New York, "Accepted Points," File—Governor's Commission on Epidemic Influenza (New York): Notes, Membership Lists, Reference Materials, 1918–1919, Box 79, Series III, Charles-Edward Amory Winslow Papers, Sterling Library, Yale University.
51. Rupert Blue, "Epidemic Influenza and the U.S. Public Health Service," *MH* 11 (December 1918): 425–426; Evans et al., "A Working Program Against Influenza," 7, 12.
52. Letter from Edwin W. Kopf, Chairman, Committee on Statistical Study of the Influenza Epidemic, American Public Health Association, and John W. Trask, Chairman, Section on Vital Statistics, American Public Health Association, to Chas. E. A. Winslow, Yale School of Medicine, Department of Public Health, November 23, 1918, "Governor's Commission on Epidemic Influenza (New York): Correspondence, 1918–1919," Series III: Box 79, Charles-Edward Amory Winslow Papers, Sterling Library, Yale University.

53. "Resolutions on the Statistical Study of the Influenza Epidemic of 1918 (Being Resolutions and Discussion before the Section on Vital Statistics, December 11, 1918, at Chicago, Ill., together with Notes of Subsequent Committee Work)," *AJPH* 9 (February 1919): 140.

54. "Epidemic Influenza ('Spanish Influenza'). Prevalence in the United States," *PHR*, 33 (September 27, 1918): 1625–1626; "Epidemic Influenza. Prevalence in the United States," *PHR*, 33 (October 4, 1918): 1677–1679; "Epidemic Influenza. Prevalence in the United States," *PHR* 33 (October 11, 1918): 1729–1731.

55. Evans et al., "A Working Program Against Influenza," 1.

56. "Brief Outline of Activities of the Public Health Service in Combating the Influenza Epidemic—1918–1919." Box 145, File 1622, RG 90, NA.

57. Ibid.; Blue, "Epidemic Influenza and the U.S. Public Health Service," 423.

58. "Brief Outline of Activities of the Public Health Service in Combating the Influenza Epidemic—1918–1919"; Blue, "Epidemic Influenza and the U.S. Public Health Service," 423; Dorothy Pettit and Janice Bailie, *A Cruel Wind: Pandemic Flu in American 1918–1920* (Murfreesboro, TN: Timberlane Books, 2008), 79–80.

59. "Measures for the Prevention of the Introduction of Epidemic Influenza," 1540–44.

60. "Editorial—Weapons Against Influenza," 788.

61. Blue, "Epidemic Influenza and the U.S. Public Health Service," 424.

62. Ibid.

63. Letter from Surgeon General to Chairman, War Council, American Red Cross, October 1, 1918, File 803.02: Epidemics—Influenza—Cooperating Organizations, Box 688, RG 200, NA; "Plan for Combatting [*sic*] the Influenza Epidemic," File 803: Epidemic Influenza—1918—Divisions, Box 688, RG 200, NA; Memo from W. Frank Persons, Chairman, Red Cross National Committee on Influenza to All Division, Managers, "General Instructions (First night letter from Chairman of National Committee)," October 5, 1918, which includes a copy of October 3 memo from Persons, File 803.02: Epidemics—Influenza—Cooperating Organizations, Box 688, RG 200, NA.

64. Blue, "Epidemic Influenza and the U.S. Public Health Service," 424–425; memo from W. Frank Persons, Chairman, Red Cross National Committee on Influenza to All Division, Managers, "General Instructions (First night letter from Chairman of National Committee)," October 5, 1918, File 803.02: Epidemics—Influenza—Cooperating Organizations, Box 688, RG 200, NA; "Brief Outline of Activities of the Public Health Service in Combating the Influenza Epidemic—1918–1919," 3–4.

65. "Brief Outline of Activities of the Public Health Service in Combating the Influenza Epidemic—1918–1919," 5; Marian Moser Jones, "The American Red Cross and Local Response to the 1918 Influenza Pandemic: A Four-City Case Study," *PHR* 125 (2010, Supplement 3): 93.

66. "Brief Outline of Activities of the Public Health Service in Combating the Influenza Epidemic—1918–1919," 4.

67. Ibid., 5.

68. "Plan for Combatting [*sic*] the Influenza Epidemic," File 803: Epidemic Influenza—1918—Divisions, Box 68, RG 200, NA.

69. "Plan of Organization of Red Cross Nursing Resources to Combat Influenza"; Influenza—1918—Divisions, File 803: Epidemics, Box 688, RG 200, NA.

70. Memo from Alfred Fairbank, Chairman, Southwestern Division Red Cross Committee on Influenza to all the Chapters, "Influenza Letter No. 4," October 12, 1918, File 803.08: Influenza Epidemic—Reports and Statistics—Southwestern Division, Box 688, RG 200, NA.

71. Elizabeth Ross, Director, Bureau of Nursing, New England Division, American Red Cross to All Organizations, October 3, 1918, File 803: Epidemics—Influenza—1918—Divisions, Box 688, RG 200, NA.

72. Blue, "Epidemic Influenza and the U.S. Public Health Service," 424–425.

73. Ibid., 425.

74. Nancy Tomes, "'Destroyer and Teacher': Managing the Masses During the 1918–1919 Influenza Pandemic," *PHR* 125 (2010, Supplement 3): 52.

75. Blue, "Epidemic Influenza and the U.S. Public Health Service," 427; Louise Drew Perry, "Control of Epidemics in Factories," *PHN* 10 (October 1918): 159; "Epidemic Influenza and the United States Public Health Service," *PHR* 33 (October 25, 1918): 1821.

76. M. G. Parsons, Assistant Sanitary Engineer in Charge, West Point, Mississippi, to the Surgeon General, October 13, 1918, File 1622, Box 144, RG 90, NA; "Influenza Warning from the Academy of Medicine," *NYMJ* (October 19, 1918): 682.

77. Blue, "Epidemic Influenza and the U.S. Public Health Service," 425.

78. Evans et al., "A Working Program Against Influenza," 10–11.

79. Blue, "Epidemic Influenza and the U.S. Public Health Service," 425.

80. Ibid.

81. "Droplet Infection Explained in Pictures," *PHR* 33 (November 15, 1918): 1969.

82. "Red Cross Bulletin—Spanish Influenza," File 803.7: Epidemics—Influenza—Publicity and Publications, Box 688, RG 200, NA.

83. Alfred W. Crosby, *America's Forgotten Pandemic: The Influenza of 1918* (New York: Cambridge University Press, 1989), 49.

84. Townsend, "United States Public Health Service—Spanish Influenza," 6.

85. Charles Richard, Acting Surgeon General, US Army, "MEMORANDUM to all Camp and Division Surgeons; Commanding Officers of Base and General Hospitals Surgeons, Independent Posts and Stations; Department Surgeons; Surgeons all Special Camps," September 27, 1918, File 710: Influenza—1918, Box 394, Decimal 710, Entry 29, RG 112, NA.

86. Townsend, "United States Public Health Service—Spanish Influenza," 6.

87. Evans et al., "A Working Program Against Influenza," 3.

88. "Red Cross Bulletin—Spanish Influenza," File 803.7: Epidemics—Influenza—Publicity and Publications, Box 688, RG 200, NA.

89. Evans et al., "A Working Program Against Influenza," 3.

90. Memo from Lieutenant Commander J. R. Phelps, Medical Corps, USN to Dr. Biggs, in reference to the memo of November 6 from the Governor's Commission on Epidemic Influenza, Box 79, Series 3, Manuscript Group #749, Charles-Edward Amory Winslow Papers, Sterling Library, Yale University; "Guarding Against Influenza," *PHR* 33(20 December 1918): 2259; "Red Cross Bulletin—Spanish Influenza," File 803.7: Epidemics—Influenza—Publicity and Publications, Box 688, RG 200, NA.

91. Rupert Blue, "'Spanish Influenza' 'Three-Day Fever' 'The Flu,'" *PHR* (September 28, 1918, Supplement 34): 4.

92. Ibid.

93. "Red Cross Bulletin—Spanish Influenza," File 803.7: Epidemics—Influenza—Publicity and Publications, Box 688, RG 200, NA.

94. "It's Up To You," USPHS circular, #1622, Box 144, RG 90, NA.

95. Blue, "'Spanish Influenza' 'Three-Day Fever' 'The Flu,'" 4.

96. Charles Richard, Acting Surgeon General, US Army, "MEMORANDUM to all Camp and Division Surgeons; Commanding Officers of Base and General Hospitals Surgeons, Independent Posts and Stations; Department Surgeons; Surgeons all Special Camps," September 27, 1918, File 710: Influenza—1918, Box 394, Decimal 710, Entry 29, RG 112, NA.

97. "Red Cross Bulletin—Spanish Influenza," File 803.7: Epidemics—Influenza—Publicity and Publications, Box 688, RG 200, NA.

98. Blue, "Epidemic Influenza and the U.S. Public Health Service," 426; Evans et al., "A Working Program Against Influenza," 5.

99. "Influenza Warning from the Academy of Medicine," 682; Blue, "Epidemic Influenza and the U.S. Public Health Service," 426; Letter "To All Organizations" from Paul W. Kimball, Director, Department of Development, American Red Cross, New England Division, October 3, 1918, File 803: Epidemics—Influenza—1918—Divisions, Box 688, RG 200, NA.

100. Blue, "Epidemic Influenza and the U.S. Public Health Service," 426; J. J. McShane, "The Attempt to Control Influenza in Illinois," *Illinois Medical Journal* (hereafter *IMJ*) 37 (January 1920): 19; memo from Lieutenant Commander J.R. Phelps to Dr. Biggs, November 9, 1918, in reference to the memo of November 6 on Governor's Commission on Influenza, Governor's Commission on Epidemic Influenza (New York)—Memoranda, 1918, Box 79, Series III, Charles-Edward Amory Winslow Papers, Sterling Library, Yale University; W. L. Holt, Charles V. Craster and Colonel Cumming in "Proceedings—Influenza Discussions," *AJPH* 9 (February 1919): 137.

101. Dr. W. L. Holt in "Proceedings—Influenza Discussions," 137; memo from Lieutenant Commander J.R. Phelps to Dr. Biggs, November 9, 1918.

102. Heman Spalding, "Public Health Measures Against Influenza," *Proceedings of the Institute of Medicine of Chicago* 2 (1918–1919): 169.

103. Blue, "'Spanish Influenza' 'Three-Day Fever' 'The Flu'"; Evans et al., "A Working Program Against Influenza," 2, 4; Telegram Blue to Sweeny, Fayetteville, NC, October 4, 1918, #1622, Box 144, RG 90, NA; Telegram Blue to Geiger, Little Rock, October 5, 1918, #1622, Box 144, RG 90, NA.

104. Evans et al., "A Working Program Against Influenza," 4.

105. Ibid.

106. Dr. Robertson in "Discussion" following McShane, "The Attempt to Control Influenza in Illinois," 21.

107. Evans et al., "A Working Program Against Influenza," 5; F. E. Harrington, USPHS, document partially lifting restrictions in Forrest County, Mississippi, attached to letter from Harrington to Surgeon General, November 2, 1918, #1622, Box 144, RG 90, NA.

108. See for instance "Order from the Board of Health," Quitman, Georgia, December 13, 1918, #1622, Box 145, RG 90, NA; "Controlling the Influenza Epidemic in Ohio," *Ohio Public Health Journal* 9 (November 1918): 453.

109. Blue, "Epidemic Influenza and the U.S. Public Health Service," 425.

110. Telegram from Perry, Acting, USPHS to G.M. Corput, New Orleans, January 11, 1919, Box 145, RG 90, NA.

111. Evans et al., "A Working Program Against Influenza," 4–5.

112. V. C. Vaughan to Dr. Royal S. Copeland, October 11, 1918, in response to Copeland's telegram of October 10, 1918, File F: (States and Cities)—New York, New York City, Subseries 1917–1927, Box 348, Entry 29, RG 112 NA.

113. Dr. Robertson in "Discussion" following McShane, "The Attempt to Control Influenza in Illinois," 21.

114. Letter from Rupert Blue, Surgeon General to Dr. C. Hampson Jones, Chief, Bureau of Communicable Diseases, Department of Health, Maryland, January 21, 1919, Box 145, File #1622, RG 90, NA; letter from C. Hampson Jones to the Surgeon General, December 28, 1918, Box 145, RG 90, NA.

115. Telegram from Rupert Blue, Surgeon General to Henry W. Peabody and Co., NYC, February 17, 1919, #1622, Box 145, 1622, RG 90, NA.

116. Evans et al., "A Working Program Against Influenza," 11–12.

117. Dr. Robertson in "Discussion" following McShane, "The Attempt to Control Influenza in Illinois," 21.

118. R. A. O'Neill, C. St. Clair Drake, and J. O Cobb, "The Work of the Illinois Influenza Commission," *AJPH* 9 (January 1919): 24.

119. John Barry, *The Great Influenza: The Epic Story of the Deadliest Plague in History* (New York: Viking, 2004), 356.

120. Alfred W. Crosby, *Epidemic and Peace, 1918* (Westport, CT: Greenwood Press, 1976), 100–101.

121. C. Y. White, "Influenza Vaccine," in "What the Health Department Has Done to Curb the Epidemic of Influenza," *Monthly Bulletin of The Department of Public Health and Charities of the City of Philadelphia* 3 (October–November 1918): 21; Crosby, *America's Forgotten Pandemic*, 84.

122. White, "Influenza Vaccine," 21.

123. On San Francisco, see Crosby, *America's Forgotten Pandemic*, 101.

124. Ibid., 84, 239.

125. Dr. Robertson in "Discussion" following McShane, "The Attempt to Control Influenza in Illinois," 21.

126. John Barry suggests such efforts ultimately frightened the public who recognized their dissonance with surrounding realities. Barry, *The Great Influenza*, 335–336.

127. Blue, "'Spanish Influenza' 'Three-Day Fever' 'The Flu.'"

128. "Editorial—Weapons Against Influenza," 787.

129. Spalding, "Public Health Measures Against Influenza," 167.

130. Elizabeth Ross, Director, Bureau of Nursing, New England Division, Red Cross, "To All Organizations," October 3, 1918, Box 688, File 803: Epidemic—Influenza—1918—Divisions, RG 200, NA. The Public Health Committee of the New York Academy of Medicine also relied on the language of danger, suggesting in their recommendations that "the public should be warned of the danger," in particular of the risk of infection among crowds. "Influenza Warning from the Academy of Medicine," 682.

131. C. E. Turner, "Organizing an Industry to Combat Influenza," *Journal of Industrial Hygiene* 1 (January 1920): 448.

132. "Mayor Puts Ban on All Gatherings to Check 'Flu,'" *Tacoma News Tribune*, October 8, 1918, 1.

133. City Health Officer Dr. Robert D. Wilson, quoted in "Two Cases of 'Flu' Reported in City," *Tacoma News Tribune*, October 10, 1918, 5.

134. William C. Woodward, Health Commissioner, "City of Boston. Health Department. Influenza and Pneumonia. Advice as to Care of Patients, and as to Prevention of these Diseases." File 803: Epidemics—Influenza—1918—Divisions, Box 688, RG 200, NA.

135. "Spanish Influenza Here, Ship Men Say," *NYT*, August 14, 1918, 1.

136. "No Quarantine Here Against Influenza," *NYT*, August 15, 1918, 6.

137. Ibid.

138. "Health Head Calls Influenza Inquiry," *NYT*, August 16, 1918, 16; "Orders Fight on Influenza," *NYT*, August 17, 1918, 5; "Epidemic Guard for Port," *NYT*, August 19, 1918, 5; "Spanish Influenza Found in 'Mild Form,'" *NYT*, August 20, 1918, 20.

139. "Influenza is Halted, Health Reports Show," *NYT*, October 1, 1918, 24.

140. "Tells of Vaccine to Stop Influenza," *NYT*, October 2, 1918, 10.

141. Ibid.

142. "Gains Slightly Here," *NYT*, October 3, 1918, 24.

143. "New Gains in Grip Here," *NYT*, October 4, 1918, 24.

144. "Drastic Steps Taken to Fight Influenza Here," *NYT*, October 5, 1918, 1, 6; "Revise Timetable in Influenza Fight," *NYT*, October 6, 1918, 1, 8.

145. "Editorial—The Spanish Influenza," *NYT*, October 7, 1918, 12.

146. "Asks Experts' Aid to Check Epidemic," *NYT*, October 13, 1918, 18.

147. "INFLUENZA: How to Avoid it—How to Care for Those Who Have It," Bound volume—Pennsylvania, vols. I and II, File 494.2—Division Bulletins, Box 521, Entry 27130D, RG 200, NA.

148. "Influenza frequently complicated with pneumonia," Chicago Department of Health, 1918, Images from the History of Medicine, NLM.

149. USPHS circular, West Point, Mississippi, "IT'S UP TO YOU," #1622, Box 144, RG 90, NA. Bold in original.

150. R. C. Williams, Assistant Surgeon, United States Public Health Service, "Public Health Bulletin No. 98—Health Almanac for 1919," (Washington, DC: Government Printing Office, 1919), 3.

151. Ibid., 4.

152. Townsend, "United States Public Health Service—Spanish Influenza," 6.

153. "Nurses," call for aid from Red Cross, File 803.3: Epidemics—Influenza—Personnel, Box 688, RG 200, NA; Memo from D. C. Dougherty, Lake Division Director of Publicity to Chapter Chairmen and Chairmen of Chapter Committees on Influenza, Subject: Influenza and Local Publicity, October 9, 1918, "What to Do with 'Flu' Leaflets we are Sending," File 803.08: Epidemics—Influenza—Reports and Statistics—Lake Division, Box 688, RG 200, NA.

154. For the use of this strategy in Seattle, see Nancy Rockafellar, "'In Gauze We Trust': Public Health and Spanish Influenza on the Home Front, Seattle, 1918–1919," *Pacific Northwest Quarterly* (1986): 108.

155. Illustration from *Illinois Health News*, October 1918, included in Karen A. Walters, "McLean County and the Influenza Epidemic of 1918–1919," *Journal of the Illinois State Historical Society* 74 (Summer 1981): 130.

156. Quoted in Richard H. Peterson, "The Spanish Influenza Epidemic in San Diego, 1918–1919," *Southern California Quarterly* 71 (1989): 96.

157. Townsend, "United States Public Health Service—Spanish Influenza," 6.
158. Public Resolution No. 42—65th Congress, included in "Brief Outline of Activities of the Public Health Service in Combating the Influenza Epidemic—1918–1919," Box 145, File 1622, RG 90, NA; Blue, "Epidemic Influenza and the U.S. Public Health Service," 423.
159. "Editorial—Weapons Against Influenza," 788.
160. J. Prentice Murphy, "Meeting the Scourge—How Massachusetts Organized to Fight Influenza Told for the Benefit of Other States," *Survey* 41 (October 26, 1918): 97.
161. "The Work of the Illinois Influenza Commission," *AJPH* 9 (January 1919): 21.
162. Oscar Jewell Harvey, *The Spanish Influenza Pandemic of 1918: An Account of Its Ravages in Luzerne County, Pennsylvania, and the Efforts Made to Combat and Subdue It* (Wilkes-Barre, PA: n.p., 1920), 6–7.
163. Mary E. Lent, "The Extent and Control of Influenza in Washington D.C.," *PHN* 10 (December 1918): 296–299.
164. Charles V. Aiken, "Influenza in South Carolina, 1918," *Journal of the South Carolina Medical Association* 15 (January 1919): 347; Crosby, *America's Forgotten Pandemic*, 93; "High Lights on Epidemic Influenza" in "What the Health Department Has Done to Curb the Epidemic of Influenza," 2; John Dill Robertson and Gottfried Koehler, "Preliminary Report on the Influenza Epidemic in Chicago," *AJPH* 8 (November 1918): 850.
165. Royal S. Copeland, quoted in "Negligent Doctors Arouse Copeland," *NYT*, October 27, 1918, 14.
166. Aiken, "Influenza in South Carolina, 1918," 347.
167. "Spanish Influenza," *LD* 58 (September 14, 1918): 21–22; "How to Fight Spanish Influenza," *LD* 59 (October 12, 1918): 13–14; "How Influenza Got In," *LD* 59 (November 30, 1918): 23; "How the 'Flu' Mask Traps the Germ," *LD* 59 (December 21, 1918): 21; "Expert Medical Advice on Influenza," *LD* 59 (December 28, 1918): 23, 117; "How the Hand Spreads Influenza," *LD* 60 (March 1, 1919): 24–25.
168. "Plagues in Europe and America," *Survey* 40 (September 28, 1918): 720; "Spanish Influenza and Its Control," *Survey* 41 (October 12, 1918): 45; "The Effects and Cost of Influenza," *Survey* 41 (November 16, 1918): 194; "A Program to Combat Influenza," *Survey* 41 (December 28, 1918): 408–409.
169. "Editorial—Keep Healthy," *Wallace Press-Times*, October 11, 1918, 6.
170. "Editorial—Avoid Panic and Take Precautions," *Wallace Press-Times*, October 22, 1918, 4.
171. "Wallace Under Influenza Ban," *Wallace Press-Times*, October 11, 1918, 1.
172. "Editorial—Avoid Panic and Take Precautions," 4.
173. "Make Your Own Mask; It Is a Simple Task," *Wallace Press-Times*, November 2, 1918, 1.
174. "Editorial—Keep Healthy," 6.
175. "Editorial—Stop Spread of Influenza," *Wallace Press-Times*, November 2, 1918, 1.
176. "Editorial—The Spanish 'Flu,'" *Tacoma News Tribune*, October 10, 1918, 8. See also "Editorial—Don't Help the Plague," *Tacoma News Tribune*, October 11, 1918, 14.
177. "Dr. A. Wilberforce Williams Talks on Preventive Measures, First Aid Remedies, Hygienics [*sic*] and Sanitation," *Chicago Defender*, October 5, 1918, 16; "Dr. A. Wilberforce Williams Talks on Preventive Measures, First Aid Remedies, Hygienics [*sic*] and Sanitation," *Chicago Defender*, October 12, 1918, 16; "Dr. A. Wilberforce Williams Talks on Preventive Measures, First Aid Remedies, Hygienics [*sic*] and Sanitation," *Chicago Defender*, October 19, 1918, 16.
178. See for instance "Editorial—Influenza Masks," *Daily Californian* (University of California, Berkeley), October 22, 1918, 2; A. H., "Editorial—Do Your Duty," *Daily Californian*, October 28, 1918, 2; "Editorial—Wear Your Masks," *Daily Californian*, January 20, 1919, 2.
179. "Order from the Board of Health," attached to letter, Sam T. Harrell, Secretary, Quitman Board of Health to Hon. Rupert Blue, December 21, 1918, #1622, Box 145, RG 90, NA.
180. "Order from the Board of Health," and "SUPPLEMENTAL RULES," attached to letter from Sam T. Harrell, Secretary, Quitman Board of Health to Hon. Rupert Blue, December 21, 1918, #1622, Box 145, RG 90, NA.
181. Judith Walzer Leavitt, *The Healthiest City: Milwaukee and the Politics of Health Reform* (Madison, Wisconsin: University of Wisconsin Press, 1996), 229–238.
182. Crosby, *America's Forgotten Pandemic*, 70.
183. Ibid., 70–73.

184. "City Provides Free Medical Service for Poor during the Epidemic," in "What the Health Department Has Done to Curb the Epidemic of Influenza," 19.

185. "Editorial Comment—Epidemic Influenza," in "What the Health Department Has Done to Curb the Epidemic of Influenza," 22–23.

186. Ibid., 22–23.

187. Crosby, *America's Forgotten Pandemic*, 70, 71; Barry, *The Great Influenza*, 321.

188. Crosby, *America's Forgotten Pandemic*, 75–84.

189. Ibid., 82–84.

190. "Deaths from Influenza and Pneumonia in Cities. 25 Weeks—September 8, 1918, to March 1, 1919," *PHR* 34 (March 14, 1919): 505.

191. "Editorial—The Influenza," *NYT*, October 3, 1918, 12.

192. James Colgrove, *State of Immunity: The Politics of Vaccination in Twentieth-Century America* (Berkeley: University of California Press, 2006), 2, 9, chap. 2.

193. Letter from John H. Faulkner to Hon. Newton D. Baker, Secretary of War, 1(4) September 1918, File 720.3: Vaccination—September and October 1918, Box 413, Decimal 720.3, Subseries 1917–1927, Entry 29, RG 112, NA.

194. File 720.3 Vacc./September and October 1918, Box 413, Decimal 720.3, Entry 29—Subseries 1917–1927, Record Group 112, National Archives. This file, as well as the file for November and December, contains a number of letters articulating opposition to the use of inoculation in army training camps, and a more general belief that forced immunization was not only dangerous, but undemocratic.

195. Rupert Blue, quoted in Crosby, *America's Forgotten Pandemic*, 74.

196. State Emergency Committee, quoted in Murphy, "Meeting the Scourge," 98.

197. Blue, "Epidemic Influenza and the U.S. Public Health Service," 426; Aiken, "Influenza in South Carolina, 1918," 346; "Controlling the Influenza Epidemic in Ohio," *Ohio Public Health Journal* 9 (November 1918): 453; McShane, "The Attempt to Control Influenza in Illinois," 18–19.

198. Alexandra Minna Stern, Mary Beth Reilly, Martin S. Cetron and Howard Markel, "'Better Off in School': School Medical Inspection as a Public Health Strategy During the 1918–1919 Influenza Pandemic in the United States," *PHR* 125 (2010, Supplement 3): 64–70.

199. "The Work of the Illinois Influenza Commission," *AJPH* 9 (January 1919): 22.

200. Stern et al., "'Better Off in School,'" 68.

201. S. Josephine Baker, *Fighting for Life* (New York: MacMillan Company, 1939), 154–56; Stern et al., "'Better Off in School,'" 67–68; Francesco Aimone, "The 1918 Influenza Epidemic in New York City: A Review of the Public Health Response," *PHR* 125 (2010, Supplement 3): 76.

202. Frank B. Cooper, quoted in "Ban Gatherings in an Effort to Halt Influenza," *Seattle Post-Intelligencer*, October 6, 1918, 1.

203. Murphy, "Meeting the Scourge," 98.

204. "The Flu and the School," *Deer Creek Mirror* (Minnesota), October 24, 1918, 1; "Spanish Influenza Hits This Community," *Deer Creek Mirror*, November 7, 1918, 1.

205. Aiken, "Influenza in South Carolina, 1918," 348.

206. "The Work of the Illinois Influenza Commission," 22.

207. "Dr. Keen Upholds Closing Order on Churches," in "What the Health Department Has Done to Curb the Epidemic of Influenza," 14.

208. "Timely Topics—The Churches and the 'Flu,'" *Washington Bee*, November 2, 1918, 4.

209. "Local Paragraphs," *Rathdrum Tribune*, December 13, 1918, 3.

210. "Influenza Lid Clamped Tight All Over City," *Minneapolis Morning Tribune*, October 13, 1918, 1.

211. "Social Events in Fog of Influenza," *Tacoma News Tribune*, October 19, 1918, Society Page.

212. "Quarantine Lifted Inside Camp and Men May Enter City in Very Near Future," *Camp Dodger* (Camp Dodge, Des Moines, IA), October 25, 1918, 1.

213. "City Shops Lose Soldier Dollars as 'Flu' Result," *Camp Dodger* (Camp Dodge, Iowa), October 4, 1918.

214. Letter from M. G. Parsons to Surgeon-General, "RE INFLUENZA," October 26, 1918, #1622, Box 144, RG 90, NA.

215. Richard Koszarski, "Flu Season: *Moving Picture World* reports on pandemic influenza, 1918–19," *Film History* 17 (2005): 466–485.
216. "Medicolegal—Board of Health Closing Schools for Influenza," *JAMA* 72 (June 21, 1919): 1864.
217. "Closing of Moving Picture Shows for Influenza," *JAMA* 73 (1919): 1007.
218. Ibid.
219. Koszarski, "Flu Season," 481–83.
220. All information on the San Francisco masking situation comes from Crosby, *America's Forgotten Pandemic*, chap. 7.
221. Ad in *Chronicle*, October 22, 1918, quoted in Crosby, *America's Forgotten Pandemic*, 102.
222. Quoted in Crosby, *America's Forgotten Pandemic*, 103.
223. Ibid., 108.
224. Ibid., 108–112.
225. "Guarding Against Influenza," *PHR* 33 (December 20, 1918): 2258.
226. Minutes of the First Meeting of the Commission on Influenza Appointed by Gov. Whitman, October 30, 1918, C. E. A. Winslow Papers, Folder 79–1205, Box 79, Sterling Memorial Library, Yale University.
227. Editorial opinion of *Scientific American*, quoted in "How Influenza Got In," *LD* 59 (November 30, 1918): 23.
228. Hermann M. Biggs, "The Recent Epidemic of Influenza," *American Review of Reviews* 59 (January 1919): 69.
229. Biggs, "The Recent Epidemic of Influenza," 70.
230. "Editorial Comment—Epidemic Influenza," in "What the Health Department Has Done to Curb the Epidemic of Influenza," 23.
231. Elizabeth J. Davies, "The Influenza Epidemic and How We Tried to Control It," *PHN* 11 (1919): 47.
232. "Current Comment—The Present Epidemic of Influenza," *JAMA* 71 (October 12, 1918): 1223.
233. Ibid.
234. Ibid.
235. Katherine Ott, *Fevered Lives: Tuberculosis in American Culture Since 1870* (Cambridge, MA: Harvard University Press, 1996), 121; Sheila Rothman, *Living in the Shadow of Death: Tuberculosis and the Social Experience of Illness in American History* (Baltimore: Johns Hopkins University Press, 1995), 183.

Chapter 4

1. Army School of Nursing, *Annual, 1921*, 177. From the History of Nursing Archives General Collection, Howard Gotlieb Archival Research Center at Boston University.
2. J. J. Waller, "Spanish Flu," *Journal of the Tennessee State Medical Association* 11 (December 1918): 298.
3. "Oral memoir of Stanhope Bayne-Jones," History of Medicine Division, National Library of Medicine (hereafter NLM). Bayne-Jones was early in his career in scientific medicine when he left for service in World War I. He would go on to a distinguished career as a bacteriologist. Albert E. Cowdrey, *War and Healing: Stanhope Bayne-Jones and the Maturing of American Medicine* (Baton Rouge: Louisiana State University Press, 1992), 36–72.
4. J. M. Perret, "A Brief Study of Influenza," *Journal of the Florida Medical Association* 6 (July, 1919): 1. See also Loy McAfee, "Epidemic Influenza in the Medical and Surgical History of the Civil War," in "Social Medicine, Medical Economics and Miscellany," *JAMA* 72 (February 8, 1919): 445; D. S. Bonar, "Influenza," *Kentucky Medical Journal* (hereafter *KMJ*) 18 (August, 1920): 288; James J. Walsh, "Influenza Therapeutics in History," *New York Medical Journal* (hereafter *NYMJ*) 109 (March 15, 1919): 442.
5. "Epidemic Influenza," in "Therapeutics," *JAMA* 71 (October 5, 1918): 1136.
6. William M. Donald, "Spanish Influenza," *Medical Review of Reviews* (hereafter *MRR*) 25 (1919): 79; A. W. Hewlett and W. M. Alberty, "Influenza at Navy Base Hospital in France," *JAMA* 71 (September 28, 1918): 1058.

7. Bernard Frankel, "Prophylaxis of Spanish Influenza," *NYMJ* 108 (November 23, 1918): 894.

8. E. B. Rogers, "The Influenza Pandemic," *Southwestern Medicine* 2 (November 1918): 6. See also "Paris Letter—Did Grip of 1890 Confer Immunity?" *JAMA* 71 (November 9, 1918): 1595; Ralph A. Kinsella, "The Bacteriology of Epidemic Influenza and Pneumonia," *JAMA* 72 (March 8, 1919): 717; Hewlett and Alberty, "Influenza at Navy Base Hospital in France," 1058; J. Heyward Gibbes, "Interesting Aspects of the Recent Epidemic of Influenza," *Journal of the South Carolina Medical Association* 15 (May 1919): 453.

9. Rufus Ivory Cole, "The Etiology and Prevention of Influenza," a lecture presented at the Practitioners' Society of New York, February 1, 1946, Rufus Cole Papers (B/C671), American Philosophical Society.

10. J. J. Keegan, "The Prevailing Pandemic of Influenza," *JAMA* 71 (September 28, 1918): 1051.

11. Donald, "Spanish Influenza," 78; S. J. McGraw, "Spanish Influenza," *Journal of the Arkansas Medical Society* 16 (October 1919): 102; E. O. Jordan, quoted in "The Institute of Medicine of Chicago—Symposium on Influenza," in "Society Proceedings," *JAMA* 72 (March 1, 1919): 674; Joseph D. Lehman, "Clinical Notes on the Recent Epidemic of Influenza," *Monthly Bulletin of The Department of Public Health and Charities of the City of Philadelphia* 4 (March, 1919): 37; Walter F. Boggess, "Some Phases of the Recent Influenza Epidemic," *KMJ* 17 (February, 19191): 72, 73; J. R. Morrison, quoted in the discussion following Boggess, "Some Phases of the Recent Influenza Epidemic," 77.

12. H. N. Street, "Personal Experience in Epidemic Influenza," *Journal of the Arkansas Medical Society* 16 (October 1919): 100.

13. "Observations on the Present Epidemic of So-Called Influenza in Europe," in "Editorials," *JAMA* 71 (November 9, 1918): 1580.

14. For a broad and international discussion of the debates surrounding Pfeiffer's bacillus, see Eugenia Tognotti, "Scientific Triumphalism and Learning from Facts: Bacteriology and the 'Spanish Flu' Challenge of 1918," *Journal of the Society for the Social History of Medicine* 16 (2003): 102–105. For American discussions, see for instance "The Influenza Pandemic," *JAMA* 71 (August 10, 1918): 485; O. T. Avery, "A Selective Medium for B. Influenzae—Oleate-Hemoglobin Agar," *JAMA* 71 (December 21, 1918): 2050; Guthrie McConnell, "The Blood Picture of Those Inoculated with Influenza Vaccine," *JAMA* 72 (May 17, 1919): 1457; T. C. Brackeen, "Spanish Influenza," *JNMA* 11 (October–December 1919): 146. The *JNMA* was the journal for the National Medical Association, the national organization for African American physicians who were excluded from membership in the American Medical Association. The organization was founded in 1895, and the journal began publication in 1909. Both the association and the journal continue their work today.

15. W. H. Park, "Anti-Influenza Vaccine as Prophylactic," *NYMJ* 108 (October 12, 1918): 621, abstracted in "Current Medical Literature," *JAMA* 71 (November 2, 1918): 1517; L. S. Medalia, "Influenza at Camp McArthur," abstracted in "Current Medical Literature," *JAMA* 72 (April 5, 1919): 1029; Keegan, "The Prevailing Pandemic of Influenza," 1055.

16. Park, quoted in John Barry, *The Great Influenza: The Epic Story of the Deadliest Plague in History* (New York: Viking, 2004), 279. See Barry for a full accounting of the research of Park, Williams, and others.

17. See "The Influenza Outbreak," in "Editorials," *JAMA* 71 (October 5, 1918): 1138; V.C.V. (Victor C. Vaughan was editor in chief of the journal), "The Bacteriology of Influenza," in "Editorials," *Journal of Laboratory and Clinical Medicine* (hereafter *JLCM*), 4 (November 1918): 85; Alfred Friedlander et al., "The Epidemic of Influenza at Camp Sherman, Ohio," in "Military Medicine and Surgery," *JAMA* 71 (November 16, 1918): 1656; S. G. Dabney, in discussion following Boggess, "Some Phases of the Recent Influenza Epidemic," 78; F. H. Rapoport, "The Complement Fixation Test in Influenzal Pneumonia," *JAMA* 72 (March 1, 1919): 636; P. G. W., "Transmission of Influenza," in "Editorials," *JLCM* 4 (March 1919): 372–373; "The Etiology of Influenza," in "Editorials," *JAMA* 72 (April 5, 1919): 1000–1001.

18. "Fact and Opinion on the Present Epidemic of Respiratory Disease," in "Editorials," *JAMA* 71 (December 21, 1918): 2074.

19. Frederick T. Lord, Arthur C. Scott, Jr., and Robert N. Nye, "Relation of Influenza Bacillus to the Recent Epidemic of Influenza," *JAMA* 72 (January 18, 1919): 190.

20. "The Influenza Outbreak," in "Editorials," *JAMA* 71 (October 5, 1918): 1138; letter from Surgeon General Rupert Blue to Senator Charles E. Townsend, September 15, 1919, Box 146, File 1622, RG 90, NA; William H. Park, "Bacteriology of Recent Pandemic of Influenza and Complicating Infections," *JAMA* 73 (August 2, 1919): 321; Reminiscences of A. R. Dochez (1957), 77, in the Oral History Collection of Columbia University.

21. "Observations on the Present Epidemic of So-Called Influenza in Europe," in "Editorials," *JAMA* 71 (November 9, 1918): 1580; John P. Turner, "Epidemic Influenza and the Negro Physician," *JNMA* 19 (October–December, 1918): 184.

22. W. L. Somerset, "Clinical Notes on the Influenza Epidemic," *Monthly Bulletin of the Department of Health, City of New York* 8 (December 1918): 278.

23. "Unsuccessful Attempts to Transmit Influenza Experimentally," in "Current Comment," *JAMA* 72 (January 25, 1919): 281.

24. Kinsella, "The Bacteriology of Epidemic Influenza and Pneumonia," 720; W. G. MacCallum, "Pathology of the Pneumonia Following Influenza," *JAMA* 72 (March 8, 1919): 723.

25. P. G. W., "Transmission of Influenza," 372; "The Etiology of Influenza," 1000, 1001; K. F. Meyer, "A Review of Our Knowledge Concerning the Etiology of Influenza," *California State Journal of Medicine* (hereafter *CSJM*) 17 (July 1919): 216. Significant efforts were undertaken to discover the causal agent by many of the country's leading bacteriologists and medical scientists. These efforts are well chronicled in Barry, *The Great Influenza*, Parts VII–X.

26. Franklin C. Gram, "The Influenza Epidemic and Its After-Effects in the City of Buffalo," *JAMA* 73 (September 20, 1919): 887.

27. "The Present Epidemic of Influenza," in "Current Comment," *JAMA* 71 (October 12, 1918): 1223.

28. Gibbes, "Interesting Aspects of the Recent Epidemic of Influenza," 456.

29. Ibid., 456–457.

30. T. C. Brackeen, "Spanish Influenza," *JNMA* 11 (October–December 1919): 147.

31. Ibid., 147.

32. Ernest W. Goodpasture, "Bronchopneumonia Due to Hemolytic Streptococci Following Influenza," *JAMA* 72 (March 8, 1919): 725; Solomon Strouse and Leon Bloch, "Notes on the Present Epidemic of Respiratory Disease," *JAMA* 71 (November 9, 1918): 1571.

33. "Epidemic Influenza," in "Therapeutics," 1137; "Quarantine and Isolation in Influenza," *JAMA* 71 (October 12, 1918): 1220; Alfred Friedlander et al., "The Epidemic of Influenza at Camp Sherman, Ohio," 1655; Bernard Fantus, "Clinical Observations on Influenza," *JAMA* 71 (November 23, 1918): 1736–1737.

34. "Epidemic Influenza," in "Therapeutics," 1137; Strouse and Bloch, "Notes on the Present Epidemic of Respiratory Disease," 1570; Alfred Friedlander et al., "The Epidemic of Influenza at Camp Sherman, Ohio," 1655; H. A. Klein, "The Treatment of 'Spanish Influenza,'" in "Correspondence," *JAMA* 71 (November 2, 1918): 1510.

35. "Influenza at the Camp Brooks Open Air Hospital," in "Medical Mobilization and the War," *JAMA* 71 (November 23, 1918): 1747. Many drug names have altered their spellings since 1918. Spellings are in the original here.

36. "Influenza Therapeutics in History," in "Editorial Notes and Comments," *NYMJ* 108 (November 2, 1918): 778–779. Also opposing coal tar see Albert C. Geyser, "Physiological Therapy in Influenza," *NYMJ* 111 (May 1, 1920): 768. In support of coal tar, see Fantus, "Clinical Observations on Influenza," 1738.

37. Strouse and Bloch, "Notes on the Present Epidemic of Respiratory Disease," 1571; Martin J. Synnott and Elbert Clark, "The Influenza Epidemic at Camp Dix," *JAMA* 71 (November 30, 1918): 1819; Walter V. Brem et al., "Pandemic 'Influenza' and Secondary Pneumonia at Camp Fremont, Calif.," *JAMA* 71 (December 28, 1918): 2142–2143; Perret, "A Brief Study of Influenza," 7; A. D. Rood, "Influenzal Pneumonia," abstracted in "Current Medical Literature," *JAMA* 72 (April 5, 1919): 1033; J. A. Nydegger, Surgeon, to Surgeon General, October 11, 1918, File #1622, Box 144, RG 90, NA.

38. Strouse and Bloch, "Notes on the Present Epidemic of Respiratory Disease," 1570; Synnott and Clark, "The Influenza Epidemic at Camp Dix," 1819; Geyser, "Physiological Therapy in Influenza," 767; H. E. Tuley, in Boggess, "Some Phases of the Recent Influenza Epidemic—Discussion," 76.

39. Thomas C. Ely, Letter to the Editor, "Alkalis in the Treatment of Influenza," in "Correspondence," *JAMA* 71 (October 26, 1918): 1431.

40. H. A. Klein, "The Treatment of 'Spanish Influenza,'" in "Correspondence," *JAMA* 71 (November 2, 1918): 1510

41. W. L. Mann, "Use of Calomel in Treatment of Influenza," abstracted in "Current Medical Literature," *JAMA* 72 (February 22, 1919): 606; C. W. Ross and Erwin J. Hund, "Treatment of the Pneumonic Disturbance Complicating Influenza: The Transfusion of Citrated Immune Blood," *JAMA* 72 (March 1, 1919): 640–645; May Farinholt Jones, Acting Assistant Surgeon, United States Public Health Service, letter of report to Medical Officer in Charge, Extra Cantonment Zone, Camp Shelby, Mississippi, February 1, 1919, Box 144, #1622, Record Group 90, National Archives.

42. See for instance "Editorial—Influenza," *JNMA* 10 (July–September, 1918): 127; "Influenza and Pneumonia in Philadelphia During the Recent Epidemic," *JNMA* 11 (January–March 1919): 20; "Epidemic Influenza," in "Therapeutics," 1137; Archibald Dixon, "Hospitalization of Influenza Patients by the Department of Health," *Monthly Bulletin of the Department of Health, City of New York* VIII (December 1918): 281; Boggess, "Some Phases of the Recent Influenza Epidemic," 74 and F. C. Simpson in ibid., "Discussion," 78; Joseph J. France, "Clinical Notes on the Influenza Epidemic," *JNMA* 11 (April–June 1919): 40; P. F. Straub, "Editorial—Lessons from Our Recent Epidemic," *Medical Surgeon* (hereafter *MS*) 44 (January 1919): 73.

43. Strouse and Bloch, "Notes on the Present Epidemic of Respiratory Disease," 1571.

44. Dr. A. J. McLaughlin, Assistant Surgeon General, USPHS, in "The Role of the Hand in the Distribution of Influenza—Discussion," part of the American Public Health Association Proceedings, December 8–11, 1918, reprinted in "Society Proceedings," *JAMA* 71 (December 28, 1918): 2174.

45. "The Influenza Outbreak," in "Editorials," *JAMA* 71 (October 5, 1918): 1138.

46. Col. Ravenel, Minutes, January 8, 1919, Meeting of the Advisory Board, Hygienic Laboratory, USPHS, Simon Flexner Papers (B/F 365), American Philosophical Society.

47. L. W. McGuire and W. R. Redden, "Treatment of Influenza Pneumonia by the Use of Convalescent Human Serum," *JAMA* 71 (October 19, 1918): 1311, 1312.

48. L. W. McGuire and W. R. Redden, "Treatment of Influenzal Pneumonia by the Use of Convalescent Human Serum: Second Report," *JAMA* 72 (March 8, 1919): 713. See also Admiral E. R. Stitt, in "Society Proceedings—American Public Health Association Meeting, December 8–11, 1918," *JAMA* 71 (December 21, 1918): 2098; John J. O'Malley and Frank W. Hartman, "Treatment of Influenzal Pneumonia with Plasma of Convalescent Patients," *JAMA* 72 (January 4, 1919): 34–37.

49. Barry, *The Great Influenza*, 279–287.

50. "Vaccines in Influenza," in "Current Comment," *JAMA* 71 (October 19, 1918): 1317.

51. "Serums and Vaccines in Influenza," in "Editorials," *JAMA* 71 (October 26, 1918): 1408. See also Gram, "The Influenza Epidemic and Its After-Effects in the City of Buffalo," 891; letter from W. F. Reasner, Acting Assistant Surgeon to Medical Officer in Charge, USPHS, Hattiesburg, Mississippi, December 30, 1918, Box 145, File 1622, RG 90, NA.

52. George M. Price, "Influenza—Destroyer and Teacher," *Survey* 41 (December 21, 1918): 368.

53. Reminiscences of Benjamin Earle Washburn (September 17, 1970 session), 13–14, 11, Oral History Collection of Columbia University.

54. Reminiscences of Connie Guion (1958), 103, Oral History Collection of Columbia University.

55. Letter from Roy to Burt, September 29, 1918, "Primary Resources: A Letter from Camp Devins [*sic*], MA.," Influenza, 1918, WGBH American Experience, available online at http://pbs.org/wgbh/americanexperience/features/primary-resources/influenza-letter/.

56. "Influenza Therapeutics in History," 778, 779.

57. Price, "Influenza—Destroyer and Teacher," 368.

58. Gibbes, "Interesting Aspects of the Recent Epidemic of Influenza," 454.

59. Reminiscences of Dana W. Atchley (1964), 95, in the Oral History Collection of Columbia University.

60. T. C. Brackeen, "Spanish Influenza," *JNMA* 11 (October–December 1919): 147.

Notes to Pages 131–133 237

61. James J. Walsh, "Influenza Therapeutics in History," *NYMJ* 109 (March 15, 1919): 444.
62. Tognotti, "Scientific Triumphalism and Learning from the Facts," 106.
63. Irving P. Lyon, Charles F. Tenney, Leopold Szerlip, "Some Clinical Observations on the Influenza Epidemic at Camp Upton," *JAMA* 72 (June 14, 1919): 1726. For at least one physician this sense of failure was overwhelming, and apparently led to his suicide. Colonel Charles B. Hagadorn, Acting Commander of Camp Grant, Illinois, shot himself as soldiers died under his watch. Carol R. Byerly, *Fever of War: The Influenza Epidemic in the U.S. Army During World War I* (New York: New York University Press, 2005), 85–86.
64. Oral history of Dr. Warren F. Draper (1976), 25, in the Oral History Collection of Columbia University.
65. Anna C. Jamme, "Conclusions Based on a Series of Inspections of Camp Hospitals in the United States," *Proceedings of the Twenty-fifth Annual Convention of the National League of Nursing Education Held at Chicago, Illinois, June 24 to June 28, 1919* (Baltimore: Williams and Wilkins Co., 1919), 188, 189. From the History of Nursing Archives General Collection, Howard Gotlieb Archival Research Center at Boston University.
66. Eunice H. Dyke, "Influenza Experiences and What They Taught," *PHN* 11 (November 1919): 891.
67. Miss Condell, "Personal experiences during the epidemic," Student nurse epidemic accounts, Folder 1, Box 8, RG 22.1, Academic Departments—Department of Nursing, College Archives, Simmons College.
68. Certainly some nurses painted the scenes of the epidemic only in horrific colors. See, for instance, Ellen D. Baer, "Letters to Miss Sanborn: St. Vincent's Hospital Nurses' Accounts of World War I," *Journal of Nursing History* 2 (April 1987): 26, 27.
69. "Report of the Director" in Visiting Nurse Association of Boston, "Thirty-Third Annual Report, The Instructive District Nursing Association, Boston, Year Ending December 31, 1918," 34. From the History of Nursing Archives General Collection, Howard Gotlieb Archival Research Center at Boston University.
70. "Annual Report of the Superintendent," from *Report of the Board of Managers of the Visiting Nurse Society of Philadelphia, January 1–December 31, 1918*, p. 13, Folder 12—Annual Reports, Box 3, Visiting Nurse Society of Philadelphia Records (MC5), Barbara Bates Center for the Study of the History of Nursing, School of Nursing, University of Pennsylvania.
71. Reminiscences of Isabel Maitland Stewart (1961), 235, in the Oral History Collection of Columbia University.
72. "Annual Report of the Superintendent," from *Report of the Board of Managers of the Visiting Nurse Society of Philadelphia, January 1–December 31, 1918*, 13.
73. "How the Red Cross Met the Influenza Epidemic," Illustrated Supplement, *Potomac Division Bulletin* 1 (November 22, 1918): available in a bound volume, *Potomac Division, 1918*, File 494.2—Div. Bulletins, Box 521, Entry 27130D, Record Group 200, National Archives.
74. Ibid.
75. Miss Franklin, "Personal experiences during the epidemic," student nurse epidemic accounts, Folder 1, Box 8, RG 22.1, Academic Departments—Department of Nursing, College Archives, Simmons College.
76. Miss Steinberg, "Personal experiences during the epidemic," student nurse epidemic accounts, Folder 1, Box 8, RG 22.1, Academic Departments—Department of Nursing, College Archives, Simmons College.
77. Mrs. Richard E. Morton, Chairman of the Department of Instruction, Report on Nurses' Aids, reprinted in "Southeastern Pennsylvania Chapter of the American Red Cross in the Influenza Epidemic, September–October, 1918," File 803.11, Epidemic—Influenza—Pennsylvania, Box 689, RG 200, NA. See also Lillian D. Wald, "Influenza: When the City Is a Great Field Hospital," *Survey* 43 (February 14, 1920): 579; Clara D. Noyes, "The Red Cross Nursing Service At Home and Abroad," *Proceedings of the Twenty-fifth Annual Convention of the National League of Nursing Education, Held at Chicago, Illinois, June 24 to June 28, 1919*, 142. From the History of Nursing Archives General Collection, Howard Gotlieb Archival Research Center at Boston University.

78. Mrs. Lydia F. Griffin, president, Gloucester District Nursing Association, Gloucester, Massachusetts, quoted in "War-Reports from the Influenza Front," *Literary Digest* (hereafter *LD*) 60 (February 22, 1919): 62, 67.

79. Letter from Mrs. W. R. Mercer, Chairman, to the Board of Directors of the Southeastern Pennsylvania Chapter of the American Red Cross on the work in Coatesville, Pennsylvania, October 27, 1918, reprinted in "Southeastern Pennsylvania Chapter of the American Red Cross in the Influenza Epidemic, September–October 1918."

80. Extract from a letter from the Chief Nurse of the Great Lakes Naval Hospital, Chicago, Illinois, quoted in the American Red Cross, *The Mobilisation of the American National Red Cross During the Influenza Epidemic 1918–1919* (Printing Office of the Tribune De Geneve, 1920), 11–12, File 803.8—Reports and Statistics, Box 688, File 803—Epidemics, Influenza, 1918, Divisions, RG, NA.

81. Nora E. Thompson, Superintendent, Army Nurse Corps, "How the Army Nursing Service Met the Demands of the War," *Proceedings of the Twenty-fifth Annual Convention of the National League of Nursing Education, Held at Chicago, Illinois, June 24 to June 28, 1919*, from the History of Nursing Archives General Collection, Howard Gotlieb Archival Research Center at Boston University.

82. Letter from Etelka Weiss, Director of Social Service, Hebrew Hospital, Baltimore, published under "Some Side Lights on the Influenza Epidemic," *PHN* 11 (April 1919): 301.

83. Volunteer nurse quoted in Bradford Luckingham, *Epidemic in the Southwest, 1918–1919* (El Paso: Texas Western Press, 1984), 10.

84. "Red Cross Care of Influenza Epidemic throughout Southern Division," File 803.8—Epidemics, Influenza—Reports and Statistics—Southern Division, Box 688, RG 200, NA.

85. Miss O'Donnell, "Personal Experiences During the Epidemic," Folder 1, Box 8, RG 22.1, Department of Nursing, Academic Departments, College Archives, Simmons College.

86. Gertrude Weld Peabody, President, "Report on Behalf of the Board of Managers," in the *33rd Annual Report, The Instructive District Nursing Association, Boston, Year Ending December 31*, 13–14. From the History of Nursing Archives General Collection, Howard Gotlieb Archival Research Center at Boston University.

87. Darlene Clark Hine, *Black Women in White: Racial Conflict and Cooperation in the Nursing Profession, 1890–1950* (Bloomington: Indiana University Press, 1989), xv.

88. Hine, *Black Women in White*, 102–103, 104. See also Darlene Clark Hine, "The Call That Never Came: Black Women Nurses and World War I, An Historical Note," *Indiana Military History Journal* 8 (January 1983): 23–27.

89. Vanessa Northington Gamble, "'There Wasn't a Lot of Comforts in Those Days:' African Americans, Public Health, and the 1918 Influenza Epidemic," *PHR* 125 (2010, Supplement 3): 119; Byerly, *Fever of War*, 145.

90. Bessie B. Hawse, Class of 1918, account included in John A. Kenney, "Some Facts Concerning Negro Nurse Training Schools and Their Graduates," *JNMA* 11 (April–June, 1919): 66.

91. Ibid.

92. Kenney, "Some Facts Concerning Negro Nurse Training Schools and Their Graduates," 53.

93. Ibid., 54.

94. Ibid., 53, 56.

95. The existence of female physicians and male nurses certainly complicated this scenario on the level of individuals. And yet the power of the professions to socialize their members was enormous at this time and medicine socialized to male norms. Regina Morantz-Sanchez, *Conduct Unbecoming a Woman: Medicine on Trial in Turn-of-the-Century Brooklyn* (New York: Oxford University Press, 1999), 8.

96. Paul Starr, *The Social Transformation of American Medicine: The Rise of a Sovereign Profession and the Making of a Vast Industry* (New York: Basic Books, 1984), 32–33, 39–40.

97. James H. Cassedy, *Medicine in America: A Short History* (Baltimore: Johns Hopkins University Press, 1991), 33–39; Thomas Neville Bonner, *To the Ends of the Earth: Women's Search for Education in Medicine* (Cambridge, MA: Harvard University Press, 1992), 15–16.

98. Cassedy, *Medicine in America*, 86–96; Kenneth M. Ludmerer, *Learning to Heal: The Development of Medical Education* (New York: Basic Books, 1985); Kenneth Ludmerer, *Time to Heal: American Medical Education from the Turn of the Century to the Era of Managed Care*

(New York: Oxford University Press, 1999), chap. One; Lester S. King, *Transformations of American Medicine: From Benjamin Rush to William Osler* (Baltimore: Johns Hopkins University Press, 1991), 210–214.

99. Mary Roth Walsh, *Doctors Wanted—No Women Need Apply: Sexual Barriers in the Medical Profession, 1835–1975* (New Haven: Yale University Press, 1977), chap. 6; Regina Markell Morantz-Sanchez, *Sympathy and Science: Women Physicians in American Medicine* (New York: Oxford University Press, 1985), chap. 9; Bonner, *To the Ends of the Earth*, 136–156; Starr, *The Social Transformation of Medicine*, 117–124.

100. Ellen S. More, Elizabeth Fee and Manon Parry, "Introduction: New Perspectives on Women Physicians and Medicine in the United States, 1849 to the Present," in *Women Physicians and the Cultures of Medicine*, ed. Ellen S. More, Elizabeth Fee and Manon Parry (Baltimore: Johns Hopkins University, 2009): 4–5.

101. John Harley Warner, *The Therapeutic Perspective: Medical Practice, Knowledge, and Identity in America, 1820–1885* (Princeton, NJ: Princeton University Press, 1997), 15; Walsh, *Doctors Wanted*, 249.

102. Sandra Beth Lewenson, *Taking Charge: Nursing, Suffrage, and Feminism in America, 1873–1920* (New York: Garland Publishing, 1993), xiii–xiv, chaps. 1 and 2; Susan Reverby, *Ordered to Care: The Dilemma of American Nursing, 1850–1945* (New York: Cambridge University Press, 1987), chaps. 7–9.

103. Reverby, *Ordered to Care*, 2.

104. Walsh, *Doctors Wanted*, 246; Margarete Sandelowski, *Devices and Desires: Gender, Technology, and American Nursing* (Chapel Hill: University of North Carolina Press, 2000), 45.

105. Hine, *Black Women in White*, xviii, xix.

106. This is not to suggest that there were no female doctors but only that the broader culture measured the performance of doctors and nurses according to closely gendered standards. On the evolution of women's position in medicine over the last century and a half, see Ellen S. More, *Restoring the Balance: Women Physicians and the Profession of Medicine, 1850–1995* (Cambridge, MA: Harvard University Press, 1999).

107. "The Health Department Nurse," *AJPH* 4 (December 1914): 1181.

108. Quoted in Barbara Melosh, *"The Physician's Hand": Work Culture and Conflict in American Nursing* (Philadelphia: Temple University Press, 1982), 3.

109. N. J. Atkinson, "Influenza," *JNMA* 13 (January–March, 1921): 21.

110. Byerly, *Fever of War*, 127–128. For a comprehensive discussion see chapter 5, "Postmortem: The Trauma of Failure, 1918–1919."

111. Vanessa Northington Gamble, *Making a Place for Ourselves: The Black Hospital Movement 1920–1945* (New York: Oxford University Press, 1995), 10–11.

112. Ibid., chap. 1.

113. Turner, "Epidemic Influenza and the Negro Physician," 184.

114. Ibid.

115. Ibid.

116. "DEATH GRIP OF EPIDEMIC BROKEN, FOLLOWING TOLL OF 483 DEAD AND 1438 SERIOUS," *Camp Sherman News*, October 9, 1918, 1; George M. Price, "Mobilizing Social Forces Against Influenza," *Survey* 41 (October 26, 1918): 96; letter from M. G. Parsons, Assistant Sanitary Engineer to the Surgeon General, October 22, 1918, Box 144, File 1622, Record Group 90, National Archives; letter from Peter Reinberg, quoted in Grace Fay Schryver, *A History of the Illinois Training School for Nurses, 1880–1929* (Chicago: Illinois Training School for Nurses, 1930), 108–109, from the History of Nursing Archives General Collection, Howard Gotlieb Archival Research Center at Boston University; Questionnaire of Corporal Walter J. Baker, U.S. Air Service, 2nd Construction Company, AEQC, WWORP, USAMHI; letter from Assistant Attorney General Thomas Parran, Jr. to the Surgeon General from Florence, Alabama, October 19, 1918, Box 146, #1622, RG 90, NA.

117. See for instance "Controlling the Influenza Epidemic in Ohio," *Ohio Public Health Journal* 9 (November 1918): 455.

118. "Wonderful Work Accomplished by Camp Crane Officers in Fight Against 'Flu' in Hard Coal Regions of Pa.," *Camp Crane News*, November 2, 1918, 1. See also "Sacrifices Life to

Help Fight the Influenza—Lieut. Louis Katze., M. C. Gives All After Volunteering Services," *Camp Crane News*, November 2, 1918, 1.

119. See for instance "Base Hospital Flurries," *Camp Jackson Click*, October 19, 1918, 1; "Influenza No Longer an Epidemic; Efficiency Keynote to Success," *Camp Crane News*, November 9, 1918, 1; letter from Dr. Amos Carter, reprinted in ARC, "Praise Work of Red Cross During 'Flu,'" *The Lake Division News* I (November 25, 1918): 7.

120. "WONDERFUL WORK ACCOMPLISHED BY CAMP CRANE OFFICERS," 1.

121. "Wear Your Mask," *Wallace Press-Times*, November 6, 1918, 2.

122. Typewritten document, no title, Folder 2: Histories 1919, Series II, Box 14, Visiting Nurse Society of Philadelphia Records (MC5), Barbara Bates Center for the Study of the History of Nursing, School of Nursing, University of Pennsylvania.

123. Volunteer at Aoy School, in El Paso, Texas, which was converted into a hospital during the epidemic, quoted in Gina Kolata, *Flu: The Story of the Great Influenza Pandemic of 1918 and the Search for the Virus That Caused It* (New York: Farrar, Straus and Giroux, 1999), 25.

124. Margaret Nutting, Director, Bureau of News, Department of Publicity, Southern Division, American Red Cross, to M. G. Scheitlin, November 15, 1918, File 803.08—Epidemics, Influenza—Reports and Statistics, Southern Division, Box 688, RG 200, NA.

125. Alfred Stengel, Professor of Medicine, in "Messages from 'Our Chiefs,'" *The Nurses' Record, 1919* (Philadelphia: Class of 1919 of the University of Pennsylvania Training School for Nurses by Patterson and White Co., n.d.), 26, in Box 22, Hospital of the University of Pennsylvania School of Nursing Records (MC94), Barbara Bates Center for the Study of the History of Nursing, School of Nursing, University of Pennsylvania.

126. "The Epidemic Over," *Red Cross Clippings*, December 5, 1918, 7, available as a bound volume, Pennsylvania vols. 1–2, Box 521, File 494.2—Division Bulletins, Entry 27130D, RG 200, NA; Dr. R. G. Hall, quoted in Rae Richen, *To Serve Those Most in Need: A History of the Albertina Kerr Centers* (Portland, OR: Albertina Kerr Centers, 1997), 38; "Minute Adopted by the Board of Trustees at a Meeting Held October 29, 1918," *59th Annual Report of the Lankenau Hospital* (Philadelphia: Edward Stern and Co., Inc., 1919), 56, Folder 9: LH: Annual Reports, Box 1, Lankenau Hospital School of Nursing Records (MC#98), Center for the Study of the History of Nursing, School of Nursing, University of Pennsylvania; "Hospital X-Ray," *Camp Jackson Click*, November 16, 1918, 4. See also "War-Reports from the Influenza Front," 62; Sister Georgiana Ennisson, President, "Report of St. Ann's Infant Asylum," August 13, 1919, in Volume 1: Miscellaneous Reports, *Annual Report of the Commissioners of the District of Columbia, Year Ended June 30, 1919* (Washington, D.C.: Government Printing Office, 1919), 516.

127. Mildred Lum, "Work of Volunteer Nurses During the Epidemic, *Monthly Bulletin of the Department of Health, City of New York* VIII (December 1918): 290–291.

128. Dora Christianson, "Your Chance," *American Journal of Nursing* (hereafter *AJN*) 19 (January 1919): 275.

129. Harry Lee, "Night in the Hospital," *Survey* 41 (November 23, 1918): 214.

130. "157 Nurses Give Healing and Spirit of Cheer," *Over-the-Top* (Camp Taylor, Kentucky), January 22, 1919, 2.

131. Homer Folks, "War, Best Friend of Disease," *Harper's* 140 (March 1920): 456.

132. Editorial page, *WN*, November 22, 1918, 6.

133. "Science Has Failed to Guard Us," *NYT*, October 17, 1918, 14.

134. Ibid.

135. "Prevention Seemingly Achieved," *NYT*, October 24, 1918, 12.

136. Ad for the Allen Remedy Co., St. Louis, Mo., Box 146, #1622, RG 90, NA (emphasis in the original).

137. *Pittsburgh Leader*, quoted in Kenneth A. White, "Pittsburgh in the Great Epidemic of 1918," *The Western Pennsylvania Historical Magazine* 68 (July 1985): 225.

138. Richard Collier, *Plague of the Spanish Lady: The Influenza Pandemic of 1918–1919* (New York: Atheneum, 1974), 162–163.

139. Jane Brox, *Five Thousand Days Like This One: An American Family History* (Boston: Beacon Press, 1990), 102; Miss Franklin, "Personal experiences during the epidemic," student nurse epidemic accounts, Folder 1, Box 8, RG 22.1, Academic Departments—Department of Nursing, College Archives, Simmons College.

140. Letter from "A lover of our Boys" to Head Surgeon, Camp Custer, October 14, 1918, Box 22, Camp Custer, Michigan, Correspondence 1918–1920, Decimal 710—Influenza, Records of U.S. Army Continental Commands, 1821–1920, RG 393, NA.

141. Russell R. Elliott, "Influenza Epidemic of 1918–1919," *Halcyon* 14 (1992): 255–256. Reports claimed that the Navajo also relied on their own traditional remedies and ceremonies to combat the epidemic. See Albert B. Reagan, "The Influenza and the Navajo," reprinted from Proceedings of the Indiana Academy of Science for 1919 (August 1921): 247.

142. Mrs. Ann Olds Woodson, September 29, 1918, "SIMPLE INFLUENZA REMEDY," in File 710 (Influenza, September 1918), Box 394, Decimal 710, Entry 29, RG 112, NA.

143. Letter from J. J. C. Elliott, Superintendent of Methodist Hospitle [*sic*] to Woodrow Wilson, September 28, 1918, File 710 (Influenza, September 1918), Box 394, Decimal 710, Entry 29, RG 112, NA.

144. Letter from Mr. Wm. B. Scott to Surgeon General, U.S. Army, September 27, 1918, File 710 (Influenza, September 1918), Box 394, Decimal 710, Entry 29, RG 112, NA; Robert S. McPherson, "Influenza Epidemic of 1918: A Cultural Response," *Utah Historical Quarterly* (Spring 1990):190; William J. Doherty, "A West Virginia County's Experience with the 1918 Influenza Epidemic," *West Virginia History* 38 (1977): 140. Suggesting the popularity of these "cures," an editorial in the *Baltimore Afro-American* acknowledged their prevalence and urged the public to avoid them. See "Camphor and the Flu," *AA*, October 18, 1918, 4.

145. "Prevent Influenza," ad for Sherwin-Williams Products, *LAT*, November 12, 1918, 14.

146. "Help Your Health Board Conquer Spanish Influenza by Disinfecting Your Home," ad for Lysol, *LAT*, October 25, 1918, II, 3.

147. "In this Time of Danger of Infection from Influenza," ad for Kolynos Company, *LAT*, October 11, 1918, 17.

148. Chapin, quoted in James H. Cassedy, *Charles V. Chapin and the Public Health Movement* (Cambridge, MA: Harvard University Press, 1962), 190.

149. McPherson, "Influenza Epidemic of 1918: A Cultural Response," 188; Gabriel W. Kirkpatrick, "Influenza 1918: A Maine Perspective," *Maine Historical Society Quarterly* 25 (1986): 172; "Tells How Influenza Patients Quickly Regain Their Strength—Had Spanish Flu; Feels Fine Now," *WN*, December 20, 1918, 3; "Before or After the Influenza," ad for Dr. Pierce's medicines, *LAT*, November 19, 1918, 113.

150. Kirkpatrick, "Influenza 1918," 172; Ad for Allen Remedy Co., Box 146, File 1622, Record Group 90, NA.

151. Letter from Professor Albert F. Porta to Surgeon General, June 6, 1919, with accompanying study, "THE EPIDEMIC OF INFLUENZA CONNECTED WITH THE MOTION OF THE PLANET JUPITER," Box 144, #1622, RG 90, NA.

152. The open hostility of members of several of these sects during the epidemic stands in stark contrast to the rapprochement between the regulars and some of the sectarians that historians describe in the period from 1870 to 1915. Norman Gevitz, "Three Perspectives on Unorthodox Medicine," in *Other Healers: Unorthodox Medicine in America*, ed. Norman Gevitz (Baltimore: Johns Hopkins University Press, 1988), 22.

153. Gevitz, "Three Perspectives on Unorthodox Medicine," 17–19, 22.

154. "Editorial—The Epidemic of Influenza," *Hahnemannian Monthly* (hereafter *HM*) 53 (September 1918): 561; Wallace McGeorge, "Influenza Remedies" (read before the Philadelphia County Homeopathic Medical Society) *NAJH* 67 (1919): 139; Crawford R. Green, "The Treatment of Influenza in Children," *NAJH* 68 (October 1920): 915; Bernarr McFadden, "Could Drugless Doctors Have Saved These Four Hundred Thousand Lives?" *NAJH* 67 (1919): 115–116; Eldridge C. Price, "Therapeutic Efficiency in the Treatment of Epidemic Influenza," *HM* 54 (December 1919): 725. For one depressed and defeated response see William A. Haman, "Influenzal Broncho-Pneumonia: Its Prophylaxis and Jugulation," *HM* 55 (September 1920): 540.

155. Price, "Therapeutic Efficiency in the Treatment of Epidemic Influenza," 726; O. S. Haines, "The Medicinal Management of Uncomplicated Influenza by the Methods of Homoeopathy," *HM* 54 (December 1919): 729; J. W. W., "Homeopathy's Great Opportunity in the Existing Medical Confusion," *NAJH* 67 (1919): 111.

156. McGeorge, "Influenza Remedies," 139.

157. "Editorial and Special Contributions—Influenza an Ancient Disease," *NAJH* 66 (October 1918): 902.

158. G. H. W., "Editorial—The Epidemic of Influenza," *HM* 53 (September 1918): 561.

159. Price, "Therapeutic Efficacy in the Treatment of Epidemic Influenza," 724–726.

160. W. D. Bayley, "Editorial—The Medical Profession and the War," *HM* 54 (August 1919): 512.

161. Ibid.

162. J. W. W., "Homeopathy's Great Opportunity in the Existing Medical Confusion," 111.

163. Ibid., 112 (emphasis in the original).

164. Ibid., 112.

165. Ibid., 112–113.

166. Ibid., 114.

167. Norman Gevitz, *The D.O.'s: Osteopathic Medicine in America* (Baltimore: Johns Hopkins University Press, 1991), 4–17; James C. Whorton, *Nature Cures: The History of Alternative Medicine in America* (New York: Oxford University Press, 2004), 141–158.

168. C. C. Reid, "Prevention and Treatment of Influenza," *Journal of the American Osteopathic Association* (hereafter *JAOA*) 18 (January 1919): 209; Gevitz, *The D.O.'s*, 72. For a few descriptions of the practices employed by osteopaths during the epidemic, see "Editorial—The Treatment of Influenza," *JAOA* 18 (October 1918): 83–85; L. K. Tuttle, with discussion and report of 106 cases, by Robert W. Rogers, "Influenza and Pneumonia Treatment," *JAOA* 18 (January 1919): 211–214; "Experiences with the Influenza," *JAOA* 18 (January 1919): 247–248; "Experiences with the Epidemic," *JAOA* 18 (February 1919): 277–278; Earl A. Bush, "Care of Influenza and Pneumonia in an Army Base Hospital," *JAOA* 18 (March 1919): 333–335; "Experiences with the Epidemic," *JAOA* 18 (March 1919): 335–338.

169. "Editorial—Our New Enemy," *JAOA* 18 (October 1918): 86.

170. Bush, "Care of Influenza and Pneumonia in an Army Base Hospital," 333.

171. W. L. Buster, "Influenza and Pneumonia," *JAOA* 18 (April 1919): 392.

172. Charles Hangsea, of the APHA, quoted in C. C. Reid, "Prevention and Treatment of Influenza," 211. Though Hangsea was not an osteopath, his words were quoted by Reid, who was.

173. L. K. Tuttle, with discussion and report of 106 cases, by Robert W. Rogers, "Influenza and Pneumonia Treatment," 211. Note the use of the term "impotent" here, which seems to suggest the failure of MDs not only as doctors, but as men.

174. "Editorial—Our New Enemy," 86.

175. Buster, "Influenza and Pneumonia," 393.

176. "Editorial—The Drug Evils and Economic Reform," *JAOA* 18 (January 1919): 230–232; Whorton, *Nature Cures*, 156–163. At the time of the epidemic, osteopathy was enduring a significant split in its ranks over the use of drug-based therapies, a feud that would last until 1929, when training in drug therapy was accepted by resolution as a component of training by the American Osteopathic Association.

177. L. K. Tuttle, with discussion and report of 106 cases, by Robert W. Rogers, "Influenza and Pneumonia Treatment," 213.

178. "For Your Local Newspaper—Influenza Deaths Unnecessary," *JAOA* 19 (November 1919): 115; "Editorial—Making the World Safe for Osteopathy," *JAOA* 18 (February 1919): 279–282; L.K. Tuttle, with discussion and report of 106 cases, by Robert W. Rogers, "Influenza and Pneumonia Treatment," 214; George W. Riley, "Osteopathic Success in the Treatment of Influenza and Pneumonia," *JAOA* 18 (August 1919): 567.

179. Gevitz, *The D.O.'s*, 72.

180. Buster, "Influenza and Pneumonia," 392.

181. J. Byron LaRue, "Pneumonia," *JAOA* 18 (January 1919): 208.

182. Bush, "Care of Influenza and Pneumonia in an Army Base Hospital," 334; Charles McFadden, contributor to "Experiences with the Influenza," *JAOA* 18 (January 1919): 247.

183. Bush, "Care of Influenza and Pneumonia in an Army Base Hospital," 334; "Editorial—Service," *JAOA* 18 (September 1918): 24–26.

184. "Editorial—Making the World Safe for Osteopathy," 279.

185. Riley, "Osteopathic Success in the Treatment of Influenza and Pneumonia," 569.

186. Buster, "Influenza and Pneumonia," 392–393.

187. Geo. Moffett, in "Experiences with the Influenza," *JAOA* 18 (February 1919): 278; R. M. Wolf and C. W. Starr, "Experiences with the Influenza," *JAOA* 18 (January 1919): 248. See also A. L. Evans, "Editorial—The Osteopathic Service League," *JAOA* 19 (July 1920): 432; "Editorial—Make Educators," *JAOA* 18 (January 1919): 234.

188. "Editorial—Making the World Safe for Osteopathy," 279–280.

189. "Editorial—Has the Epidemic Convinced Us?" *JAOA* 18 (February 1919): 287.

190. See for instance "Editorial—Making the World Safe for Osteopathy," 279–282; Albert C. Johnson in "Experiences with the Epidemic," *JAOA* 18 (February 1919): 278; Buster, "Influenza and Pneumonia," 392–393; "Editorial—Has the Epidemic Convinced Us," 287.

191. Whorton, *Nature Cures*, 165–190; Gevitz, *The D.O.'s*, 58–60; Walter I. Wardwell, "Chiropractors: Evolution to Acceptance," in *Other Healers*, ed. Gevitz, 157–191.

192. Whorton, *Nature Cures*, 171.

193. Whorton, *Nature Cures*, 176–182; Gevitz, *The D.O.'s*, 59.

194. Letter from Julius C. Leve to Secretary of War Baker, September 28, 1918, File 710—Influenza September 1918, Box 394, Decimal 710, Entry 29, RG 112, NA.

195. Ibid. For other examples see for instance, Elliott, "Influenza Epidemic of 1918–1919," 255; Philip C. Ensley, "Indiana and the Influenza Pandemic of 1918," *Indiana Medical History Quarterly* 9 (1983): 12.

196. No title, inset box featuring advertisement by Chiropractor James F. McGinnis, from the *Jackson Sentinel* of Maquoketa, Iowa, with editorial comment, published in *JAMA* 71 (November 23, 1918): 1764. The advertisement appears as part of a critique of chiropractic (emphasis in the original).

197. Though Christian Science practitioners were medical practitioners of a sort, their legal protection increasingly required their definition as members of a religion. Rennie B. Schoepflin, "Christian Science Healing in America," in *Other Healers*, ed. Gevitz, 204–207.

198. Eddy was not the first to use the term "Christian Science." Rather, she owed a substantial debt to Phineas Quimby who coined the name "Christian Science" for his belief that "Christ and Science were synonymous." Whorton, *Nature Cures*, 118–120.

199. The central text in Christian Science, alongside the Bible, is Mary Baker Eddy, *Science and Health with Key to the Scriptures* (Boston: Trustees, Church of Christ, Scientist, 1934 [1875]). For a useful presentation of Christian Science for the non-practitioner, see Robert Peel, *Health and Medicine in the Christian Science Tradition* (New York: Crossroad Publishing Company, 1988).

200. "Mind or Matter?" *Christian Science Monitor* (hereafter *CSM*), September 27, 1918, 16.

201. "Campaign Against Fear Is Advocated," *CSM*, October 22, 1918, 6. See also "Commission Rejects Gauze Mask Ruling," *CSM*, October 26, 1918, 8; "Closing Order Meets with Protest," *CSM*, November 19, 1918, 5; "Inoculations Fail to Prevent Disease," *CSM*, November 20, 1918, 1; "New York City and Health Issue," *CSM*, November 29, 1918, 9.

202. Whorton, *Nature Cures*, 123.

203. "A Mad World," *CSM*, October 8, 1918, 16.

204. "Mind or Matter?" 16.

205. "Tyrants' Thrones," *CSM*, April 30, 1919, 17.

206. Letter from Victor W. Jones to his mother, October 28, 1918, 166th Depot Brigade, 8th (45th) Co., Camp Lewis, AEQC, WWORP, USAMHI.

207. Collier, *The Plague of the Spanish Lady*, 199.

208. "A Mad World," 16; "People Ordered to Don Gauze Masks," *CSM*, November 1, 1918, 1; "Doctors Disagree on Influenza Issue," *CSM*, December 13, 1918, 1; "Germ Theory and Common Sense," Letter to the Editor, *CSM*, May 20, 1919, 3; "Inoculations Fail to Prevent Disease," *CSM*, November 20, 1918, 1; "Typhoid Inoculation and the Influenza," *CSM*, December 23, 1918, 9; "Objection to Reports of Contagion," Letter to the Editor, *CSM*, October 4, 1918, 3; "Campaign Against Fear Is Advocated," *CSM*, October 22, 1918, 6; "Press Attitude on Epidemic Condemned," *CSM*, October 29, 1918, 1; "Influence Seen of Fear on Disease," *CSM*, December 31, 1918, 8; "Mental Conditions and Disease," Letter to the Editor, *CSM*, March 6, 1919, 3; "Health Official Tells of Work During Epidemic," *CSM*, April 5, 1919, 1.

209. "Mental Conditions and Disease," 3.
210. "Inconsistencies of Allopathy," Letter to the Editor, *CSM*, November 13, 1918, 3; "Inconsistency of Health Rule Seen," *CSM*, December 27, 1918, 5;
211. "Medical Bills for Washington State," *CSM*, February 26, 1919, 5; "School 'Weighing Issue in California," *CSM*, April 24, 1919, 1; "Inconsistencies of Allopathy," 3.
212. "What '2' Do—You want to know when there is no specific for Influenza," *Jackson Sentinel*, Maquoketa, Iowa, insert with commentary, *JAMA* 71 (November 23, 1918): 1764.
213. "Figures Never Lie," in "Current Comment," *JAMA* 72 (March 8, 1919): 731.
214. C. B. Burr, Letter to the Editor, "Attitude of Christian Scientists in the Present Epidemic of Influenza," *JAMA* 71 (October 19, 1918): 1337.
215. Rupert Blue, "'Spanish Influenza' 'Three-Day Fever' 'The Flu,'" *PHR* (September 28, 1918, Supplement No. 34): 4.
216. "Sure Cures for Influenza," *PHR* 33 (November 8, 1918): 1931–1933. See also John McMullen, "The U.S. Public Health Service and Influenza," *KMJ* 17 (July 1919): 277.
217. "No Specific 'Cure' for Influenza," *JAMA* 71 (November 2, 1918): 1489; Kirkpatrick, "Influenza 1918," 173; "Advice to Persons Who Have Had Influenza or Pneumonia—General Advice—Patent Medicines," *Weekly Bulletin of the Department of Health, City of New York* New Series, Vol. VII (December 7, 1918): 383. This criticism was not new. Gevitz, "Three Perspectives on Unorthodox Medicine," 9–10; James Harvey Young, *The Toadstool Millionaires: A Social History of Patent Medicines in America Before Federal Regulation* (Princeton, NJ: Princeton University Press, 1961), 224–225 and chap. 14.
218. "Try Them on the Dog," *The Bulletin*, 3 (October 21, 1918), Folder 3:5, Box 3, Minneapolis Family and Children's Services, Social Welfare History Archives, University of Minnesota.
219. Simon Flexner, "Epidemiology and Recent Epidemics," *Science* 50 (October 3, 1919): 315.

Chapter 5

1. Mazyck P. Ravenel, "Preventive Medicine and War" (lecture before the Public Health Administration Section, APHA Annual Meeting, October 28, 1919), *AJPH* 10 (January 1920): 27.
2. Ibid., 28.
3. Ibid., 28.
4. Ibid., 30.
5. Mazyck P. Ravenel, "The American Public Health Association, Past, Present, Future" (Presidential Address, APHA, November 14, 1921), *AJPH* 11 (December 1921): 1031–1041.
6. Ibid., 1039.
7. Ibid. Amalthea, a figure from both Greek and Roman mythology, was the goat that nursed Zeus/Jupiter. One of the horns of this goat was called the "cornucopia," and filled with whatever the owner desired. This is the source of the notion of a "horn of plenty," and of the term "cornucopia" implying abundance.
8. Ibid., 1040.
9. Lillian Kancianich, interview with the author, August 8, 2003. Kancianich described her situation with a smile and perhaps a hint of humor. Her words as recorded may present a more tragic account than she intended.
10. Resolution of the Section on Industrial Medicine and Surgery of the American Medical Association to Congress on appropriation for USPHS to Conduct Influenza Research, June 13, 1919, Harold Lindsay Amoss Papers, American Philosophical Society.
11. Attachment to letter from Dr. Otto P. Geier, Secretary, Miscellaneous Topics Section on Industrial Medicine and Surgery, American Medical Association to Dr. Harold Amos [sic], 29 July 1919, Harold Lindsay Amoss Papers, American Philosophical Society.
12. See for instance C.W. Ross and Erwin J. Hund, "Treatment of the Pneumonic Disturbance Complicating Influenza," *JAMA* 72 (March 1, 1919): 640.
13. Rufus Cole, "Endemic Influenza" (paper presented at the New York Clinical Society, January 27, 1922), B/C671, American Philosophical Society. See also Colonel Deane C. Howard and Major Albert G. Love, "Influenza—US Army," *MS* 46 (May 1920): 522.
14. William M. Donald, "Spanish Influenza," *Medical Review of Reviews* (hereafter *MRR*) 25 (1919): 79.

15. Milton J. Rosenau, "Experiments to Determine Mode of Spread of Influenza," *JAMA* 73 (August 2, 1919): 313.

16. James B. Herrick, "Treatment of Influenza by Means Other Than Vaccines and Serums," *JAMA* 73 (August 16, 1919): 483; Louis A. Turley, "The Etiology and Pathology of the Spanish Influenza," *Journal of the Oklahoma State Medical Association* 12 (November 1919): 311; "Lipovaccines as a Prophylactic in Influenza," in "Correspondence," *JAMA* 73 (November 29, 1919): 1716–1717.

17. J. Frank Points, "The Evolution of a Successful Treatment for the Complicated Cases of Influenza," *New Orleans Medical and Surgical Journal* 72 (January 1920): 408. See also "Editorial—The Present Status of our Knowledge Concerning the Etiology of Influenza," *JLCM* 5 (May 1920): 543.

18. See for instance "The Cause of Influenza," in "Editorials," *JAMA* 76 (February 19, 1921): 523–524; "The Status of Vaccination Against Influenza," in "Current Comment," *JAMA* 76 (May 28, 1921): 1503.

19. See for instance Francis G. Blake, "The Relation of the Influenza Bacillus to Influenza," in "Society Proceedings—New York Academy of Medicine, February 19, 1920," *JAMA* 74 (March 6, 1920): 697; Dr. Tice in discussion following Albert J. Croft, "Influenza Versus the Epidemic: An Etiologic Resume" (paper presented before the Douglas Park Branch, Chicago Medical Society, January 21, 1919), *Illinois Medical Journal* 35 (February 1919): 83; "Cyanosis in Influenza," in "Current Comment," *JAMA* 72 (May 31, 1919): 1620; Cole, "Endemic Influenza"; "The Cause of Influenza," in "Current Comment," *JAMA* 79 (October 21, 1922): 1431; Leland O. Mauldin, "Some Results of Influenza with Special Reference to Eye, Ear, Nose and Troat [*sic*] Diseases," *The Journal of the South Carolina Medical Association* 15 (May 1919): 441; Victor C. Vaughan and George T. Palmer, "Communicable Disease in the United States Army During the Summer and Autumn of 1918," *Journal of Laboratory and Clinical Medicine* (hereafter *JLCM*) 4 (July 1919): 599; "The Cause of Influenza and Its Bearing on Treatment," in "Current Comment," *JAMA* 73 (November 1, 1919): 1368; "More About War Gases and Influenza," in "Editorials," *JAMA* 77 (30 July 1921): 382.

20. "Interepidemic Influenza," in "Editorials," *JAMA* 79 (October 21, 1922): 1430.

21. Douglas Symmers in collaboration with Morris Dinnerstein and A. D. Frost, "Differences in Pathology of Pandemic and Recurrent Forms of So-Called Influenza," *JAMA* 74 (March 6, 1920): 646; "Influenza," *JAMA* 78 (February 4, 1922): 354.

22. "Editorial—Interepidemic Influenza," *JAMA* 79 (October 21, 1922): 1429.

23. Peter K. Olitsky and Frederick L. Gates, "Investigations on the Bacteriology of Epidemic Influenza," *Science* 57 (February 9, 1923): 164; "Quotations—The Virus of Influenza," reprinted from *The British Medical Journal* in *Science* 57 (February 23, 1923): 236–237.

24. "Subject Index," *JAMA* 82 (June 28, 1924): 2174; "Subject Index," *JAMA* 83 (December 27, 1924): 2143.

25. "Editorial—Experimental Human Influenza," *JAMA* 85 (August 15, 1925): 520. For a full account of the ongoing research into the influenza virus, see John Barry, *The Great Influenza: The Epic Story of the Deadliest Plague in History* (New York: Viking, 2004), Part X.

26. "The World's Health," in "Current Comment," *JAMA* 84 (January 10, 1925): 123.

27. Ibid.; See also "Forecasting Epidemics," *LD* 89 (April 10, 1926): 21.

28. Certainly there were exceptions to this triumphalism, and influenza continued to prove a troubling subject for some. See George H. Bigelow, "Epidemics and the Community," *The Independent* 117 (July 10, 1926): 38; "The Influenza Epidemic in Europe," *Science* (March 4, 1927, Supplement 65): xii.

29. "How Influenza Kills," *LD* 93 (May 14, 1927): 22.

30. John McMullen, "The U.S. Public Health Service and Influenza," *KMJ* 17 (July 1919): 277.

31. "Discussion" following J. J. McShane, MD, PhD, "The Attempt to Control Influenza in Illinois," *Indiana Medical Journal* (hereafter *IMJ*) 37 (January 1920): 20; C. E. Turner, Sanitary Engineer, USPHS, "Spanish Influenza: A Report Upon Preventive Measures Adopted in New England Shipyards of the Emergency Fleet Corporation," Box 144, #1622, RG 90; letter from Rupert S. Blue, Surgeon General to G. Prather Knapp, Manager of Publicity, Mississippi Valley Trust Co., February 1, 1919, Box 145, #1622, RG 90, NA.

32. "Combine to Hunt Influenza Germ," *NYT*, September 21, 1919, 25.

33. See for instance John Dill Robertson and Gottfried Koehler, "Preliminary Report on the Influenza Epidemic in Chicago," *AJPH* 8 (November 1918): 854; letter from May Farinholt Jones, Acting Assistant Surgeon, USPHS to Medical Officer in Charge, Extra Cantonment Zone, Camp Shelby, February 1, 1919, Box 144, #1622, RG 90, NA; Sherman C. Kingsley, Director, Welfare Federation of Cleveland, "Cleveland and the 'Flu,'" *PHN* 10 (December 1918): 314, 316.

34. "Brief Outline of the Activities of the Public Health Service in Combating the Influenza Epidemic—1918–1919," 8, Box 145, #1622, RG 90, NA.

35. George M. Price, "Influenza—Destroyer and Teacher: A General Confession by the Public Health Authorities of a Continent," *Survey* 41 (December 21, 1919): 367.

36. Ibid., 368.

37. Ibid., 368.

38. See for instance "Influenza—Relative to a Possible Recurrence of the Epidemic during the Fall or Winter," *PHR* 34 (September 19, 1919): 2105.

39. William L. Moss, "Epidemiological Activities in Base Section No. 2," in *The History of U.S. Army Base Hospital No. 6 and Its Part in the American Expeditionary Forces 1917–1918* (Boston: Massachusetts General Hospital, 1924), 108.

40. Major George A. Soper, "The Lessons of the Pandemic," *Science* 49 (May 30, 1919): 501.

41. Lee K. Frankel, "The Future of the American Public Health Association," *AJPH* 9 (February 1919): 91, 92.

42. Louis I. Harris, "The Ultimate Benefits to Be Derived from the Epidemic," *AJPH* 9 (January 1919): 43.

43. Ibid., 41. See also Paul Mason, "Cincinnati Survey of the After Effects of Influenza," *Modern Medicine* 2 (April 1920): 305.

44. "Influenza Discussions" (report on discussions at the APHA meeting, December 1918), *AJPH* 9 (February 1919): 133–139; "Proceedings and Discussions of the American Public Health Association at New Orleans, LA., October 27–30, 1919," *AJPH* 9 (December 1919): 968–971.

45. "Influenza. Relative to a Possible Recurrence of the Epidemic During the Fall or Winter," *PHR* 34 (September 19, 1919): 2105.

46. "Editorials—National Epidemic Detector," *AJPH* 9 (June 1919): 450; J. Prentice Murphy, "The Aftermath of Influenza," *Survey* 41 (November 23, 1918): 213; Soper, "The Lessons of the Pandemic," 505; Harris, "The Ultimate Benefits to Be Derived from the Epidemic," 41–43.

47. "Symposium on the Health Center," *AJPH* 11 (March 1921): 212–233; Livingston Farrand, "Public Health and the Nurse," in "Department of Red Cross Nursing," *AJN* 20 (September 1920): 981–984; James G. Cumming, "Influenza-Pneumonia as Influenced by Dishwashing in Three Hundred and Seventy Public Institutions," *AJPH* 9 (November 1919): 849–852; James G. Cumming, "Influenza-Pneumonia as Influenced by Dishwashing in 370 Public Institutions (Concluded)," *AJPH* 10 (July 1920): 576–582; William H. Peters, "American Red Cross Health Crusade—After Effects of Influenza in Cincinnati," *AJPH* 9 (December 1919): 929.

48. Allen W. Freeman, "Administrative Measures Against Influenza," *AJPH* 9 (December 1919): 919.

49. Ibid., 919, 922–923.

50. "Ten Million Deaths in 'Flu' Plague a Year Ago," *NYT*, February 1, 1920, xxxi.

51. Letter from Rupert Blue, Surgeon General to Charles E. Townsend, US Senator, September 15, 1919, Box 146, #1622, RG 90, NA.

52. Dorothy A. Pettit and Janice Bailie, *A Cruel Wind: Pandemic Flu in America, 1918–1920* (Murfreesboro, TN: Timberlane Books, 2008), 199.

53. Lida Hafford, "Red Cross and Influenza," *KMJ* 17 (July 1919): 280.

54. Ibid., 280.

55. "To Defend City's Health—Dr. Copeland Suggests Organization of Agencies and Citizens," *NYT*, November 5, 1918, 13. See also Price, "Influenza—Destroyer and Teacher," 369.

56. Eugene R. Kelley and B. W. Carey, "Centralized Health and Relief Agencies in an Influenza Epidemic," *AJPH* 8 (October 1918): 744.

57. Charles V. Aiken, "Influenza in South Carolina, 1918," *Journal of the South Carolina Medical Association* 15 (January 1919): 350.

58. Harris, "The Ultimate Benefits to Be Derived from the Epidemic," 42; Rupert Blue, Surgeon General, "Epidemic Influenza and the U.S. Public Health Service," *MH* 11 (December 1918): 427.

59. Ravenel, "Preventive Medicine and War," 30.

60. Frank Overton, "Some Epidemiological Points Regarding Acute Respiratory Diseases," *AJPH* 10 (May 1920): 431.

61. Dr. J. W. Duke, discussant following Walton Forest Dutton, MD, "Prevention of Influenza and Allied Diseases" (paper presented at Section on General Medicine, Annual State Meeting, May 1919), reprinted in *Journal of the Oklahoma State Medical Association* 12 (November 1919): 328.

62. Ibid.

63. H. L. Rockwood, "Some Ways of Preventing Influenza," *PHN* 11 (November 1919): 850–851.

64. J. Alvin Jefferson, "Public Health Education" (paper presented before the Twenty-First Annual Session of the National Medical Association, Newark, 1919), reprinted in *JNMA* 11 (October–December 1919): 144.

65. H. T. Price, discussant following Dutton, "Prevention of Influenza and Allied Diseases," 327.

66. Lee K. Frankel, "The Future of the American Public Health Association" (address before the General Sessions, APHA, at Chicago, Illinois, December 10, 1918), reprinted in *AJPH* 9 (February 1919): 88.

67. Ibid.

68. Ibid., 90.

69. Ravenel, "Preventive Medicine and War," 32.

70. Grace Niles, "Some Bugs," *PHN* 14 (November 1922): 575–576.

71. Harris, "The Ultimate Benefits to Be Derived from the Epidemic," 42.

72. Freeman, "Administrative Measures Against Influenza," 922–923.

73. "Will the Flu Return?" HEALTH NEWS—Issued by the United States Public Health Service, For release Sunday, September 14, 1919, p. 5, Box 146, File 1622, RG 90, NA; letter from Acting Surgeon General to Dr. J. C. Price, State Director of Health, New Jersey, February 6, 1920, Box 146, #1622, RG 90, NA; letter from Rupert Blue, Surgeon General to Charles E. Townsend, US Senator, September 15, 1919, Box 146, # 1622, RG 90, NA.

74. "Editorial—Influenza and the Coming Annual Meeting," *AJPH* 8 (November 1918): 861.

75. "Public Health: A Live, Progressive Force," *AJPH* 10 (January 1920): 75. See also Rockwood, "Some Ways of Preventing Influenza," 854; W. S. Rankin, "The American Public Health Association, Past, Present, Future," *AJPH* 10 (April 1920): 300.

76. Presentation of Mr. Fess, *Congressional Record*, 65th Congress, 3rd Session, 1919, vol. 57, pt. 5: 4372.

77. "Symposium on How to Further Progress in Health Education and Publicity" (an account of the principal discussions given at the second session of the Health Education and Publicity Group, Fiftieth Annual Meeting, American Public Health Association, New York City, November 15, 1921,) *AJPH* 12 (April 1922): 279–289; Hibbert W. Hill, "What Is the Matter with Public Health?" *AJPH* 10 (August 1920): 673–675; Charles T. Nesbitt, "Relative Functions of Health Agencies—III. What Is the Matter with Public Health?" *AJPH* 10 (December 1920): 953–955.

78. See for instance "Editorial—The Organization of Public Health Nursing," *AJPH* 12 (September 1922): 775; "Editorial—The President's Message a Disappointment," 14 (February 1924): 138–139.

79. John Duffy, *The Sanitarians: A History of American Public Health* (Chicago: University of Illinois Press, 1990), 244–249.

80. "Symposium on the Health Center—V. The American Red Cross Health Center," *AJPH* 11 (March 1921): 227.

81. Elizabeth Ross, "Health Centers as Seen by a Public Health Nurse," *AJPH* 11 (October 1921): 915, 917.

82. Algernon Brashear Jackson, "Public Health and the Negro," *JNMA* 15 (October–December 1923): 257, 259. See also "Editorial—Public Health Work and Prolongation of Life," *AJPH* 14 (December 1924): 1061.

83. Adelaide Nutting, "The Outlook in Nursing," *PHN* 12 (September 1920): 765.

84. Katherine Tucker, "Annual Report of the Superintendent," *Report of the Board of Managers of the Visiting Nurse Society of Philadelphia, January 1–December 31, 1918*, 14–15, Folder 12—Annual Reports, Box 3, Visiting Nurse Society of Philadelphia Records (MC5), Center for the Study of the History of Nursing, School of Nursing, University of Pennsylvania.

85. Christopher G. Parnall, "The Future of Nursing Service and Nursing Education," *AJN* 20 (August 1920): 897–901; Christopher G. Parnall, "Nursing and the Health of the Future," *PHN* 13 (November 1921): 573–578.

86. "Some Sidelights on the Influenza Epidemic," *PHN* 11 (May 1919): 376.

87. Livingston Farrand, "Public Health and the Nurse," *AJN* 20 (September 1920): 981; F. B., "Nurses from a Patient's Standpoint," *AJN* 21 (December 1920): 157, 158.

88. Damon B. Pfeiffer, "The Position of the Nursing Profession Today" (an address to the nurses of the Presbyterian Hospital, Philadelphia, May 6, 1920), reprinted in *AJN* 21 (October 1920): 26.

89. Pfeiffer, "The Position of the Nursing Profession Today," 26. See also Clara D. Noyes, "Department of Red Cross Nursing—Great Need for Nurses for United States Public Health Service," *AJN* 20 (August 1920): 904.

90. "Editorial—The Production of Public Health Nurses," *PHN* 10 (December 1918): 295.

91. B. F. Thomson, quoted in "War-Reports from the Influenza Front," *Literary Digest* 60 (February 22, 1919): 67. See also Albert Howe, "Secretary's Report," *Twenty-eighth Annual Report of the Hampton Training School for Nurses and Dixie Hospital*, 7, University Archives, Hampton University; Minutes of November 7, 1918, in notebook with label "Compositions," no other label, which contains handwritten minutes, Folder 8: MVNA—Minutes of Monthly Meetings, 1914–1924, Series 1, Box 1, Moorestown Visiting Nurse Association Records (MC66), Center for the Study of the History of Nursing, School of Nursing, University of Pennsylvania; Helen Bell Upton, Superintendent of the King's Daughters' District Nursing Association of Louisville, "Influenza in Louisville, Kentucky," *PHN* 11 (January 1919): 49; "Teaching the People How to Keep Well," *NYT*, January 26, 1919, 72.

92. "Editorial Comment—Rank for American Nurses," *AJN* 19 (May 1919): 577–585; "Letters to the Editor—Rank for Nurses," *AJN* 19 (July 1919): 796–800; Helen Hoy Greeley, Counsel, National Committee to Secure Rank for Nurses, "Rank for Nurses," *AJN* 19 (July 1919): 840–853. See also Susan Zeiger, *In Uncle Sam's Service: Women Workers with the American Expeditionary Forces, 1917–1919* (Philadelphia: University of Pennsylvania Press, 2004).

93. Anna C. Jamme, "Address of the President of the National League of Nursing Education," *AJN* 22 (September 1922): 996; Nutting, "The Outlook in Nursing," 754.

94. Susan Reverby, *Ordered to Care: The Dilemma of American Nursing, 1850–1945* (New York: Cambridge University Press, 1987), 160.

95. Letter from "Organizer" to Mrs. Robert T. Reinman, President, Twentieth Century Club, March 5, 1919, Folder 1: "Special Committee on Public Health Nursing correspondence, Public Health Nursing Association of Pittsburgh; By-Laws, Correspondence, Reports, 1918–1920," Box 1, Visiting Nurse Association of Allegheny County Records (MC106), Barbara Bates Center for the Study of the History of Nursing, School of Nursing, University of Pennsylvania; Eunice H. Dyke, "Influenza Experiences and What They Taught," *PHN* 11 (November 1919): 890.

96. Lillian D. Wald, "Influenza: When the City Is a Great Field Hospital," *Survey* 43 (February 14, 1920): 580.

97. Lillian D. Wald, "The Work of the Nurses' Emergency Council," *PHN* 19 (December 1918): 311.

98. Nutting, "The Outlook in Nursing," 755–758.

99. Reverby, *Ordered to Care*, 159–164.

100. "From the Report of the Committee on Nursing Education," *AJN* 22 (August 1922): 882.

101. Ibid., 882–884; Reverby, *Ordered to Care*, 164–166.

102. "Editorial Comment—Report of the Committee on Nursing," *AJN* 22 (August 1922): 879.
103. Reverby, *Ordered to Care*, 166–168.
104. Jamme, "Address of the President of the National League of Nursing Education," 996, 998.
105. Elizabeth G. Fox, "Address of the President of the National Organization for Public Health Nursing," *AJN* 22 (September 1922): 1005.
106. Clara D. Noyes, "Address of the President of the American Nurses' Association," *AJN* 22 (September 1922): 994.
107. Ibid., 995.
108. "Fighting on Two Fronts! At Home and 'Over There,'" *Supplement to the Gulf Division Bulletin* (November 1, 1918), File 803.7—"Epidemics, Influenza, Publicity and Publications," Box 688, RG 200, NA.
109. "Red Cross Care of Influenza Epidemic throughout Southern Division," Southern Division, Reports and Statistics, Epidemics—Influenza, File 803.08, Box 688, RG 200, NA; "Report of the Activities of the Chapters and Branches of the Atlantic Division of the American Red Cross during the Epidemic of Spanish Influenza, December 20, 1918," Atlantic Division, Reports and Statistics, Epidemics—Influenza, File 803.08, Box 688, RG 200, NA; Earl Kilpatrick, Division Manager, "Practical and Constructive Suggestions to Red Cross Workers for Adequate Preparation Against Influenza," *Bulletin of the American Red Cross—Northwestern Division* III (January 31, 1920): 1 in File 803.7—Epidemics, Influenza, Publicity and Publications, Box 688, RG 200, NA.
110. Handwritten note at the conclusion of "Red Cross Care of Influenza Epidemic Throughout Southern Division," presented by Mrs. Arkwright, Southern Division, Reports and Statistics, Epidemics—Influenza, File 803.08, Box 688, RG200, NA.
111. Report of the Southern Division, attached to letter from Margaret Nutting, Director, Bureau of News, Department of Publicity to M.G. Scheitlin, Director, News Service. File 803.08, EPIDEMICS, INFLUENZA—Reports and Statistics, Southern Division, Box 688, RG 200, NA.
112. "Report of the Department of Civilian Relief July 1—December 31, 1918," attached to letter from Starr Cadwallader, Division Director, Civilian Relief, Lake Division to James L. Fieser, Associate Director General, National Headquarters, August 22, 1919, Lake Division, Civilian Relief Reports: July–December 1918, File 149.18, Box 216, Entry 27130D, RG 200, NA.
113. American Red Cross, *The Mobilisation of the American Red Cross during the Influenza Pandemic 1918–1919* (Geneva: Printing Office of the Tribune de Geneve, 1920), 24–25.
114. *Southeastern Pennsylvania Chapter of the American Red Cross in the Influenza Epidemic September–October 1918*, Pennsylvania, Epidemics—Influenza, File 803.11, Box 689, RG 200, NA.
115. Pettit and Bailie, *A Cruel Wind*, 184–186.
116. "The Great Plague," *Independent* 101 (February 21, 1920): 292; "Death Rate Far Below a Year Ago," *NYT*, November 1919, E1; "Red Cross Starts Drive for Members," *NYT*, November 2, 1919, E1.
117. "Flu Jumped Death Rate," *LAT*, 13 July 1919, II:10; "The Influenza Plague Spread Terror and Death in the South Seas," *LD* 61 (May 24, 1919): 52, 54.
118. "Influenza—A Foe to Genius," *LD* 97 (April 21, 1928): 21.
119. "Look out for the 'Flu!'" *Independent* 199 (October 4, 1919): 6; Charles A. L. Reed, "The War Against Germs," *Review of Reviews* 70 (July 1924): 80.
120. See for instance "Will the 'Flu' Return?" *LD* 63 (October 11, 1919): 26; "Believe Flu Is to Come Again," *LAT*, September 10, 1919, I:1; "Warns of Influenza," *NYT*, August 15, 1919, 6.
121. "Will the 'Flu' Return?" 26.
122. "Mutual Life's Report," *NYT*, January 31, 1919, 14; "Our Death Losses in Battle 57 Per 1,000," *NYT*, February 16, 1919, 11; "Influenza Spoiled City Health Record," *NYT*, May 25, 1919, 23; "Death Rate Far Below a Year Ago," *NYT*, November 16, 1919, E1.
123. "Ten Million Deaths in 'Flu' Plague A Year Ago," *NYT*, February 1, 1920, XXX1.
124. "Bank President a Suicide," *NYT*, January 24, 1919, 4; "A Misnomer Should be Avoided," *NYT*, March 17, 1919, 14; "Best Health Report for City in 53 Years," *NYT*, January 4, 1920, 20; "1919 Health Record Good," *NYT*, January 12, 1920, 8; "5,634 Get Fresh-Air Trips," *NYT*, August 31, 1919, 7.
125. "Happier Days for 'Hundred Neediest,'" *NYT*, May 18, 1919, 25.

126. Ibid.

127. Ibid.

128. Case 15, "New York's 100 Neediest Cases," *NYT*, December 14, 1919, XXX1.

129. Ibid.

130. Ibid., XXX2; "Families Aided by Times Appeal," *NYT*, May 2, 1920, E1.

131. "Influenza Virus Found," *NYT*, February 6, 1919, 14; "Discoveries Abounding in Promise," *NYT*, February 7, 1919, 14; "Influenza Germ Elusive," *NYT*, June 14, 1919, 13; "Combine to Hunt Influenza Germ," *NYT*, September 21, 1919, 25; "Best Health Report for City in 53 Years," *NYT*, January 4, 1920, 20; "1919 Health Record Good," *NYT*, January 12, 1920, 8; "Says He Found Grip Germ," *NYT*, January 24, 1920, 4; "Fighting Epidemics," *Survey* 49 (November 15, 1922): 247; "Forecasting Epidemics," *LD* 89 (April 10, 1926): 21; "Another Flu Epidemic?" *LD* 92 (January 29, 1927): 12; "How Influenza Kills," *LD* 93 (May 14, 1927): 22.

132. Homer Folks, "War, Best Friend of Disease," *Harper's* 140 (March 1920): 456; "The Great Plague," *Independent* 101 (February 21, 1920): 292; "The 'Flu' at Its Work Again," *LD* 64 (January 1920): 13.

133. "Their Task Far From Fully Done," *NYT*, February 7, 1919, 14.

134. Ibid.

135. "Topics of the Times—Discoveries Abounding in Promise," *NYT*, February 7, 1919, 14.

136. Ibid.

137. See for instance "This Year's 'Flu,'" *LD* 76 (March 3, 1923): 26–27; Charles A. L. Reed, "The War Against the Germs," *Review of Reviews* 70 (July 1924): 80–82.

138. *Congressional Record*, 65th Cong., 3d sess., 1919, 57, pt. 4:3320.

139. *Congressional Record*, 65th Cong., 3d sess., 1919, 57, pt. 4:4107.

140. *Congressional Record*, 65th Cong., 3d sess., 1919, 57, pt. 5:5018.

141. *Congressional Record*, 66th Cong., 1st sess., 1919, 58, pt. 3:2574, 3083.

142. Alfred W. Crosby, *America's Forgotten Pandemic: The Influenza of 1918* (New York: Cambridge University Press, 1989), 314.

143. *Congressional Record*, 65th Cong., 3d sess., 1919, 57, pt. 4:4107.

144. *Congressional Record*, 65th Cong., 3d sess., 1919, 57, pt. 4:3320. The arguments of Congressman Fess of Ohio mirrored those of his state congress. See *Congressional Record*, 65th Cong., 3d sess., 1919, 57, pt. 5: 4372.

145. See for instance the comments of Mr. France, Mr. Townsend, and Mr. Norris, *Congressional Record*, 66th Cong., 2d sess., 1920, 59, pt. 2: 2044–2045.

146. See Mr. Smith of Carolina, *Congressional Record*, 66th Cong., 2d sess., 1920, 59, pt. 2: 2045.

147. *Congressional Record*, 66th Cong., 2d sess., 1920, 59, pt. 2: 2045.

148. Ibid.

149. Ibid.

150. Ibid.

151. Ibid., 2043.

152. *Congressional Record*, 65th Cong., 3d sess., 1919, 57, pt. 5: 4372.

153. Carter Glass, quoted in Crosby, *America's Forgotten Pandemic*, 313.

154. See for instance the speech of Mr. King, *Congressional Record*, 66th Cong., 2d sess., 1920, 59, pt.2: 2043–2044.

155. Ibid., 2044.

156. See speech of Mr. Phelan, *Congressional Record*, 66th Cong., 2d sess., 1920, 59, pt. 2: 2046–2047.

157. Ibid., 2044.

158. Ibid., 2045.

159. Ibid., 2044.

160. Essie Jenkins, "1919 Influenza Blues," *Blues with a Message* (El Cerrito, CA: Arhoolie Records, 2005), available at http://www.rhapsody.com/album/blues-with-a-message [accessed June 18, 2009].

161. Blind Willie Johnson, "Jesus Is Coming," *Complete Recordings of Blind Willie Johnson* (Sony, 1993), lyrics available at http://blueslyrics.tripod.com/artistswithsongs/blind_willie_johnson_1.htm [accessed on December 28, 2008].

162. Letter from William G. McAdoo to Nona, his daughter, November 7, 1918, William G. McAdoo Papers, Manuscript Division, Library of Congress.

163. Letter from Joseph P. Tumulty to Hon. Robert W. Woolley, January 20, 1919, Container 83, Joseph P. Tumulty Papers, Manuscript Division, Library of Congress.

164. Letter Joseph P. Tumulty to Major E. F. Kinkead ("Gene"), January 25, 1919, Container 83, Joseph P. Tumulty Papers, Manuscripts Division, Library of Congress.

165. Letter from Harold Bowman to Herbert W. Fisher, January 8, 1919, Folder 324, Correspondence—Family: Vol. 6—1918–1920, Series 1—Box 20, Irving Fisher Papers, MSS Group 212, Sterling Memorial Library, Yale University.

166. Pettit and Bailie, *A Cruel Wind*, 228.

167. Ibid., 129.

168. Crosby, *America's Forgotten Pandemic*, 317–318.

169. Katherine Anne Porter, "Pale Horse, Pale Rider," *Pale Horse, Pale Rider: Three Short Novels* (New York: Harcourt, Brace, Jovanovich, 1967 [1936]), 141.

170. Ibid., 142–143. The title of the novella comes from an African American spiritual, as the characters note at one point as they sing the song during Miranda's illness. In the song, the singer laments the loss not only of their lover but also of others: "There's a lot more to it than that,' said Adam, 'about forty verses, the rider done taken away mammy, pappy, brother, sister, the whole family besides the lover." Miranda notes, though, that the singer is not taken. "Death always leaves one singer to mourn," she explains (189, 190). The spiritual, of course, references one of the four horsemen of the apocalypse, Death, who rode a pale horse in the Book of Revelations, the final book of the New Testament.

171. Ibid., 173, 175, 176, 177, 178.

172. Ibid., 154, 157.

173. Ibid., 162–163.

174. Ibid., 141, 143, 148, 161.

175. Ibid., 170.

176. Ibid., 178.

177. Ibid., 182, 183.

178. Ibid., 184.

179. Ibid., 181, 183–184, 185–186

180. Ibid., 187–188.

181. Ibid., 198.

182. Ibid., 200.

183. Crosby, *America's Forgotten Pandemic*, 319.

184. Porter, *Pale Horse, Pale Rider*, 200–204.

185. Ibid., 204–205.

186. Ibid., 205.

187. Ibid., 207.

188. Ibid., 207–208.

189. Ibid., 208.

190. Ibid., 208.

191. William Maxwell, *They Came Like Swallows* (New York: Vintage, 1997 [1937]), 8–9.

192. Ibid., 62, 121, 163.

193. Ibid., 129, 160.

194. Ibid., 167.

195. Ibid., 135.

196. Ibid., 169, 171–172.

197. Ibid., 173.

198. William Maxwell, interview with Terry Gross, first aired on March 29, 1995, Fresh Air, Public Broadcasting Service, available at http://www.npr.org/templates/story/story.php?storyId=18413172 [accessed September 14, 2011].

199. Francis B. Fourvier, PFC, Company H, 341st Infantry, 86th Division, AEQC, WWORP, USAMHI.

200. Clarence M. Bodner, 343rd Infantry, 86th Division and Louis Brooks, 42nd Infantry, 12th Division, both in AEQC, WWORP, USAMHI.

201. Merle E. Swanger, 68th Infantry, 18th Infantry Brigade, 9th Division, AEQC, WWORP, USAMHI.
202. Private Orville Holman, Camp Funston, AEQC, WWORP, USAMHI.
203. Grant M. Church, 14th Division, AEQC, WWORP, USAMHI.
204. Melvin Lynn Frank, "Reminiscences: 'Sawmill City Boyhood,'" 59, undated, Minnesota Historical Society.
205. Ibid., 79.
206. Ibid., 79.
207. Ibid., 79.
208. Ibid., 79.
209. Ibid., 80.
210. Ibid., 80
211. Mary McCarthy, *Memories of a Catholic Girlhood* (New York: Harcourt, Brace, Jovanovich, 1957 [1946]), 29–30.
212. Thomas Wolfe, *Look Homeward, Angel: A Story of the Buried Life* (New York: Charles Scribner's Sons, 1929), 537–557.
213. Ibid., 538, 550.
214. Ibid., 541–542. Another writer of fiction, Willa Cather, captured the horror of an influenza death scene in her World War I novel, *One of Ours*, but concluded her description with the patient dying "in perfect dignity." That Cather's account of an influenza death can end so differently from Wolfe's may reflect a different personal relationship to the epidemic. Willa Cather, *One of Ours* (New York: Alfred A. Knopf, 1922), 300–301.
215. Wolfe, *Look Homeward Angel*, 543.
216. Ibid., 543.
217. Ibid., 548–549.
218. Ibid., 538–539.
219. Ibid., 544–545.
220. Ibid., 545.
221. Victor C. Vaughan, *A Doctor's Memories* (New York: Bobbs-Merrill Co., 1926), chaps. 7, 10, 11.
222. Col. Victor C. Vaughan in "Discussion" following "Prophylactic Inoculation in Pneumonia and Influenza," in "Society Proceedings—American Public Health Association, December 8–11, 1918," *JAMA* 71 (December 21, 1918): 2099.
223. Victor C. Vaughan and George Palmer, "Communicable Disease in the United States Army during the Summer and Autumn of 1918," *JLCM* 4 (July 1919): 591, 592.
224. Vaughan, *A Doctor's Memories*, 432.
225. Ibid., 382.
226. Ibid., 383–384.
227. Colonel V. C. Vaughan, quoted in Price, "Influenza—Destroyer and Teacher," 367.

Conclusion

1. Edward T. Linenthal, *The Unfinished Bombing: Oklahoma City in American Memory* (New York: Oxford University Press, 2001), chap. 2, 53.
2. Susan Urbach, quoted in ibid., 70. See also ibid., 53–70.
3. Ibid., 70, 71–80.
4. Edward T. Linenthal, "Epilogue: Reflections," *Slavery and Public History: The Tough Stuff of American Memory*, ed. James Oliver Horton and Lois E. Horton (Chapel Hill: University of North Carolina Press, 2006), 214.
5. Ibid., 214.
6. Manning Marable, *Living Black History: How Re-imagining the African-American Past Can Remake America's Racial Future* (New York: Basic Civitas Books, 2006), chap. 1.
7. John Bodnar, *The "Good War" in American Memory* (Baltimore: Johns Hopkins University Press, 2010).
8. Leigh Raiford and Renee C. Romano, "Introduction: The Struggle over Memory," *The Civil Rights Movement in American Memory*, ed. Leigh Raiford and Renee C. Romano (Athens: University of Georgia Press, 2006), xvii.

9. See for instance William Langewiesche, *American Ground: Unbuilding the World Trade Center* (New York: North Point Press, 2002), 8; David Simpson, *9/11: The Culture of Commemoration* (Chicago: University of Chicago Press, 2006), 43.

10. Linenthal, *The Unfinished Bombing*, 46–47.

11. Carol R. Byerly, *Fever of War: The Influenza Epidemic in the U.S. Army During World War I* (New York: New York University Press, 2005), 185–190.

12. David W. Blight, "Epilogue: Southerners Don't Lie; They Just Remember Big," in *Where These Memories Grow: History, Memory, and Southern Identity*, ed. W. Fitzhugh Brundage (Chapel Hill: University of North Carolina Press, 2000), 350.

13. Thanks to David Rosner for calling my attention to the importance of this conflict between the narratives of individuals and the progressive narratives of their broader communities.

14. Jamie Kalven, *Working with Available Light: A Family's World after Violence* (New York: W.W. Norton and Co., 1999), 292–293.

15. Linenthal, *The Unfinished Bombing*, 89–91, 94–96.

16. Errol Laborde, "Bringing Closure to a Word with a Pop Psychological Spin," quoted in ibid., 95.

17. Susan J. Brison, *Aftermath: Violence and the Remaking of a Self* (Princeton, NJ: Princeton University Press, 2002), x–xi.

18. Ilana Lowy, "Comment: Influenza and Historians: A Difficult Past," in *Influenza and Public Health: Learning from Past Pandemics*, ed. Tamara Giles-Vernick and Susan Craddock (London: Earthscan, 2010), 91. For historical works see for instance Gina Kolata, *Flu: The Story of the Great Influenza Pandemic of 1918 and the Search for the Virus That Caused It* (New York: Farrar, Straus and Giroux, 1999); Lynette Iezzoni, *Influenza, 1918* (New York: TV Books, 1999); Pete Davies, *The Devil's Flu: The World's Deadliest Influenza Epidemic and the Scientific Hunt for the Virus That Caused It* (New York: Henry Holt and Company, 2000); Howard Phillips and David Killingray, ed., *The Spanish Influenza Pandemic of 1918–19: New Perspectives* (London: Routledge, 2003); John Barry, *The Great Influenza: The Epic Story of the Deadliest Plague in History* (New York: Viking, 2004); Byerly, *Fever of War*; W. Jones Esyllt, *Influenza 1918: Disease, Death and Struggle in Winnipeg* (Toronto: University of Toronto Press, 2007); Tom Quinn, *Flu: A Social History of Influenza* (London: New Holland Publishers, 2008); Dorothy A. Pettit and Janice Bailie, *A Cruel Wind: Pandemic Flu in America, 1918–1920* (Murfreesboro, TN: Timberlane Books, 2008); Tamara Giles-Vernick and Susan Craddock, *Influenza and Public Health: Learning from Past Pandemics* (London: Earthscan, 2010). Perhaps the clearest indication that the epidemic has fully entered the culture is its increasing appearance in fiction. In 2000 David Getz published a children's book on the epidemic, *Purple Death: The Mysterious Flu of 1918* (New York: Henry Holt and Co., 2000). More recently, the epidemic has made several appearances, for instance playing a central role in the creation of one of the main characters in Stephenie Meyer's bestselling teen novel series, *The Twilight Saga*. The influenza outbreak also serves as the central narrative event for Thomas Mullen's *The Last Town on Earth*, and as the backdrop for the 2011 Newberry Prize winner *Moon over Manifest*. See Stephenie Meyer, *Twilight* (New York: Little, Brown and Company, 2005), 287; Thomas Mullen, *The Last Town on Earth: A Novel* (New York: Random House, 2007); Clare Vanderpool, *Moon over Manifest* (New York: Delacorte Books, 2010).

19. Kolata, *Flu*, chaps. 7 and 9.

20. See for instance James Stevens et al., "Structure of the Uncleaved Human H1 Hemagglutinin from the Extinct 1918 Influenza Virus," *Science* 303 (March 19, 2004): 1866–1870; S. J. Gamblin et al., "The Structure and Receptor Binding Properties of the 1918 Influenza Hemagglutinin," *Science* 303 (March 19, 2004): 1838–1842; Edward C. Holmes, "1918 and All That," *Science* 303 (March 19, 2004): 1787–1788; Terrence M. Tumpey et al., "Characterization of the Reconstructed 1918 Spanish Influenza Virus," *Science* 310 (October 7, 2005): 77–80; Jeffery K. Taubenberger et al., "Capturing a Killer Virus," *Scientific American* 292 (January 2005): 62–71; Jeffery K. Taubenberger et al., "Initial Genetic Characterization of the 1918 'Spanish' Influenza Virus," *Science* 275 (March 21, 1997): 1793–1796.

21. Jeffery K. Taubenberger and David M. Morens, "1918 Influenza: The Mother of All Pandemics," *Emerging Infectious Disease* 2 (January 2006): 16; Taubenberger and Morens, "Influenza: The Once and Future Pandemic," 19-21.

22. Jeffery K. Taubenberger and David M. Morens, "Influenza: The Once and Future Pandemic," 19–21. Evolutionary biologist Paul Ewald offers an alternative explanation for its virulence, pointing to the conditions of trench warfare and the movement of troops caused by World War I, and the opportunities for constant infection and adaptation such conditions offered. See Byerly, *Fever of War*, 92–96.

23. Robert G. Wallace et al., "Are Influenzas in Southern China Byproducts of the Region's Globalizing Historical Present?" in *Influenza and Public Health: Learning from Past Pandemics*, ed. Tamara Giles-Vernick and Susan Craddock (London: Earthscan, 2010), 102.

24. Susan Craddock and Tamara Giles-Vernick, "Introduction," in *Influenza and Public Health: Learning from Past Pandemics*, 1.

25. S. Harris Ali, "Globalized Complexity and the Microbial Traffic of New and Emerging Infectious Disease Threats," in *Influenza and Public Health*, ed. Giles-Vernick and Craddock 22.

26. Cleve Jones, "Prologue: A Vision of the Quilt," *Remembering the AIDS Quilt*, ed. Charles E. Morris III (East Lansing: Michigan State University Press, 2011), xiv.

27. NAMES Project Foundation website, http://www.aidsquilt.org/history.htm [accessed September 15, 2011].

28. John D'Emilio, "The Names Project Quilt: A People's Memorial," in *Making Trouble: Essays on Gay History, Politics, and the University* (New York: Routledge, 1992), 218, 217.

29. Jones, "Prologue: A Vision of the Quilt," xxi.

30. Charles E. Morris III, "The Mourning After," in *Remembering the AIDS Quilt*, ed. Morris III, xlv–l. Morris's book is an excellent example of the ongoing scholarly interest in the Quilt.

31. Richard Kim, quoted in Morris III, *Remembering the AIDS Quilt*, xlvi.

32. Alice Dautry, "Foreword," in *Influenza and Public Health*, ed. Giles-Vernick and Craddock xiv.

SELECTED BIBLIOGRAPHY

ARCHIVAL RECORDS

American Philosophical Society
   Harold Lindsay Amoss Papers
   Rufus Ivory Cole Papers
   Simon Flexner Papers
   Victor George Heiser Papers
   Peter K. Olitsky Papers
   Eugene Lindsay Opie Papers
Armed Forces Institute of Pathology
Bancroft Library, University of California, Berkeley
   Clemens Max Richter Collection (BANC MSS 71/57c)
Barbara Bates Center for the Study of the History of Nursing, University of
   Pennsylvania School of Nursing
Columbia University, Oral History Collection
   A. R. Dochez
   Warren F. Draper
   Connie M. Guion
   Gardner Jackson
   Isabel Maitland Stewart
   Benjamin Earle Washburn
District of Columbia Public Library
   Annual Reports of the Commissioners of the District of Columbia
Hampton University
   University Archives
Hazel A. Braugh Records Center of the American Red Cross
   Division Bulletins
Howard Gotlieb Archival Research Center, Boston University
   History of Nursing Archives General Collection
Idaho State Historical Society
   Visiting Nurse Association (Boise, Idaho) Papers
Indiana Historical Society
   Haughville Collection, Photographs (P0069)
Indiana State Library
   Hugh Arthur Barnhart Manuscript Collection
   Harold Standish Barr Manuscript Collection
   Urban C. Stover Manuscript Collection

Library of Congress, Manuscript Division
　Newton D. Baker Papers
　Helen Culver Kerr Papers
　William G. McAdoo Papers
　Joseph P. Tumulty Papers
　WPA Federal Writers' Project Collection
Minnesota Historical Society
　Melvin Lynn Frank, "Sawmill City Boyhood"
　Oscar Jewell Harvey, "The Spanish Influenza Pandemic of 1918; an account of its ravages in
　　Luzerne County, Pennsylvania, and the efforts made to combat and subdue it"
　Albert B. Reagan, "Wild or Indian Rice."
　Carl R. and Erwin J. Jones and Family Papers
　Max Winkel and Family Papers
Moorland Spingarn Research Center, Manuscript Division, Howard University
　Francis James Grimke Collection
National Archives and Records Administration, Pacific-Alaska Region,
Seattle
　Record Group 75: Records of the Bureau of Indian Affairs
National Archives and Records Administration, San Francisco
　Record Group 75: Records of the Bureau of Indian Affairs
National Archives and Records Administration, Washington, D.C. and College Park, Maryland
　Record Group 90: Records of the Public Health Service
　Record Group 112: Records of the Surgeon General of the Army
　Record Group 200: Records of the American Red Cross
　Record Group 393: Records of U. S. Army Continental Commands, 1821–1920
　Record Group 407: Records of the Office of the Adjutant General
　Still Picture Branch
National Library of Medicine (NLM), History of Medicine Division
　Stanhope Bayne-Jones Oral History
　Shields Warren Oral History
　Martin Franklin, Diary, 1914–1919
New York City Municipal Reference and Research Center
　Annual Report of the Department of Health of the City of New York for the Year 1918
　Annual Report of the Department of Health of the City of New York for the Year 1919
　Monthly Bulletin of the Department of Health, City of New York, 1918
　Weekly Bulletins of the Department of Health, City of New York, 1918
　School Health News, Department of Health, New York City, 1918–1919
　Minutes of the Board of Health, New York City
Philadelphia College of Physicians
　City of Philadelphia Department of Public Health and Charities Monthly Bulletins
Schlesinger Library, Radcliffe Institute for Advanced Study, Harvard University
　Kenneth Griggs Merrill Papers, 1918–1919 (A/M571)
Social Welfare History Archives, University of Minnesota
　Henry Street Visiting Nurse Service (SW63)
　Minneapolis Family and Children's Services (SW75)
　Minneapolis Family and Children's Services Case Records, 1895–1945 (SWF19)
U.S. Army Military History Institute, Carlisle Barracks
　Medical Historical Unit Collection, Chester Oliver Davidson Papers
　Army Experiences Questionnaire Collection, World War One Research Project
University of Virginia Special Collections Department
　William B. Bean Oral History (RG26/4-#4)
　Ella Katherine Fife Freudenberg Papers (#5943-e)
　Gregory-Whitmore Family Papers (MSS#10754-d)
　"Help Fight the Grippe" (Broadside 1918 H44)

Yale University, Manuscripts and Archives, Sterling Library
    Irving Fisher Papers
    Arthur T. Hadley Papers
    James M. Howard Papers
    William Kent Family Papers
    Charles-Edward A. Winslow Papers

GOVERNMENT PUBLICATIONS
    United States Congress. Congressional Record, Hearings, and Documents, 1917–1919

NEWSPAPERS
    Atlanta Constitution (electronic—NewspaperARCHIVE)
    Baltimore Afro-American
    Camp Bowie Pass-in-Review
    Camp Crane News
    Camp Devens News
    Camp Dodger
    Camp Jackson Click
    Camp Logan Reveille
    Camp Sherman News
    Cavalier Daily (University of Virginia)
    Chicago Tribune (electronic— NewspaperARCHIVE)
    Christian Science Monitor (electronic—ProQuest Historical Newspapers)
    Daily Astorian (Oregon)
    Salem Daily Statesman
    Deer Creek Mirror (Minnesota)
    Des Moines Daily News (electronic—NewspaperARCHIVE)
    Des Moines Homestead (electronic—NewspaperARCHIVE)
    Eastern Oregon Republican
    Los Angeles Times (electronic—ProQuest Historical Newspapers)
    Marshall Daily Chronicle (Michigan) (electronic—NewspaperARCHIVE)
    Minnesota Daily (University of Minnesota)
    Morning Oregonian
    Nevada State Journal (electronic—NewspaperARCHIVE)
    Newark Daily Advocate (Ohio) (electronic—NewspaperARCHIVE)
    New York Age
    New York Times (electronic—ProQuest Historical Newspapers)
    Oregon Statesman
    San Antonio Daily Express (electronic—NewspaperARCHIVE)
    San Antonio Daily Light (electronic—NewspaperARCHIVE)
    Shenandoah Valley (New Market, Virginia)
    Trench and Camp (Camp Greene, Camp Cody)
    World News (Roanoke, Virginia)

JOURNALS
    American Journal of Nursing
    American Journal of Public Health
    Climatologist
    Hahnemannian Monthly
    Journal of the American Medical Association
    Journal of the American Osteopathic Association
    Journal of the National Medical Association
    North American Journal of Homeopathy
    Public Health Bulletin
    Public Health Nurse
    Public Health Reports

PUBLISHED PRIMARY SOURCES: ARTICLES AND BOOKS

Aiken, Charles V. "Influenza in South Carolina, 1918." *Journal of the South Carolina Medical Association* 15 (August 1919): 346–349.

Allen, George. "Cases of Insanity Following La Grippe." *NAJH* 6 (1891): 718–721.

Allen, P. M. and Hudson, P. L. "The Present Influenza Epidemic in New York." *Journal of the South Carolina Medical Association* 12 (February 1916): 47–51.

Althaus, J. "Influenza: Its Origin and Mode of Spreading." *Contemporary Review* 62 (August 1892): 225–239.

American Red Cross, *The Mobilisation of the American Red Cross During the Influenza Pandemic, 1918–1919*. Geneva: Printing Office of the Tribune de Geneve, 1920.

Anders, J. M. "Clinical Features of the Present Epidemic of Influenza." *Medical and Surgical Reporter* 66 (1892): 445–448.

"Another Flu Epidemic?" *LD* 92 (January 29, 1927): 12.

Baker, S. Josephine. *Fighting for Life*. New York: MacMillan Company, 1939.

Bigelow, H. "Epidemics and the Community." *Independent* 117 (July 10, 1926): 36–38.

Biggs, H. M. "Recent Epidemic of Influenza." *Review of Reviews* 59 (January 1919): 69–71.

Bird, R. L. "The Symptoms, Diagnosis and Treatment of Influenza." *KMJ* 18 (1920): 291–293.

Blue, Rupert. "Epidemic Influenza." *Memphis Medical Monthly* 39 (August 1, 1918): 169–171.

———. "Epidemic Influenza and the U.S. Public Health Service." *Modern Hospital* 11 (December 1918): 423–427.

———. "'Spanish Flu' 'Three-Day Fever' 'The Flu.'" *PHR* (September 25, 1918, Supplement 34).

Boggess, Walter F. "Some Phases of the Recent Influenza Epidemic." *KMJ* 17 (1918): 72–78.

Brewer, Isaac W. "The Control of Communicable Diseases in Camps." *AJPH* 8 (February 1918): 121–124.

———. "Report of Epidemic of Spanish Influenza, Which Occurred at Camp A.A. Humphreys, Va., during September and October, 1918." *JLCM* 4 (1918–1919): 87–111.

Brooks, W. A. "Out-door Treatment of Spanish Influenza." *Modern Hospital* 11 (December 1918): 427–429.

Brown, George S. "Clinical Lessons from 343 Cases of Influenza and 49 Cases of Pneumonia." *Journal of the Arkansas Medical Society* 16 (October 1918): 98–100.

Buckler, T. H. "Influenza from a Sanitary Point of View." *Maryland Medical Journal* 27 (1892): 575–584.

Bush, Earl A. "Care of Influenza and Pneumonia in an Army Base Hospital." *JAOA* 18 (March 1919): 333–335.

Buster, W. L. "Influenza and Pneumonia." *JAOA* 18 (April 1919): 392–396.

Cather, Willa. *One of Ours*. New York: A.A. Knopf, 1922.

Chandler, G. C. "Lessons Learned and Results Accomplished During the Influenza Epidemic." *New Orleans Medical and Surgical Journal* 72 (1919–1920): 124–129.

Chaney, W. C. "The Treatment of Fifty-one Selected Cases of Influenza in the Epidemic of 1920." *Minnesota Medicine* 3 (1920): 436–439.

"Controlling the Influenza Epidemic in Ohio." *Ohio Public Health Journal* 9 (November 1918): 452–456.

Coolidge, Emelyn Lincoln. "The Young Mother's Guide: The Sick Child—Influenza or Grip." *Ladies Home Journal* 26 (November 1919): 68.

Croft, Albert J. "Influenza Versus the Epidemic." *Illinois Medical Journal* 35 (1919): 80–85.

Curtin, R. G. and E. W. Watson. "Epidemic of Influenza in Philadelphia in 1889, '90, '91." *Climatologist* 2 (1892): 77–94.

Cushing, Harvey. *From a Surgeon's Journal 1915–1918*. Boston: Little, Brown and Co., 1936.

Davidson, A. C. "La Grippe: Its Etiology, Clinical History and History." *Southern Medical Record* 21 (1891): 469–479.

Davies, Elizabeth J. "The Influenza Epidemic and How We Tried to Control It." *PHN* 11 (January 1919): 45–47.

"Deaths from Influenza and Pneumonia in Cities. 25 Weeks—September 8, 1918, to March 1, 1919." *PHR* 34 (March 14, 1919): 505.

Dock, Lavinia et al. *History of American Red Cross Nursing.* New York: MacMillan Co., 1922.

Donald, William. M. "Spanish Influenza." *Medical Review of Reviews* 25 (1919): 78–85.

Doty, Permelia Murnan. "A Retrospect of the Influenza Epidemic." *PHN* 11 (December 1919): 949–957.

"Dr. Richardson on Chloroform and Influenza (summary)," *Review of Reviews* 5 (June 1892): 598–599.

Duncan, C. H. "A Remedy of Precision in Influenza." *Medical Standard* 39 (1916): 97–99.

Dyke, Eunice H. "Influenza Experiences and What They Taught." *PHN* 11 (November 1919): 888–891.

Eddy, Mary Baker. *Science and Health with Key to the Scriptures.* Boston: Trustees, Church of Christ, Scientist, 1934 [1875].

"Editorial: An Explosive Epidemic of Influenzal Disease at Fort Oglethorpe." *JLCM* 3 (June 1918): 560–564.

"Editorial: Making the World Safe for Osteopathy." *JAOA* 18 (February 1919): 279–282.

Edson, C. "Defenses Against Epidemic Disease." *Forum* 9 (June 1980): 475–481.

Eichelberger, Wm. Wirt. "The Study of a Few Cases of Psychoses Following Influenza." *Maryland Psychiatric Quarterly* 9 (April 1920): 90–96.

Emerson, C. P. "Clinical Manifestations and Sequelae in Influenza." *Journal of the Indiana State Medical Association* 13 (1920): 155–157 and discussion, 161–166.

"Epidemic of Spanish Influenza." *Science* 48 (September 20, 1918): 289.

Evans, W. A. et al. (Editorial Committee of the American Public Health Association). "A Working Program Against Influenza." *AJPH* 9 (January 1919): 1–13.

"Experiences with the Epidemic." *JAOA* 18 (February 1919): 277–278, 299.

"Experiences with the Influenza." *JAOA* 18 (January 1919): 247–248.

"Expert Medical Advice on Influenza." *LD* 59 (December 28, 1918): 23, 117.

"Extent and Control of the Influenza Epidemic." *Survey* 41 (October 19, 1918): 63–64.

"Extent and Cost of Influenza." *Survey* 41 (November 16, 1918): 194.

Farrand, Livingston. "Public Health and the Nurse." *AJN* 20 (September 1920): 981–984.

"Fighting Epidemics." *Survey* 49 (November 15, 1922): 247.

Fisher, Irving. "Health and War." *AJPH* 8 (August 1918): 559–563.

Flexner, Simon. "Epidemiology and Recent Epidemics." *Science* 50 (October 3, 1919): 313–319.

"The 'Flu' at Its Work Again." *LD* 64 (January 31, 1920): 13.

Folks, Homer. "War, Best Friend of Disease." *Harper's* 140 (March 1920): 451–459.

"Forecasting Epidemics." *LD* 89 (10 April 1926): 21.

Fox, Elizabeth G. "Address of the President of the National Organization for Public Health Nursing." *AJN* 22 (September 1922): 999–1005.

Francis, F. D., M.W. Hall and A. R. Gaines. "Early Use of Convalescent Serum in Influenza." *MS* (August 1920): 177–179.

Friedlander, Alfred, Carey P. McCord, Frank J. Sladen and George W. Wheeler. "The Epidemic of Influenza at Camp Sherman, Ohio." *JAMA* 71 (November 16, 1918): 1652–1656.

"From the Report of the Committee on Nursing Education." *AJN* 22 (August 1922): 882–884.

Frost, W. H. "The Epidemiology of Influenza." *JAMA* 73 (August 2, 1919): 313–318.

"Germs of Influenza and Yellow Fever." *Science* 49 (April 18, 1919): 372–374.

Gibbes, J. Heyward. "Interesting Aspects of the Recent Epidemic of Influenza." *Journal of the South Carolina Medical Association* 15 (May 1919): 452–458.

Gram, Franklin C. "The Influenza Epidemic and Its After-Effects in the City of Buffalo." *JAMA* 73 (September 20, 1919): 886–891.

"Great Plague." *Independent* 101 (February 21, 1920): 292.

Greenberg, D. "Two Historic World-Pestilences Robbed of Their Terrors by Modern Sanitation." *Scientific Monthly* 4 (June 1917): 554–566.

Grumm, C. C. "Results of Public Health Work in Fort Worth." *American City* 19 (November 1918): 413–415.

"Guarding Against Infection from War Epidemics." *Review of Reviews* 51 (February 1915): 231–232.

Hafford, Lida. "Red Cross and Influenza." *KMJ* 17 (1919): 277–280.

Hall, Holworthy. "Grippe." *McClure's Magazine* 46 (January 1916): 24–26.

Hall, M. W. "A Note on the Epidemiology of Influenza." *Military Surgeon* 46 (May 1920): 564–569.

Hamilton, J. H. "Control of Influenza Epidemics." *Journal of the Iowa State Medical Society* 10 (1920): 38–42.

Harris, I. "War and Influenza." *Survey* 47 (December 3, 1921): 365–366.

Harvey, Oscar Jewell. *The Spanish Influenza Pandemic: An Account of Its Ravages in Luzerne County, Pennsylvania, and the Efforts Made to Combat and Subdue It*. Wilkes-Barre, PA: n.p., 1920.

Haywood, F. "Brotherhood of Misericordia; Nursing Influenza Patients at the New York Municipal Lodging House." *Survey* 41 (November 9, 1918): 148–149.

Hedrich, A. W. "Army-trained Health Officers for Cities." *American City* 20 (April 1919): 371.

Hermann, E. T. "Epidemic Influenza; Report of 296 Cases at the University Hospital." *Minnesota Medicine* 3 (1920): 139–144.

Hewlett, A. W. and W. M. Alberty. "Influenza at Navy Hospital in France." *JAMA* 71 (September 28, 1918): 1056–1059.

Hinkelman, A. J. "Bacteriology of the So-Called Intestinal Influenza." *IMJ* 28 (1915): 353–358.

"History of Influenza." *Science* 49 (February 28, 1919): 216–217.

Hodgdon, A. I. "A Few Observations on the Treatment of Epidemic Influenza." *Maryland Medical Journal* 26 (1891–1892): 331.

Hogan, G. A. "Prevention and Treatment of Influenza and Influenza Pneumonia." *New Orleans Medical and Surgical Journal* 72 (1919–1920): 402–408.

Holbrook, C. S. and W. B. Terhune. "An Epidemic of La Grippe." *New Orleans Medical and Surgical Journal* 68 (1916): 638–642.

"How Influenza Got In." *LD* 59 (November 30, 1918): 23.

"How Influenza Kills." *LD* 93 (May 14, 1927): 22.

"How the Flu Mask Traps the Germ." *LD* 59 (December 21, 1918): 21.

"How the Hand Spreads Influenza." *LD* 60 (March 1, 1919): 24–25.

"How to Avoid Influenza." *Science* 49 (March 28, 1919): 311–312.

"How to Fight Influenza." *LD* 59 (October 12, 1918): 13–14.

Huber, John B. "A Doctor's Point of View–Influenza." *Colliers* 56 (March 11, 1916): 40.

Hunton, Addie W. and Kathryn M. Johnson. *Two Colored Women with the A.E.F.* 1921. Reprint, Brooklyn: Eagle Press, 1971.

"Immunity from Influenza." *Survey* 48 (April 1, 1922): 21.

"Influenza, a Foe to Genius." *LD* 97 (April 21, 1928): 21.

"Influenza and Other Communicable Diseases." *Science* 68 (November 30, 1928, Supplement 12).

"Influenza and Pneumonia." *Science* 63 (February 26, 1926, Supplement 14).

"Influenza and the Death Rate." *Science* 57 (March 9, 1923, Supplement 12).

"Influenza Epidemic." *Science* 48 (October 25, 1918): 412–413.

"Influenza Epidemic." *Science* 48 (December 13, 1918): 594.

"Influenza Epidemic." *Science* 57 (February 16, 1923, Supplement 10).

"Influenza Epidemic in Europe." *Science* 65 (March 4, 1927, Supplement 10–12).

"Influenza Plague Spread Terror and Death in the South Seas." *LD* 61 (May 24, 1919): 52–54.

"Influenza. Relative to a Possible Recurrence of the Epidemic During the Fall or Winter." *PHR* 34 (September 19, 1919): 2105–2110.

"Influenza Warning from the Academy of Medicine." *NYMJ* (October 19, 1918): 681–682.

"Influenza with a Difference." *LD* 73 (May 6, 1922): 29.

Ingals, E. F. "The Epidemics of Influenza of 1890 and 1891 in Chicago." *Climatologist* 2 (1892): 223–230.

Ingle, Dwight. *A Dozen Doctors*. Chicago: University of Chicago Press, 1963.

"In the Wake of the Flu." *Survey* 41 (February 22, 1919): 728–730.

"Investigation of Influenza in England." *Science* 66 (July 15, 1927, Supplement 12).

"Is the Influenza a Chinese Plague?" *LD* 59 (December 7, 1918): 26–27.

Jamme, Anna C. "Address of the President of the National League of Nursing." *AJN* 22 (September 1922): 995–999.

Jenkins, Essie. "1919 Influenza Blues." *Blues with a Message*. El Cerrito, CA: Arhoolie Records, 2005.

Johnson, Blind Willie. "Jesus Is Coming." Complete Recordings of Blind Willie Johnson. Sony, 1993.

Jordan, Edwin O. *Epidemic Influenza: A Survey*. Chicago: American Medical Association, 1927.

Keegan, J. J. "The Prevailing Pandemic of Influenza." *JAMA* 71 (September 28, 1918): 1051–1055.

"Keeping Down the Curves of an Epidemic." *Survey* 36 (August 5, 1916): 490–492.

"Keeping up with Public Health." *Survey* 41 (March 15, 1919): 874.

Kenney, John A. "Some Facts Concerning Negro Nurse Training Schools and Their Graduates." *JNMA* 11 (April–June 1919): 53–68.

Kernodle, Portia. *The Red Cross Nurse in Action*. New York: Harper Bros., 1949.

Kinsella, Ralph A. "The Bacteriology of Epidemic Influenza and Pneumonia." *JAMA* 71 (March 8, 1919): 717–720.

Koons, H. H. "Some Observations on the Use of Vaccines and Glucose in the Treatment of Influenza and Bronchopneumonia." *Military Surgeon* 46 (April 1920): 403–406.

Kopf, E.W. "Statistical Study of the Influenza Epidemic." *Science* 49 (March 7, 1919): 228–230.

Krusen, W. "National Efficiency Through Health." *Annals of the American Academy of Political and Social Science* 78 (July 1918): 58–60.

Lee, Benjamin. "An Analysis of the Statistics of Forty-One Thousand Five Hundred Cases of Epidemic Influenza." *JAMA* 16 (March 14, 1891): 366–368.

Lee, Harry. "Night in the Hospital." *Survey* 41 (November 23, 1918): 214.

Leeds, A. B. "Some of the Sequelae of Epidemic Influenza." *Journal of the Oklahoma State Medical Association* 12 (1919): 318–320.

Lent, Mary E. "The Extent and Control of Influenza in Washington D.C." *PHN* 10 (December 1918): 296–304.

Levy, Ernest C. "Some Public Health Lessons of the War." *AJPH* 8 (September 1918): 664–667.

"Look out for the Flu!" *Independent* 100 (October 4, 1919): 6–7.

Lyon, Irving G., Charles F. Tenney and Leopold Szerlip. "Some Clinical Observations on the Influenza Epidemic at Camp Upton." *JAMA* 72 (June 14, 1919): 1726–1731.

MacDonald, Arthur. "Confirmation of the Discovery of the Influenza Bacillus." *Science* 19 (February 19, 1892): 100.

MacDonald, Arthur. "Latest Details Concerning the Germ of Influenza." *Science* 19 (February 12, 1892): 90.

Mackenzie, Morrell. "Influenza." *Living Age* 190 (August 1, 1891): 296–302.

MacMahon, A. W. "Health Activities of State Councils of Defense." *Annals of the American Academy of Political and Social Science* 79 (September 1918): 239–245.

"Mapping the Influenza." *LD* 65 (May 29, 1920): 32.

Martin, Franklin H. *Fifty Years of Medicine and Surgery: An Autobiographical Sketch*. Chicago: Surgical Publishing Company of Chicago, 1934.

Mason, Paul. "Cincinnati Survey of the After-Effects of Influenza." *Modern Medicine* 2 (1920): 305–307.

Mathers, George. "Etiology of the Epidemic Acute Respiratory Infections Commonly Called Influenza." *JAMA* 68 (March 3, 1917): 678–680.

McCarthy, Mary. *Memories of a Catholic Girlhood*. New York: Harcourt, Brace, Jovanovich, 1957.

McGraw, S. J. "Spanish Influenza." *Journal of the Arkansas Medical Association* 26 (October 1919): 102–104.

McMullen, John. "The U.S. Public Health Service and Influenza." *Kentucky Medical Journal* 17 (1919): 275–277.

McShane, J. J. "The Attempt to Control Influenza in Illinois (and Discussion)." *IMJ* 37 (1920): 17–22.

"Measures for the Prevention of the Introduction of Epidemic Influenza." *PHR* 33 (September 13, 1918): 1540–1544.

Mills, Charles K. "The Nervous and Mental Phenomena and Sequelae of influenza." *JAMA* 18 (January 30, 1892): 121–127.

Moody, A. M. and J. A. Capps. "Notes on Grip Epidemic in Chicago." *JAMA* 66(May 27, 1916): 1696.

Moody, A.M. and J.A. Capps. "The Recent Epidemic of Grip." *JAMA* 67 (November 4, 1916): 1349–1350.

Moore, Harry H. *Public Health in the United States*. New York: Harper and Brothers Publishers, 1923.

Moseley, J. M. "Complications and Sequelae of Influenza." *New Orleans Medical and Surgical Journal* 70 (July 1917): 68–73.

Munro, John C. "The Epidemiology of Influenza." *Climatologist* 2 (1892): 231–235.

Murphy, J. Prentice. "Aftermath of Influenza." *Survey* 41 (November 23, 1918): 212–214.

———. "Meeting the Scourge: How Massachusetts Organized to Fight Influenza." *Survey* 41 (October 26, 1918): 97–100.

Murphy, Margaret. "Grip's Don'ts." *JAMA* 66 (February 5, 1916): 449.

Newton. Richard Cole. "How We Can All Avoid the Grippe." *Ladies Home Journal* 25 (October 1908): 34.

Noyes, Clara D. "Address of the President of the American Nurses' Association." *AJN* 22 (September 1922): 992–995.

———. "Department of Red Cross Nursing—Great Need for Nurses for United States Public Health Service." *AJN* 20 (August 1920): 902–904.

Nuthall, G. H. F. Letter to the Editor, "Bacillus of Influenza." *Science* 19 (1 April 1892): 193–194.

Nutting, Adelaide. "The Outlook in Nursing." *PHN* 12 (September 1920): 754–765.

Olitsky, P. K and L. Gates. "Investigations on the Bacteriology of Epidemic Influenza." *Science* 57 (February 9, 1923): 159–166.

Olson, Helene Dean. "The Flu—1918." *Kansas Quarterly* 8 (1976): 35–40.

Opie, Eugene L., Francis G. Blake, James C. Small and Thomas M. Rivers. *Epidemic Respiratory Disease: The Pneumonias and other Infections of the Respiratory Tract That Accompany Influenza and Measles*. St. Louis: C.V. Mosby Company, 1921.

Osler, William. *The Principles and Practice of Medicine: Designed for the Use of Practitioners and Students of Medicine*. New York: D. Appleton and Company, 1892.

Osler, William and Thomas McCrae. *The Principles and Practice of Medicine: Designed for the Use of Practitioners and Students of Medicine*, 8th ed. New York: D. Appleton and Company, 1912.

"Our Army's Victory over Disease." *World's Work* 33 (November 1916): 12–13.

P., J. F. "Epidemic of Influenza." *Living Age* 184 (February 22, 1890): 508–510.

Palmer, T. "Opportunities for Contact Infection." *Science* 49 (March 21, 1919): 288–291.

"Paramount Issue." *Independent* 85 (January 31, 1916): 144.

Park, William H. ""Bacteriology of Recent Pandemic of Influenza and Complicating Infections." *JAMA* 73 (August 2, 1919): 318–321.

Parker, J. T. "The Poisons of the Influenza Bacillus." *Journal of Immunology* 4 (1919): 331–357.

Parnall, Christopher G. "The Future of Nursing Service and Nursing Education." *AJN* 20 (August 1920): 897–901.

———. "Nursing the Health of the Future." *PHN* 13 (November 1921): 573–578.

"Periodicity of Influenza." *Science* 58 (October 26, 1923, Supplement 10).

Perret, J. M. "A Brief Study of Influenza." *Journal of the Florida Medical Association*. 6 (1919): 1–8.

Perry, J.C. "Military Health Dependent on Civil Health." *Annals of the American Academy of Political and Social Science* 78 (July 1918): 34–40.

Pershing, John J. *My Experiences in the World War*. 2 volumes. New York: Frederick A. Stokes Co., 1931.

Pfeiffer, Damon B. "The Position of the Nursing Profession Today." *AJN* 21 (October 1920): 24–29.

"Place of the Public Health Service." *Survey* 40 (April 6, 1918): 16–17.

"Plagues in Europe and America." *Survey* 40 (September 28, 1918): 720.

Points, J. Frank. "The Evolution of a Successful Treatment for the Complicated Cases of Influenza." *New Orleans Medical and Surgical Journal* 72 (1919–1920): 408–413.

Porter, Katherine Anne. *Pale Horse, Pale Rider: Three Short Novels.* New York: Harcourt, Brace, Jovanovich, 1967 [1936].

Porter, William. "Epidemic Influenza." *JAMA* 14 (January 25, 1890): 113–115.

Potter, Frank Hunter. "Prevention First: What the Health Department Is Doing for New York City." *Outlook* 117 (September 5, 1917): 17–18.

Pottle, Frederick. *Stretchers!* New Haven: Yale University Press, 1929.

"Practical Notes—The Treatment of Influenza." *JAMA* 14 (January 25, 1890): 137.

"Practical Notes—The Treatment of Influenza." *JAMA* 14 (February 8, 1890): 209.

Price, Eldridge C. "Therapeutic Efficiency in the Treatment of Epidemic Influenza." *HM* 54 (December 1919): 721–728

Price, George M. "Influenza—Destroyer and Teacher." *Survey* 41 (December 21, 1919): 367–369.

———. "Mobilizing Social Forces against Influenza." *Survey* 41 (October 26, 1918): 95–96.

———. "The Nationalization of Public Health: War Program of the United States Public Health Service." *Survey* 41 (October 19, 1918): 62–63.

"Program to Combat Influenza." *Survey* 41 (December 28, 1918): 408–409.

"The Progress of Science: The Control of Epidemic Diseases and the Causes of Death." *Scientific Monthly* 3 (October 1916): 410–412.

"Progress of the World." *Review of Reviews* 1 (February 1890): 87.

"Proposed Federal Health Program." *Science* 48 (August 30, 1918): 215–216.

"Public Health." *Survey* 42 (June 7, 1919): 404–405.

Radcliffe, S. J. "Epidemic Influenza, with Cases Illustrating Some of Its Peculiar Complications." *Virginia Medical Monthly* 18 (1892): 1046–1051.

Reed, A. L. "The War against the Germs." *Review of Reviews* 70 (July 1924): 80–82.

Reid, C. C. "Prevention and Treatment of Influenza." *JAOA* 18 (January 1919): 209–211.

"Report of the Committee on Nursing Education (Editorial Comment)." *AJN* 22 (August 1922): 878–880.

Richberg, Donald. *My Hero: The Indiscreet Memoirs of an Eventful but Unheroic Life: An Autobiography.* New York: G.P. Putnam's Sons, 1954.

Robertson, John Dill and Gottfried Koehler. "Preliminary Report on the Influenza Epidemic in Chicago." *AJPH* 8 (November 1918): 850.

Rogers, E. B. "The Influenza Pandemic." *Southwestern Medicine.* 2 (November 1918): 6–10.

Rosenau, Milton J. "Experiments to Determine Mode of Spread of Influenza." *JAMA* 73 (August 2, 1919): 311–313.

Ross, Elizabeth. "Health Centers as Seen by a Public Health Nurse." *AJPH* 11 (October 1921): 915–917.

Royster, Lawrence A. "Grip in Children." *JAMA* 67 (October 28, 1916): 1265–1268.

Schryver, Grace Fay. *A History of the Illinois Training School for Nurses, 1880–1920.* Chicago: Illinois Training School for Nurses, 1930.

Seymour, Gertrude. "Health of Soldier and Civilian." *Survey* 39 (December 1, 1917): 227–232.

———. "Health of Soldier and Civilian." *Survey* 39 (December 29, 1917): 363–367.

———. "Health of Soldier and Civilian." *Survey* 40 (April 27, 1918): 89–94.

———. "Health of Soldier and Civilian." *Survey* 40 (May 11, 1918): 154–158.

———. "Public Health in State and Nation." *Survey* 40 (June 22, 1918): 355.

Sheibley, E. G. "Sanitary Engineer as Health Officer." *American City* 23 (November 1920): 487.

"Some Spanish Views on Spanish Influenza." *New Orleans Medical and Surgical Journal* 71 (1918–1919): 222–234.

Soper, George A. "Influenza Pneumonia Pandemic in the American Army Camps During September and October, 1918." *Science* 48 (November 8, 1918): 451–456.

————. "Lessons of the Pandemic." *Science* 49 (May 30, 1919): 501–506.

Spalding, Heman. "Public Health Measures against Influenza (and Discussion)." *Proceedings of the Institute of Medicine of Chicago* 2 (1918-1919): 166–172.

"Spanish Influenza." *LD* 58 (September 14, 1918): 21–22.

"Spanish Influenza and Its Control." *Survey* 41 (October 12, 1918): 45.

Steele, Leola. "Your Country Needs You." *AJN* 21 (February 1921): 302–303.

Stevens, J.V. "A Clean Town; the Duties of a Health Officer in a Small Municipality." *American City* 21 (August 1919): 133–134.

St. John, Robert. *This Was My World.* Garden City, NY: Doubleday and Co., 1953.

Stockbridge, Frank Parker. "Health at Home to Help the Army." *World's Work* 35 (April 1918): 603–608.

Straub, P. F. "Lessons from our Recent Epidemic." *MS* 44 (1919): 72–74.

Street, H.N. "Personal Experience in Epidemic Influenza." *Journal of the Arkansas Medical Society* 16 (October 1919): 100–102.

Strouse, Solomon and Leon Bloch. "Notes on the Present Epidemic of Respiratory Disease." *JAMA* 71 (November 9, 1918): 1568–1571.

"Survey of City Health Departments." *Survey* 35 (February 12, 1916): 574–575.

"That Flu Stuff." *LD* 59 (December 14, 1918): 81.

"This Year's Flu." *LD* 76 (March 3, 1923): 26–27.

"Therapeutics–Cause and Treatment of the Present Epidemic of Grip." *JAMA* 66 (January 15, 1916): 189–190.

Thompson, F. D. "La Grippe, as It Prevailed in North Texas." *Virginia Medical Monthly* 18 (1891–1892): 365–369.

Townsend, J. G. "United States Public Health Service—Spanish Influenza." *Pass-in-Review* (Camp Bowie), October 5, 1918, 6.

Turner, C. E. "Organizing an Industry to Combat Influenza." *Journal of Industrial Hygiene* 1 (1919–1920): 448–451.

Turner, John P. "Epidemic Influenza and the Negro Physician." *JNMA* 19 (October–December, 1918):184.

Ulrich, C. F. "Some Vagaries of the Grippe." *JAMA* 15 (October 4, 1890): 495–497.

"United States Public Health Service and the Influenza Epidemic." *Science* 48 (November 15, 1918): 487–488.

"Vaccination Against Influenza." *LD* 59 (December 28, 1918): 25.

Vaughan, Victor C. "The Bacteriology of Influenza." *JLCM* 4 (1918–1919): 83–85.

————. *A Doctor's Memories.* Indianapolis: Bobbs-Merrill Co., 1926.

————. "An Explosive Epidemic of Influenzal Disease at Fort Oglethorpe." *JLCM* 3 (1918): 560–564.

————. "Influenza in Camp Custer." *JLCM* 4 (1918–1919): 225–228.

Vaughan, Victor C. and George Palmer. "Communicable Disease in the United States Army During the Summer and Autumn of 1918." *JLCM* 4 (July 1919): 587–623.

"Virus of Influenza." *Science* 57 (February 23, 1923): 236–237.

Wald, Lillian D. "Influenza: When the City Is a Great Field Hospital." *Survey* 43 (February 14, 1920): 579–581.

————. *Windows on Henry Street.* Boston: Little Brown, 1941.

————. "The Work of the Nurses' Emergency Council." *PHN* 10 (December 1918): 303–313.

Waller, J. J. "Spanish Flu." *Journal of the Tennessee State Medical Association.* 11 (December 1918): 298–300.

Walker, O. J. "Pathology of Influenza-Pneumonia." *Journal of Laboratory and Clinical Medicine* 5 (1919): 154–175.

Walsh, J. J. "Don't Worry about the Flu." *Independent* 101 (February 14, 1920): 245.

————. "Influenza Epidemic Again." *Independent* 96 (October 19, 1918): 86.

"War as a Life-Saver." *LD* 58 (September 21, 1918): 23–24.

Warfield, L. M. "Acute Ascending Paralysis Following Grippe." *Wisconsin Medical Journal* 14 (1916): 508.

"War-Reports from the Influenza Front." *LD* 60 (February 22, 1919): 62–67.

"Weapons Against Influenza (Editorial)." *AJPH* 8 (October 1918): 787–788.

"What Follows the Flu?" *LD* 62 (September 13, 1919): 24.

"What the Health Department Has Done to Curb the Epidemic of Influenza." *Monthly Bulletin of the Department of Public Health and Charities of the City of Philadelphia* 3 (October-November, 1918).

Wheeler, Marianna. "Influenza, or 'Grippe,' in Babies and Young Children." *Harper's Bazaar* 46 (December 1912): 620.

Whittenberg, J. I. "The Influenza Epidemic, Its Lessons." *Kentucky Medical Journal* 17(1919): 280–282.

"Will the Influenza Come Back?" *LD* 60 (January 11, 1919): 23.

"Will the Influenza Return?" *LD* 63 (October 11, 1919): 26.

Williams, E. G. "Physicians as a Factor in national Efficiency." *Annals of the American Academy of Political and Social Science* 78 (July 1918): 41–47.

"A Winding Sheet and a Wooden Box." *Navy Medicine* 77 (May-June 1986): 18–19.

Winternitz, M. C., Isabel M. Wason and Frank P. McNamara. *The Pathology of Influenza*. New Haven, CT: Yale University Press, 1920.

Winslow, C.-E. A. *The Life of Hermann Biggs, M.D., D. Sc., L.L.D: Physician and Statesman of Public Health*. Philadelphia: Lea and Febiger, 1929.

W., J. W. "Homeopathy's Great Opportunity in the Existing Medical Confusion." *NAJH* 67 (1919): 111–114.

Wolfe, Thomas. *Look Homeward, Angel: A Story of the Buried Life*. New York: Charles Scribner's Sons, 1929.

Woolley, P. G. "The Epidemic of Influenza at Camp Devens, Mass." *JLCM* 4 (1918–1919): 330–343.

Young, Filson. "Influenza." *Living Age* 277 (May 3, 1913): 306–308.

SECONDARY SOURCES

Adams, David Wallace. *Education for Extinction: American Indians and the Boarding School Experience, 1875–1928*. Lawrence: University of Kansas, 1995.

Afkhami, Amir. "Compromised Constitutions: The Iranian Experience with the 1918 Influenza Pandemic." *Bulletin of the History of Medicine* 77 (Summer 2003): 367–392.

Aimone, Francesco. "The 1918 Influenza Epidemic in New York City: A Review of the Public Health Response." *PHR* 125 (2010, Supplement 3): 71–79.

Altman, Dennis. *AIDS in the Mind of America: The Social, Political and Psychological Impact of a New Epidemic*. Garden City, NY: Anchor Press/Doubleday, 1987.

Altman, Roberta. *Waking Up, Fighting Back: The Politics of Breast Cancer*. Boston: Little, Brown, 1996.

Aronowitz, Robert A. *Making Sense of Illness: Science, Society and Disease*. Cambridge, UK: Cambridge University Press, 1998.

Arrington, Leonard J. "The Influenza Epidemic of 1918–1919 in Southern Idaho." *Idaho Yesterdays* 32 (1988): 19–29.

———. "The Influenza Epidemic of 1918–1919 in Utah." *Utah Historical Quarterly* 58 (1990): 164–182.

Baer, E. D. "Letters to Miss Sanborn: St. Vincent's Hospital Nurses' Accounts of World War One." *Journal of Nursing History* 2 (April 1987): 17–32.

———. "Nurses." In *Women, Health and Medicine in America: A Historical Handbook*, ed. Rima D. Apple, 459–475. New York: Garland Publishing, 1990.

Baird, Nancy D. "'The Spanish Lady' in Kentucky, 1918–1919." *Filson Club History Quarterly* 50 (1976): 290–301.

Baker, Paula. "The Domestication of American Politics: Women and American Political Society, 1780–1920." *American Quarterly* 89 (June 1984): 620–647.

Barry, John M. *The Great Influenza: The Epic Story of the Deadliest Plague in History*. New York: Viking, 2004.

Batt, Sharon. *Patient No More: The Politics of Breast Cancer*. Charlottesville, Canada: Gynergy Books, 1994.

Blight, David W. *Race and Reunion: The Civil War in American Memory*. Cambridge, MA: Harvard University Press, 2002.

Blythe, Jo Ann. "The Great Flu Epidemic of 1918." *Panhandle-Plains Historical Review* 66 (1993): 1–23.

Bodnar, John E. *"The Good War" in American Memory*. Baltimore: Johns Hopkins University Press, 2010.

———. *Remaking America: Public Memory, Commemoration and Patriotism in the Twentieth Century*. Princeton, NJ: Princeton University Press, 1992.

Bonnell, Sonicray. "Chemawa Indian Boarding School: The First One Hundred Years, 1880–1980." MA thesis, Dartmouth College, 1997.

Bonner, Thomas Neville. *To the Ends of the Earth: Women's Search for Education in Medicine*. Cambridge, MA: Harvard University Press, 1992.

Brandt, Allan M. and Paul Rozin, eds. *Morality and Health*. London: Routledge, 1997.

Brandt, Allan M. "AIDS and Metaphor: Toward the Social Meaning of Epidemic Disease." *Social Research* 55 (1988): 413–432.

———. *No Magic Bullet: A Social History of Venereal Disease in the United States since 1880*. New York: Oxford University Press, 1985.

Brison, Susan J. *Aftermath: Violence and the Remaking of a Self*. Princeton, NJ: Princeton University Press, 2002.

Bristow, Nancy K. *Making Men Moral: Social Engineering During the Great War*. New York: New York University Press, 1997.

———. "'It's as Bad as Anything Can Be': Patients, Identity, and the Influenza Pandemic." *PHR* 125 (2010, Supplement 3): 134–144.

———. "'You Can't Do Anything for Influenza': Doctors, Nurses and the Power of Gender during the Influenza Epidemic in the United States." In *The Spanish Influenza Pandemic of 1918—New Perspectives*, ed. Howard Phillips and David Killingray, 58–69, 262–266. London: Routledge, 2003.

Brox, Jane. "Influenza, 1918," in *Five Thousand Days Like This One: An American Family History*. Boston: Beacon Press, 1999.

Brundage, W. Fitzhugh, ed. *Where These Memories Grow: History, Memory, and Southern Identity*. Chapel Hill: University of North Carolina Press, 2000.

Buhler-Wilkerson, Karen. "False Dawn: The Rise and Decline of Public Health Nursing in America, 1900–1930." In *Nursing History: New Perspectives, New Possibilities*, ed. Ellen Condliffe Lagemann, 89–101. New York: Teachers College Press, 1983.

Burch, Marybelle. "'I Don't Know Only What We Hear': The Soldiers' View of the 1918 Influenza Epidemic." *Indiana Medical History Quarterly* 9 (1983): 23–27.

Byerly, Carol R. *Fever of War: The Influenza Epidemic in the U.S. Army During World War I*. New York: New York University Press, 2005.

Carr, Dennis J. "The Spanish Influenza Epidemic of 1918 and Berkshire County." *Historical Journal of Massachusetts* 19 (1991): 43–62.

Carter, Laura Stephenson. "Cold Comfort." *Dartmouth Medicine* (Winter 2006): 36–42, 56–57.

Cassedy, James H. *Charles V. Chapin and the Public Health Movement*. Cambridge, MA: Harvard University Press, 1962.

———. *Medicine in America: A Short History*. Baltimore: Johns Hopkins University Press, 1991.

Cayleff, Susan E. "The Politics of Disease: Contemporary Analyses of the AIDS Epidemic." *Radical History Review* 45 (1989): 172–180.

———. "Self-Help and the Patent Medicine Business." In *Women, Health and Medicine in America: A Historical Handbook*, ed. Rima D. Apple, 311–336. New York: Garland Publishing, 1990.

Child, Brenda J. *Boarding School Seasons: American Indian Families, 1900–1940*. Lincoln: University of Nebraska Press, 1998.

Colgrove, James. *State of Immunity: The Politics of Vaccination in Twentieth-Century America*. Berkeley: University of California Press, 2006.

Collier, Richard. *The Plague of the Spanish Lady: The Influenza Pandemic of 1918–1919*. New York: Atheneum, 1974.

Comaroff, J. "Medicine: Symbol and Ideology." In *The Problem of Medical Knowledge: Examining the Social Construction of Medicine*, ed. P. Write and A. Teachers, 49–69. Edinburgh, Scotland: University of Edinburgh Press, 1982.

Cowdrey, Albert E. *War and Healing: Stanhope Bayne-Jones and the Maturing of American Medicine*. Baton Rouge: Louisiana State University Press, 1992.

Craddock, Susan L. *City of Plagues: Disease, Poverty, and Deviance in San Francisco*. Minneapolis: University of Minnesota Press, 2000.

Crosby, Alfred E. *America's Forgotten Pandemic: The Influenza of 1918*. Cambridge, UK: Cambridge University Press, 1990.

Davies, Pete. *The Devil's Flu: The World's Deadliest Influenza Epidemic and the Scientific Hunt for the Virus That Caused It*. New York: Henry Holt and Company, 2000.

D'Emilio, John. "The Names Project Quilt." In *Making Trouble: Essays on Gay History, Politics, and the University*, ed. John D'Emilio, 216–219. New York: Routledge, 1992.

De Moulin, Daniel. *A Short History of Breast Cancer*. Boston: Martinus Nijhoff, 1983.

Derickson, Alan. "Federal Intervention in the Joplin Silicosis Epidemic, 1911–1916." *Bulletin of the History of Medicine* 62 (1988): 236–251.

Dexter, Madeline. *Secret Agents: The Menace of Emerging Infections*. New York: Penguin Books, 2003.

Diamond, Jared. *Guns, Germs, and Steel: The Fates of Human Societies*. New York: W.W. Norton and Company, 1997.

Doherty, William T. "A West Virginia County's Experience with the 1918 Influenza Epidemic." *West Virginia History* 38 (1977): 136–140.

Dowling, Harry F. *City Hospitals: The Undercare of the Underprivileged*. Cambridge, MA: Harvard University Press, 1982.

Duffy, John. *The Sanitarians: A History of American Public Health*. Chicago: University of Illinois Press, 1990.

Eckley, Grace. *Finley Peter Dunne*. Boston: Twayne Publishers, 1981.

Elliott, Russell R. "The Influenza Epidemic of 1918–1919." *Halcyon* 14 (1992): 247–258.

Ensley, Philip C. "Indiana and the Influenza Pandemic of 1918." *Indiana Medical History Quarterly* 9 (1983): 3–15.

Erwin, Deborah Oates. "The Militarization of Cancer Treatment in American Society." In *Encounters with Biomedicine: Case Studies in Medical Anthropology*, ed. Harold O. Baer, 201–227. New York: Gordon Breach Science Publishers, 1987.

Esyllt, W. Jones. *Influenza 1918: Disease, Death and Struggle in Winnipeg*. Toronto: University of Toronto Press, 2007.

Evans, Sara. *Born for Liberty: A History of Women in America*. New York: Free Press, 1997.

Eyler, John M. "The State of Science, Microbiology, and Vaccines Circa 1918." *PHR* 125 (2010, Supplement 3): 27–36.

Fagin, C. M. and Donna Diers. "Nursing as Metaphor." *New England Journal of Medicine* 309 (July 14, 1983): 116–117.

Ferrell, James J. *Inventing the American Way of Death, 1830–1920*. Philadelphia: Temple University Press, 1980.

Fee, Elizabeth. *Disease and Discovery: A History of the Johns Hopkins School of Hygiene and Public Health, 1916–1939*. Baltimore: Johns Hopkins University Press, 1987.

Fee, Elizabeth and Daniel M. Fox, eds. *AIDS: The Burden of History*. Berkeley: University of California Press, 1988.

———. "The Contemporary Historiography of AIDS." *Journal of Social History* 23 (1989): 303–314.

Fincher, Jack. "America's Deadly Rendezvous with the 'Spanish Lady.'" *Smithsonian* 19 (1989): 130–145.

Ford, Nancy Gentile. *Americans All! Foreign-Born Soldiers in World War I*. (College Station: Texas A & M University Press), 2001.

Galishoff, Stuart. "Germs Know No Color Line: Black Health and Public Policy in Atlanta, 1900–1918." *Journal of the History of Medicine* 40 (1985): 22–41.

————. "Newark and the Great Influenza Pandemic of 1918." *Bulletin of the History of Medicine* 43 (1969): 246–258.

Gamble, Vanessa. *Making a Place for Ourselves: The Black Hospital Movement, 1920–1945.* New York: Oxford University Press, 1995.

————. "'There Wasn't a Lot of Comforts in Those Days:' African Americans, Public Health, and the 1918 Influenza Epidemic." *PHR* 125 (2010, Supplement 3): 114–122.

Gamblin, S. J. et al. "The Structure and Receptor Binding Properties of the 1918 Influenza Hemagglutinin." *Science* 303 (March 19, 2004): 1838–1842.

Garrett, Thomas A. "Pandemic Economics: The 1918 Influenza and Its Modern-Day Implications." *Federal Reserve Bank of St. Louis Review* 90 (March/April 2008): 75–93.

Gevitz, Norman, *The D.O.'s: Osteopathic Medicine in America.* Baltimore: Johns Hopkins University Press, 1982.

————, ed. *Other Healers: Unorthodox Medicine in America.* Baltimore: Johns Hopkins University Press, 1988.

Gibson, John M. *Physician to the World: The Life of General William C. Gorgas.* Durham, NC: Duke University Press, 1950.

Giles-Vernick, Tamara and Susan Craddock, eds. *Influenza and Public Health: Learning from Past Pandemics.* London: Earthscan, 2010.

Gilman, Sandra L. *Disease and Representation: Images of Illness from Madness to AIDS.* Cornell, NY: Cornell University Press, 1988.

Hampton, Kathleen Edtl. "The 1918 Spanish Influenza: A Pandemic Strikes Cowlitz County." *Cowlitz Historical Quarterly* 38 (1996): 5–30.

Hawkins, Kenneth. "Notes on the Life of an Artist: Roswell Holt Dosch." *Oregon Historical Quarterly* 85 (1984): 55–73.

Hawkins, Peter S. Ars Memoriandi: The NAMES Project AIDS Quilt." *Facing Death: Where Culture, Religion, and Medicine Meet,* ed. Howard M. Spiro, Mary G. McCrea Curnen, and Lee Palmer Wandel. New Haven: Yale University Press, 1996.

Higgins, James. "Keystone of an Epidemic." Unpublished manuscript, 2011.

Hine, Darlene Clark. "The Call That Never Came: Black Women Nurses and World War I, An Historical Note." *Indiana Military History Journal* 15 (1983): 23–27.

————. Black Women in White: Racial Conflict and Cooperation in the Nursing Profession, 1890–1950. Bloomington: Indiana University Press, 1989.

Hoehling, A. A. *The Great Epidemic.* Boston: Little, Brown and Company, 1961.

Holmes, Edward C. "1918 and All That." *Science* 303 (March 19, 2004): 1787–1788.

Honigsbaum, Mark. "The Art of Medicine: The Patient's View: John Donne and Katherine Anne Porter." *Lancet* 374 (July 18, 2009): 194–195.

Honigsbaum, Mark. *Living with Enza: The Forgotten Story of Britain and the Great Flu Pandemic of 1918.* London: Macmillan, 2009.

Horton, James Oliver and Lois E. Horton. *Slavery and Public History: The Tough Stuff of American Memory.* Chapel Hill: University of North Carolina Press, 2006.

Hudson, Robert P. *Disease and Its Control: The Shaping of Modern Thought.* Westport, CT: Greenwood Press, 1983.

Iezzoni, Lynette. *Influenza, 1918.* New York: TV Books, 1999.

Ingle, Dwight J., ed. *A Dozen Doctors: Autobiographical Sketches.* Chicago: University of Chicago Press, 1936.

Jackson, Stanley W. "The Wounded Healer." *Bulletin of the History of Medicine* 75 (Spring 2001): 1–36.

Jacoby, Karl. *Shadows at Dawn: A Borderlands Massacre and the Violence of History.* New York: Penguin, 2008.

Johnson, Judith R. "Kansas in the 'Grippe': The Spanish Influenza Epidemic of 1918." *Kansas History* 15 (1992): 44–55.

Johnson, Niall and Juergen Mueller. "Updating the Accounts: Global Mortality of the 1918–1920 'Spanish' Influenza Pandemic." *Bulletin of the History of Medicine* 76 (Spring 2002): 105–115.

Johnston, William. *The Modern Epidemic: A History of Tuberculosis in Japan*. Cambridge, MA: Harvard University Press, 1995.

Jones, Marian Moser. "The American Red Cross and Local Response to the 1918 Influenza Pandemic: A Four-City Case Study." *PHR* 125 (2010, Supplement 3): 92–104.

Jordan, William G. *Black Newspapers and America's War for Democracy, 1914–1920*. Chapel Hill: University of North Carolina Press, 2001.

Kalven, Jamie. *Working with Available Light: A Family's World After Violence*. New York: W.W. Norton & Company, 1999.

Karlen, Arno. *Man and Microbes: Disease and Plagues in History and Modern Times*. New York: Touchstone, 1995.

Kasper, Anne S. and Susan J. Ferguson, eds. *Breast Cancer: Society Shapes an Epidemic*. New York: St. Martin's Press, 2000.

Katz, Robert S. "Influenza 1918–1919: A Study in Mortality." *Bulletin of the History of Medicine* 48 (1974): 416–422.

———. "Influenza 1918: A Further Study in Mortality." *Bulletin of the History of Medicine* 51 (1977): 617–619.

Keeling, Arlene W. "'Alert to the Necessities of the Emergency': U.S. Nursing During the 1918 Influenza Pandemic." *PHR* 125 (2010, Supplement 3): 105–112.

Kennedy, David M. *Over Here: The First World War and American Society*. New York: Oxford University Press, 1980.

Kimmel, Michael. *Manhood in America: A Cultural History*. New York: Free Press, 1996.

King, Lester S. *Transformations in American Medicine: From Benjamin Rush to William Osler*. Baltimore: Johns Hopkins University Press, 1991.

Kirkpatrick, Gabriel W. "Influenza 1918: A Maine Perspective." *Maine Historical Society Quarterly* 25 (1986): 162–177.

Klein, Kerwin Lee. "On the Emergence of Memory in Historical Discourse." *Representations* 69 (Winter 2000), Special Issue: 127–150.

Kleinman, Arthur. *The Illness Narratives: Suffering, Healing and the Human Condition*. New York: Basic Books, 1988.

———. *Patients and Healers in the Context of Culture: An Exploration of the Borderland Between Anthropology, Medicine, and Psychiatry*. Berkeley: University of California Press, 1980.

Kleinman, Arthur, Veena Das and Margaret Lock, eds. *Social Suffering*. Berkeley: University of California Press, 1997.

Knoll, Kenneth. "When the Plague Hit Spokane." *Pacific Northwesterner* 33 (1989): 1–7.

Kolata, Gina. *Flu: The Story of the Great Influenza Pandemic of 1918 and the Search for the Virus That Caused It*. New York: Farrar, Straus and Giroux, 1999.

Koszarski, Richard. "Flu Season: Moving Picture World reports on pandemic influenza, 1918–19." *Film History* 17 (2005): 466–485.

Kraut, Alan. *Huddled Masses: The Immigrant in American Society, 1880–1921*. Arlington Heights, IL: Harlan Davidson, 1982.

———. "Immigration, Ethnicity, and the Pandemic." *PHR* 125 (2010, Supplement 3): 123–133.

———. *Silent Travelers: Germs, Genes, and the "Immigrant Menace."* New York: Basic Books. 1994.

Krieg, Joann P. *Epidemics in the Modern World*. New York: Twayne Publishers, 1992.

Lagemann, Ellen Condliffe. *Nursing History: New Perspectives, New Possibilities*. New York: Teachers College Press, 1983.

Langer, Lawrence. *Admitting the Holocaust: Collected Essays*. New Haven: Yale University Press, 1995.

———. *Holocaust Testimonies: The Ruins of Memory*. New Haven: Yale University Press, 1991.

———. *Pre-empting the Holocaust*. New Haven: Yale University Press, 1998.

Lauteret, Ronald L. "Alaska's Greatest Disaster: The 1918 Spanish Influenza Epidemic." *Alaska Journal* 16(1986): 238–243.

Leavitt, Judith Walzer. *The Healthiest City: Milwaukee and the Politics of Health Reform*. Princeton: Princeton University Press, 1982.

Leavitt, Judith Walzer and Ronald L. Numbers, eds. *Sickness and Health in America: Readings in the History of Medicine and Public Health*, 3rd ed. Madison: University of Wisconsin Press, 1997.

Leopold, Ellen. *A Darker Ribbon: Breast Cancer, Women, and Their Doctors in the Twentieth Century*. Boston: Beacon Press, 1999.

Lerner, Barron H. *Breast Cancer Wars: Hope, Fear, and the Pursuit of a Cure in Twentieth-Century America*. New York: Oxford University Press, 2001.

Lewenson, Sandra Beth. *Taking Charge: Nursing, Suffrage, and Feminism in America, 1873–1920*. New York: Garland Publishing, 1993.

Linenthal, Edward T. *The Unfinished Bombing: Oklahoma City in American Memory*. New York: Oxford University Press, 2001.

Lomawaima, K. Tsianina. *They Called It Prairie Light: The Story of Chilocco Indian School*. Lincoln: University of Nebraska Press, 1994.

Long, Diana Elizabeth and Janet Golden, eds. *The American General Hospital: Communities and Social Contexts*. Ithaca, NY: Cornell University Press, 1989.

Lowy, Ilana. *Between Bench and Bedside: Science, Healing, and Interleukin-2 in a Cancer Ward*. Cambridge, Mass.: Harvard University Press, 1996.

Luckingham, Bradford. *Epidemic in the Southwest, 1918–1919*. El Paso: Texas Western Press, 1984.

———. "To Mask or Not to Mask: A Note on the 1918 Spanish Influenza Epidemic in Tucson." *Journal of Arizona History* 25 (1984): 191–204.

Ludmerer, Kenneth M. *Learning to Heal: The Development of Medical Education*. New York: Basic Books, 1985.

———. *Time to Heal: American Medical Education from the Turn of the Century to the Era of Managed Care*. New York: Oxford University Press, 1999.

Lupton, Deborah. *Medicine as Culture: Illness, Disease, and the Body in Western Societies*. London: Sage Publications, 1994.

Mack, Arien, ed. *In Time of Plague: The History and Social Consequences of Lethal Epidemic Disease*. New York: New York University Press, 1991.

Markel, Howard. *Quarantine! East European Jewish Immigrants and the New York City Epidemics of 1892*. Baltimore: Johns Hopkins University Press, 1997.

———. *When Germs Travel: Six Major Epidemics that have Invaded America Since 1900 and the Fears They Have Unleashed*. New York: Pantheon, 2004.

Markel, Howard et al. "Nonpharmaceutical Interventions Implemented by US Cities During the 1918–1919 Influenza Pandemic." *JAMA* 298 (August 8, 2007): 644–654.

McGerr, Michael. *A Fierce Discontent: The Rise and Fall of the Progressive Movement in America, 1870–1920*. New York: Free Press, 2003.

McLaurin, Ann. "The Influenza Epidemic of 1918 in Shreveport." *North Louisiana Historical Association* 13 (1982): 1–14.

McLoughlin, William G., Jr. *Billy Sunday Was His Real Name*. Chicago: University of Chicago Press, 1955.

McNeill, William H. *Plagues and Peoples*. Garden City, NY: Anchor Press, 1976.

McPherson, Robert S. "The Influenza Epidemic of 1918: A Cultural Response." *Utah Historical Quarterly* 58 (1990): 183–200.

Melosh, Barbara. *"The Physician's Hand": Work, Culture and Conflict in American Nursing*. Philadelphia: Temple University Press, 1982.

Melosi, Martin V. *Garbage in the Cities: Refuse, Reform, and the Environment*, 3rd ed. Pittsburgh: University of Pittsburgh Press, 2005.

Melzer, Richard. "A Dark and Terrible Moment: The Spanish Flu Epidemic of 1918 in New Mexico." 57 (1982): 213–236.

Morantz-Sanchez, Regina. *Conduct Unbecoming a Woman: Medicine on Trial in Turn-of-the-Century Brooklyn*. New York: Oxford University Press, 1999.

———. "Physicians." In *Women, Health and Medicine in America: A Historical Handbook*, ed. Rima D. Apple, 477–495. New York: Garland Publishing, 1990.

———. *Sympathy and Science: Women Physicians in American Medicine.* New York: Oxford University Press, 1985.

More, Ellen S. *Restoring the Balance: Women Physicians and the Profession of Medicine, 1850–1995.* Cambridge, MA: Harvard University Press, 1999.

More, Ellen S., Elizabeth Fee and Manon Perry, eds. *Women Physicians and the Culture of Medicine.* Baltimore: Johns Hopkins University Press, 2008.

Mullen, Pierce C. and Michael L. Nelson. "Montanans and 'the Most Peculiar Disease': The Influenza Epidemic and Public Health, 1918–1919." *Montana* 37 (1987): 50–61.

Navarro, Julian A. "Influenza in 1918: An Epidemic in Images." *PHR* 125 (2010, Supplement 3): 9–14.

Nealon, Eleanor. "The Bugs Bit What Bullets Bypassed in Bygone Battles." *Smithsonian* 7 (1976): 76–81.

Nelkin, Dorothy and Sander L. Gilman. "Placing Blame for Devastating Disease." *Social Research* 55 (1988): 361–378.

Noymer, Andrew. "The 1918 influenza pandemic hastened the decline of tuberculosis in the United States: An age, period, cohort analysis." *Vaccine* 29 (2011, Supplement 2): B38–B41.

Noyes, William R. "Influenza Epidemic, 1918–1919: A Misplaced Chapter in U.S. Social and Institutional History." PhD diss., University of California, Los Angeles, 1968.

Oldstone, Michael B. A. *Viruses, Plagues and History.* New York: Oxford University Press, 1998.

Olick, Jeffrey K., Vered Vinitzky-Seroussi and Daniel Levy. *The Collective Memory Reader.* New York: Oxford University Press, 2011.

Opdycke, Sandra. *No One Was Turned Away: The Role of Public Hospitals in New York City Since 1900.* New York: Oxford University Press, 1999.

Osborn, June E. *Influenza in America: 1918–1976.* New York: Prodist, 1977.

Oshinsky, David M. *Polio: An American Story. The Crusade That Mobilized the Nation Against the 20th Century's Most Feared Disease.* New York: Oxford University Press, 2005.

Ott, Katherine. *Fevered Lives: Tuberculosis in American Culture Since 1870.* Cambridge, MA: Harvard University Press, 1996.

Palmer, Susan J. "AIDS as Metaphor." *Society* 26 (1989): 44–50.

Patterson, James T. *The Dread Disease: Cancer and Modern American Culture.* Cambridge, MA: Harvard University Press, 1987.

Patterson, K. and Gerald F. Pyle. "The Geography and Mortality of the 1918 Influenza Pandemic." *Bulletin of the History of Medicine* 65 (1991): 4–21.

Peel, Robert. *Health and Medicine in the Christian Science Tradition.* New York: Crossroad Publishing, 1988.

Peterson, Alan R. and Deborah Lupton. *The New Public Health: Health and Self in the Age of Risk.* London: Sage Publications, 1996.

Peterson, Richard H. "The Spanish Influenza Epidemic in San Diego, 1918–1919." *Southern California Quarterly* 71(1989): 89–105.

Pettit, Dorothy A. "A Cruel Wind: America Experiences Pandemic Influenza, 1918–1920. A Social History." PhD diss., University of New Hampshire, 1976.

Pettit, Dorothy A. and Janice Bailie. *A Cruel Wind: Pandemic Flu in America, 1918–1920.* Murfreesboro, TN: Timberlane Books, 2008.

Phillips, Howard and David Killingray, eds. *The Spanish Influenza Pandemic of 1918–1919: New Perspectives.* London: Routledge, 2003.

Porter, Dorothy, *Health, Civilization, and the State: A History of Public Health from Ancient to Modern Times.* New York: Routledge, 1999.

———, ed. *The History of Public Health and the Modern State.* New York: Clio Medica, 1994.

Porter, Roy. *The Greatest Benefit to Mankind.* New York: W.W. Norton and Co., 1998.

———. "The Patient's View: Doing Medical History from Below." *Theory and Society* 14 (March 1985): 175–198.

Quinn, Tom. *Flu: A Social History of Influenza.* London: New Holland Publishers, 2008.

Radstone, Susanna and Bill Schwarz. *Memory: Histories, Theories, Debates.* New York: Fordham University Press, 2010.

Ranger, Terence and Paul Slack. *Epidemics and Ideas: Essays on the Historical Perception of Pestilence.* Cambridge, UK: Cambridge University Press, 1992.

Ratner, Joseph, ed. *Characters and Events: Popular Essays in Social and Political Philosophy,* vol. 2. New York: H.H. Holt, 1929.

Reid, Ann H., T. G. Fanning, J. V. Hultin and J. K. Taubenberger. "Original and Evolution of the 1918 'Spanish' Influenza Virus Hemagglutinin Gene." *Proceedings of the National Academy of Sciences of the United States of America* 96 (February 16, 1999): 1651–1656.

Reverby, Susan. *Ordered to Care: The Dilemma of American Nursing, 1850–1945.* Cambridge, UK: Cambridge University Press, 1987.

Risse, Guenter. "'A Long Pull, A Strong Pull, and All Together': San Francisco and Bubonic Plague, 1907–1908." *Bulletin of the History of Medicine* 66 (1992): 260–286.

Roberts, Samuel Kelton, Jr. *Infectious Fear: Politics, Disease, and the Health Effects of Segregation.* Chapel Hill: University of North Carolina Press, 2009.

Rockafellar, Nancy. "'In Gauze We Trust': Public Health and Spanish Influenza on the Home Front, Seattle, 1918–1919." *Pacific Northwest Quarterly* 77 (1986): 104–113.

Romano, Renee C. and Leigh Raiford, eds. *The Civil Rights Movement in American Memory.* Athens: University of Georgia Press, 2006.

Rosenberg. Charles E. *The Care of Strangers: The Rise of America's Hospital System.* New York: Basic Books, 1987.

———. *Explaining Epidemics and Other Studies in the History of Medicine.* New York: Cambridge University Press, 1992.

———. "What Is an Epidemic?: AIDS in Historical Perspective." *Daedalus* 118(1989): 1–17.

Rosenberg, Charles E. and Janet Golden. *Framing Disease.* New Brunswick, NJ: Rutgers University Press, 1991.

Rosner, David. *A Once and Charitable Enterprise: Hospitals and Health Care in Brooklyn and New York 1885–1915.* New York: Cambridge University Press, 1982.

———, ed. *Hives of Sickness: Public Health and Epidemics in New York City.* New Brunswick, NJ: Rutgers University Press, 1995.

———. "'Spanish Flu, or Whatever It Is. . . .': The Paradox of Public Health in a Time of Crisis." *PHR* (2010, Supplement 3): 38–47.

Rothman, Sheila M. *Living in the Shadow of Death: Tuberculosis and the Social Experience of Illness in American History.* New York: Basic Books, 1994.

Rothstein, David. *American Physicians in the Nineteenth Century: From Sects to Science.* Baltimore: Johns Hopkins University Press, 1972.

Rotundo, E. Anthony. *American Manhood: Transformations in Masculinity from the Revolution to the Modern Era.* New York: Basic Books, 1993

Ruth, David E. "Don't Shake—Salute!" *Chicago History* 19 (1990–1991): 4–23.

Sandelowski, Margarete. *Devices and Desires: Gender, Technology, and American Nursing.* Chapel Hill: University of North Carolina Press, 2000.

Sanford, Wayne L. "The Influenza Epidemic of 1918 and its Effects on the Military." *Indiana Medical History Quarterly* 9 (1983): 16–22.

Sarnecky, Mary T. *A History of the U.S. Army Nurse Corps.* Philadelphia: University of Pennsylvania Press, 1999.

Scott, Kim Allen. "Plague on the Homefront: Arkansas and the Great Influenza Epidemic of 1918." *Arkansas Historical Quarterly* 47 (1988): 311–344.

Shah, Nayan. *Contagious Divides: Epidemics and Race in San Francisco's Chinatown.* Berkeley: University of California Press, 2001.

Sontag, Susan. *Illness as Metaphor and AIDS and Its Metaphors.* New York: Anchor Books, 1990.

Stabiner, Karen. *To Dance with the Devil: The New War on Breast Cancer.* New York: Delacorte, 1997.

Stannard, David E. *The Puritan Way of Death: A Study of Religion, Culture and Social Change*. New York: Oxford University Press, 1977.

Starr, Paul. *The Social Transformation of American Medicine: The Rise of a Sovereign Profession and the Making of a Vast Industry*. New York: Basic Books, 1982.

Stein, Howard F. *American Medicine as Culture*. Boulder, CO: Westview Press, 1990.

Sterba, Christophe M. *Good Americans All: Italian and Jewish Immigrants during the First World War*. New York: Oxford University Press, 2003.

Stern, Alexandra Minna, Mary Beth Reilly, Martin S. Cetron and Howard Markel. "'Better Off in School': School Medical Inspection as a Public Health Strategy During the 1918–1919 Influenza Pandemic in the United States." *PHR* 125 (2010, Supplement 3): 63–70.

Stern, Alexandra Minna, Martin S. Cetron and Howard Markel. "Closing the Schools: Lessons from The 1918–19 U.S. Influenza Pandemic." *Health Affairs* 28 (November-December 2009): 1066–1078.

Stevens, James et al. "Structure of the Uncleaved Human H1 Hemagglutinin from the Extinct 1918 Influenza Virus." *Science* 303 (March 19, 2004): 1866–1870.

Stevenson, R. Scott. *Morrell Mackenzie: The Story of a Victorian Tragedy*. London: Heinemann Medical, 1946.

Taubenberger, Jeffery K. and David M. Morens. "1918 Influenza: the Mother of All Pandemics." *Emerging Infectious Diseases* 12 (January 2006): 15–22.

———. "Influenza: The Once and Future Pandemic." *PHR* 125 (2010, Supplement 3): 16–26.

Taubenberger, Jeffery K., Ann H. Reid, Amy E. Krafft, Karen E. Bijwaard and Thomas G. Fanning. "Initial Genetic Characterization of the 1918 'Spanish' Influenza Virus." *Science* 275 (March 21, 1997): 1793–1796.

Taubenberger, Jeffery K. Ann H. Reid and Thomas G. Fanning. "Capturing a Killer Flu VIRUS." *Scientific American* 292 (January 2005): 62–71.

Tognotti, Eugenia. "Scientific Triumphalism and Learning from Facts: Bacteriology and the 'Spanish Flu' Challenge of 1918." *Social History of Medicine* 16(2003): 97–110.

Tomes, Nancy. "'Destroyer and Teacher': Managing the Masses during the 1918–1919 Influenza Pandemic." *PHR* 125 (2010, Supplement 3): 48–62.

———. *The Gospel of Germs: Men, Women, and the Microbe in American Life*. Cambridge, MA: Harvard University Press, 1998.

Tumpey, Terrence M. et al. "Characterization of the Reconstructed 1918 Spanish Influenza Pandemic Virus." *Science* 310 (October 7, 2005): 77–80.

Vogel, Morris J. *The Invention of the Modern Hospital, Boston 1870–1930*. Chicago: University of Chicago Press, 1980.

Wailoo, Keith. *Dying in the City of the Blues: Sickle Cell Anemia and the Politics of Race and Health*. Chapel Hill: University of North Carolina Press, 2001.

Walsh, Mary Roth. *Doctors Wanted—No Women Need Apply: Sexual Barriers in the Medical Profession, 1835–1975*. New Haven: Yale University Press, 1977.

Walters, Karen A. "McLean County and the Influenza Epidemic of 1918–1919." *Journal of the Illinois State Historical Society* 74 (1981): 130–144.

Warner, John Harley. *The Therapeutic Perspective: Medical Practice, Knowledge, and Identity in America, 1820–1885*. Princeton: Princeton University Press, 1997.

Wells, Robert V. *Facing the "King of Terrors": Death and Society in an American Community, 1750–1990*. New York: Cambridge University Press, 2000.

WGBH, Boston. *Influenza, 1918 (American Experience)*. 1998. Transcript. http://www.pbs.org/wgbh/americanexperience/features/transcript/influenza-transcript/.

White, Kenneth. "Pittsburgh in the Great Epidemic of 1918." *Western Pennsylvania Historical Magazine* 68 (1985): 221–242.

Whorton, James C. *Nature Cures: The History of Alternative Medicine in America*. New York: Oxford University Press, 2002.

Wilkerson, Karen Buhler. "False Dawn: The Rise and Decline of Public Health Nursing in America, 1900–1930." In *Nursing History: New Perspectives, New Possibilities,* ed. Ellen C. Lagerman. New York: New York Teacher's College Press, 1983, 89–106.

Young, James Harvey. *The Toadstool Millionaires: A Social History of Patent Medicines in America before Federal Regulation.* Princeton, NJ: Princeton University Press, 1961.

Zeiger, Susan. *In Uncle Sam's Service: Women Workers with the American Expeditionary Forces, 1917–1919.* Philadelphia: University of Pennsylvania Press, 2004.

INDEX

CPSIA information can be obtained
at www.ICGtesting.com
Printed in the USA
LVHW111541280520
656842LV00009B/187